Documentation
for Physical Therapist
Assistants

FIFTH EDITION

Wendy D. Bircher, PT, EdD

Retired Program Director/Professor

San Juan College

Farmington, New Mexico

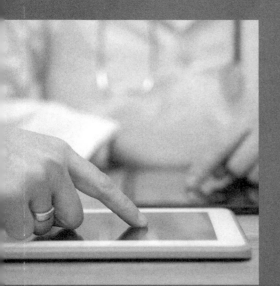
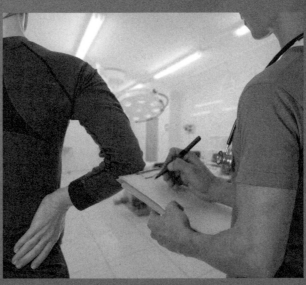
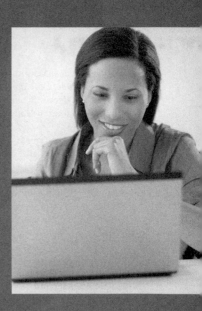

Documentation
for Physical Therapist
Assistants

FIFTH EDITION

F. A. Davis Company
1915 Arch Street
Philadelphia, PA 19103
www.fadavis.com

Copyright © 2018 by F. A. Davis Company

Printed in the United States of America

Last digit indicates print number: 10 9 8 7 6 5 4 3 2 1

Acquisitions Editor: Melissa Duffield
Director of Content Development: George W. Lang
Developmental Editor: Stephanie Kelly
Design and Illustration Manager: Carolyn O'Brien

As new scientific information becomes available through basic and clinical research, recommended treatments and drug therapies undergo changes. The author(s) and publisher have done everything possible to make this book accurate, up to date, and in accord with accepted standards at the time of publication. The author(s), editors, and publisher are not responsible for errors or omissions or for consequences from application of the book, and make no warranty, expressed or implied, in regard to the contents of the book. Any practice described in this book should be applied by the reader in accordance with professional standards of care used in regard to the unique circumstances that may apply in each situation. The reader is advised always to check product information (package inserts) for changes and new information regarding dose and contraindications before administering any drug. Caution is especially urged when using new or infrequently ordered drugs.

Library of Congress Cataloging-in-Publication Data

Names: Bircher, Wendy D., author.
Title: Documentation for physical therapist assistants / Wendy D. Bircher.
Description: Fifth edition. | Philadelphia : F.A. Davis Company, [2018] |
    Includes bibliographical references and index.
Identifiers: LCCN 2017014875 | ISBN 9780803661141
Subjects: | MESH: Forms and Records Control—methods | Physical Therapy
    Modalities—organization & administration | Physical Therapist Assistants
    | Medical Records—standards
Classification: LCC RM705 | NLM WB 460 | DDC 615.8/2—dc23
LC record available at https://lccn.loc.gov/2017014875

To my husband, John, for your patience, love, friendship, and humor.

Preface

The physical therapy profession continues to evolve with new research in clinical practice, changes in documentation procedures with the introduction of electronic health records, changes in insurance reimbursement, and coding with the initiation of the ICD-10 system. One of the most significant changes came with the introduction of the physical therapist assistant (PTA). With that introduction, there became a need to provide educational programming to enable our profession to bring the standards of care for patient treatment into the 21st century. Along with the development of additional PTA educational programs in 4-year educational institutions and community colleges, textbooks at the PTA level became essential. F.A. Davis's vision continues to ensure that the development of such textbooks remains available in a timely fashion. Along with the development of textbooks specific to the PTA student, ancillary support was also necessary for educators in PTA programs. F.A. Davis has also met that challenge.

Having practiced for more than 41 years in the pediatric, home health, outpatient, and rehabilitation settings, I have found that the changes in documentation, over time, have made it difficult for many therapists to keep current with third-party payers and their individual and specific requirements. After teaching in a PTA program for 16 years, I found that instruction in documentation is vital for the PTA student to develop suitable documentation skills and then to transfer those skills into the clinical setting, ensuring proper documentation that supports quality patient care and appropriate reimbursement.

In addition to becoming familiar with the revisions presented in this new edition, the PTA, along with the PT, must keep abreast of new developments in documentation, as outlined in APTA's *Guide to Physical Therapist Practice* (revised 2014) and the impact of the World Health Organization's International Classification of Functioning, Disability, and Health (ICF) on proper documentation and reimbursement for patient care. Information included in the *Guide to Physical Therapist Practice* provides the PTA student with essential information related to ethical practice, appropriate documentation techniques, and general guidelines for PTA supervision in any treatment setting. The *Guide* continues to be a valuable and necessary resource for any PT or PTA practicing in today's clinical setting.

With the implementation of the ICD-10 coding and billing system on October 1, 2015, which replaced the ICD-9 coding system, additional and updated changes were needed in this edition of this textbook to address those changes. For that purpose, a new chapter was added to address the initiation of the ICD-10, not because PTAs will be responsible for billing but instead to provide an understanding of that process when treating their patients. In addition, multiple reviewers have requested information be included in this revision related to electronic health records (EHR), issues related to the Commission on Accreditation in Physical Therapy Education (CAPTE), clinical performance evaluation in the clinical setting, and the differences between education provided for the PT versus the PTA. While these issues remain paramount to the education of the profession, it is not the purpose of this textbook to discuss the functionality of these issues. The main purpose of this textbook continues to be providing the information inherent in the content of the documentation process provided when treating patients receiving skilled physical therapy care, whether that information is collected on paper or in electronic form. It is hoped that the additional content that was requested is provided through the use of other textbooks, through the use of the online material provided by the American Physical Therapy Association (APTA), and through the mentorship provided in the educational and clinical settings.

For those educational programs that would like more information on the use of documentation and EHR, F.A. Davis provides a CD for programs to practice adding information in an example of an EHR. Also new to this edition and included on the instructor disk are multiple case studies that can be used in the educational setting. The case studies address multiple types of diagnoses within different clinical settings, and the instructor may use them in any way he or she chooses. Instructors are also reminded that the answers to all of the review and practice exercises are included in the instructor information and can be printed for student use and review.

While we will continue to address an ever-changing scenario for the provision of health-care services in the years to come, it is hoped that this textbook will provide those taking the journey with the skills to map their route with confidence.

—*Wendy Bircher*

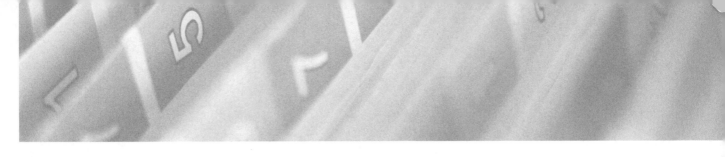

Reviewers

DENISE ABRAMS, PT, DPT, MA
Chairperson
Physical Therapist Assistant Program
SUNY Broome Community College
Binghamton, New York

TAWNY CHAMBERLAIN, PT, DPT
Program Director
Physical Therapist Assistant Program
South University
Glen Allen, Virginia

JILL DZIAK, PTA, CBIS, MEd
Adjunct Faculty
Health and Sciences
College of DuPage
Glen Ellyn, Illinois

GABRIELLA M. FERREIRA, BS, PTA
Instructor
PTA Program
Harcum College
Bryn Mawr, Pennsylvania

COSETTE HARDWICK, PT, DPT
Associate Professor
Department of Nursing and Allied Health
Missouri Western State University
St Joseph, Missouri

PATRICIA HOOKER, PTA, MA
Associate Professor
PTA Program, Health Sciences
College of Central Florida
Ocala, Florida

LINDA J. JOHNSON, PT, MS
Academic Coordinator of Clinical Education
CACHE PTA Program
Anne Arundel Community College
Arnold, Maryland

JACKI KLACZAK KOPACK, PT, DPT
PTA Program Director
PTA Program
Harcum College
Bryn Mawr, Pennsylvania

TAMMY MARCIN, PT, DPT, MBA
Chair
Physical Therapist Assistant Program
Horry Georgetown Technical College
Conway, South Carolina

BETTY T. SALAS, PT, DPT
Physical Therapist Assistant
Wharton County Junior College
Wharton, Texas

ADAM J. THOMPSON, PhD, LAT, ATC
Professor
Health and Human Performance
Indiana Wesleyan University
Marion, Indiana

Acknowledgments

Many individuals were responsible for the fifth edition of this textbook, and I would like to take this opportunity to thank them.

To Margaret Biblis and Melissa Duffield, for their continued enthusiasm, vision, patience, and confidence to ensure that each subsequent revision of this text continues to meet the stringent guidelines of F.A. Davis. You continue to be a credit to F.A. Davis and the profession of physical therapy by keeping your publications relevant to the changing times. In addition, I would also like to thank the individuals with F.A. Davis who provided their review of the completed material to ensure its consistency and accuracy in the final edition. Cindy Breuninger (Director, Content Solutions), Lisa Thompson (Production Editor), Beth Morel (Copy Editor), Sharon Lee (Production Manager) and Daniel Domzalski (Illustration Coordinator), your input was invaluable to ensure every "i" was dotted and every "t" was crossed. Thank you for your time and effort on behalf of all of the students who will have access to this textbook. For any of the individuals I have failed to mention, who work tirelessly with F.A. Davis to ensure quality publishing of medical information, I extend my thanks for your willingness to help authors in this challenging, but rewarding process.

To my editor, Stephanie Kelly, what a pleasure it was to work with you, and I so appreciated your insight and input to make this new edition as informative and supportive for physical therapist assistant education as the previous editions. Your passion, phenomenal efforts, and patience to help me improve the text, and your thoughtful and perceptive comments helped guide me where I needed to go.

To Amelia Blevins, my developmental editor, for your judicious review of the ancillary material and excellent suggestions for ensuring this material will provide the necessary support to faculty using this textbook.

To the American Physical Therapy Association (APTA) and the Commission on Education in Physical Therapy Education (CAPTE), for your persistent and innovative updates to the materials made available to physical therapists and physical therapist assistants and educational programs that provide support to these professions. Your continued diligence provides documentation support for appropriate reimbursement to treat our patients. Without your continued efforts to keep the material that we access current and available, our jobs would be much more difficult.

To Michele Tillson, Member Communications Specialist at the APTA office, for your continued assistance in obtaining permission to reprint the multiple examples of ethical and supportive material in this revision. Your assistance helped ensure the continued high quality of the information disseminated to physical therapists and physical therapist assistants and the educational programs that train such individuals.

To the reviewers of the material presented in this revision, thank you for your comments, which helped ensure that the fifth edition met program guidelines and included material appropriate for the ever-changing field of patient treatment and documentation.

To Kim Noyes, and all of her employees at Special K Fitness, for your invaluable input, corrections to material, and suggestions for revisions to the fifth edition. A simple thank you is not enough for the valuable time you provided to ensure this edition was current and would meet the ever-changing needs of our profession. Without your timely suggestions for information related to changes in billing with the implementation of the ICD-10 and review of the case studies, this revision would not have been as complete or timely to the current changes in reimbursement.

To John, my husband and soul mate, whose continued support never fails me and who is the best part of my life. Thank you for sharing my journey and for your continued encouragement in all I do. It means so very much to me, and you continue to make our lives together a true blessing!

And finally, to all the students for whom this textbook was written. It is my hope that it provides you with a map to follow in your quest to learn appropriate and accurate documentation that will support the care you provide to your patients and help ensure proper reimbursement for that care. I wish you the best of luck in your future endeavors, and I welcome you, as colleagues, to the exceptional and caring profession of physical therapy.

"Transforming society by optimizing movement to improve the human experience"
(Vision Statement from the American Physical Therapy Association)

—WDB

Contents

WK 1

WK 1

WK 2

WK 2

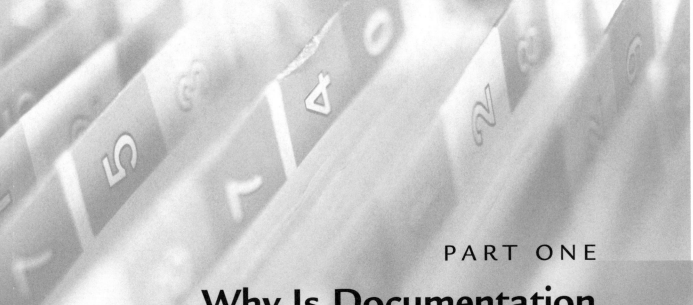

PART ONE

Why Is Documentation Important?

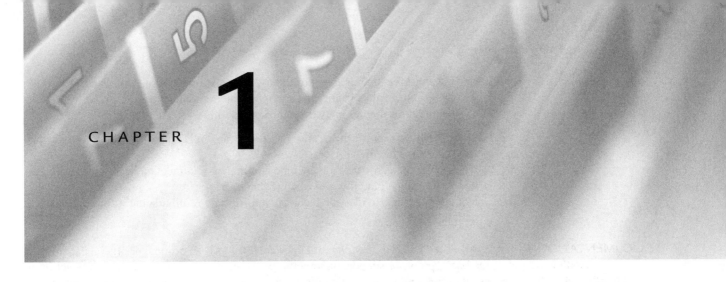

CHAPTER 1

Introduction to Documentation

LEARNING OBJECTIVES

After studying this chapter, the student will be able to:

☐ Define *documentation*

☐ Identify the significance of documentation in patient care

☐ Describe changes in the process for obtaining a referral for physical therapy that have occurred since the early 1960s

☐ Explain how changes in the process for obtaining a referral for physical therapy have affected the evolution of responsibilities for the physical therapist (PT) and physical therapist assistant (PTA)

☐ Describe the differences in classifications for documentation among the Nagi Disablement Model; the International Classification of Impairments, Disabilities, and Handicaps model; and the International Classification of Functioning, Disability and Health framework

☐ Identify the major factors that currently influence the provision of health-care services and the responsibilities of the PT and PTA

☐ Identify standards and criteria for documentation set by federal and state governments, professional associations, accrediting agencies, and health-care facilities

☐ Describe the role and discuss the importance of documentation in patient care

☐ Discuss how documentation benefits the PT and PTA professions and the patient

INTRODUCTION

Having been introduced to documentation more than 40 years ago, I have witnessed the changes that have occurred to ensure proper patient care, documentation, and reimbursement for that care. With the introduction of physical therapist assistants (PTAs) in the provision of patient care, some of the documentation responsibilities that once rested with the physical therapist (PT) have shifted to the PTA. The PTA now bears as much responsibility for proper documentation as the PT.

This book discusses the documentation tasks expected from the PTA, the importance of quality documentation, and the best way to produce thorough and proper documentation that fills the needs of the patient, the facility, and third-party payers and that addresses the legal and ethical issues that surround quality patient care. In preparing to learn proper documentation, the PT and PTA must remain cognizant of the myriad changes that continue to occur through third-party payers and changes in coding for appropriate reimbursement.

The following three themes are woven throughout this text:

1. Documentation records the quality of patient care and creates the ability to replicate that care in the treatment process.
2. Documentation constructs a legal report of patient treatment and care for the protection of the patient, facility, and treating therapist.
3. Documentation provides the basis for appropriate reimbursement for skilled patient care.

DOCUMENTATION AND ITS SIGNIFICANCE

Merriam-Webster's Online Dictionary defines *document* as "an original or official paper relied on as the basis, proof, or support of something." *Documentation* is defined as "the act or an instance of furnishing or authenticating with documents or the provision of documents in substantiation."[1]

Evidence of Patient Care

In any health-care facility, service is provided to the patient by more than one medical professional. Records or medical charts are kept to document the treatments given, services performed, and services to be provided. Medical charts provide information that authenticates the care given to the patient and the reasons for providing that care. Thus, documentation is written so legal proof exists that medical care was given to the patient, and this evidence is available for future use. If the treatment provided is not documented in the chart, it is assumed the treatment was not provided. "If it isn't written, it didn't happen" is a good rule.

Accountability for Patient Care

The written record is the mechanism through which the health-care professional is held accountable for the medical care provided to the patient. The record is reviewed by the third-party payer to determine the reimbursement value of the medical services provided, and the information is studied to measure or determine the efficacy of the treatment procedures. The reader of the medical record finds the rationale that supports the medical necessity for the treatment, the activities involved in that treatment process, and the legal basis for such treatment.

An Example of the Importance of Documentation

The impact of poorly written physical therapy documentation is illustrated by the following story based on a true experience of a PT in 1998. The situation includes some of the topics and information discussed in this and additional chapters. However, in some instances, the situation only alludes to this information. A practice exercise at the end of the chapter challenges you to identify these topics.

The Experience

A PT who worked for a home health-care agency was contacted by an attorney for the prosecution in a child abuse case that involved a patient who had previously been under the PT's care. The patient's father had been accused of shaking the patient violently enough to cause brain damage. The patient was last seen by the PT more than 3 years ago. Additionally, the PT received a phone call from the PTA who also had worked with this patient under the PT's supervision.

The PTA informed the PT that she was being called to testify by the attorney for the defense, not for the prosecution, in the same court case. The PTA was worried about the case and having to testify for the first time in a federal court because this incident occurred on an American Indian reservation (reservations are sovereign nations and subject to federal, not state, jurisdiction). Because the PT had supervised the PTA during this time, how could they present their information for opposing sides? Needless to say, both individuals were concerned about the legality of testifying against each other, especially since the PT had supervised the PTA in the care of this patient. Because 3 years had passed since this patient had received treatment, the PT hoped that the records regarding the patient's treatment were complete enough to ensure that the patient had received appropriate and skilled therapeutic intervention from the therapists and correctly documented the role of the patient's father in the patient's injury (shaken baby syndrome: ICD-9 code 995.54/ICD-10 code T74.12XA) and the patient's subsequent recovery.

The PT and PTA met with the attorneys for each side separately. They each reviewed the medical chart from the hospital where the patient had been admitted following the incident in question and the records completed by the PT and PTA while working for the home health-care agency. The patient had been 8 months old when the patient's father became angry because the baby would not stop crying. In an attempt to get the baby to be quiet, he had shaken the baby violently, causing damage to the frontal and occipital lobes. It was reported that the patient's father knew he had caused severe damage to the patient and had immediately brought him to the emergency room at a nearby hospital. The mother had been contacted at work and had arrived in the emergency room just as her husband was being arrested for child abuse. The patient initially presented with right-side paralysis, visual impairment, and increased muscle tone.

After being treated for 2 years, the patient had completely regained normal function in all areas of development and had normal vision once more. The defense for the case was attempting to keep the patient's father out of jail and return him to his family. The defense was arguing that he had paid for his mistake by realizing what he had done to the patient. The patient's father followed all the guidelines of the court, which included attending therapy sessions when he was not incarcerated and spending supervised time with the patient. There had been no further incidents of abuse, and the child appeared to have an excellent relationship with his father. The prosecution wanted the patient's father to continue with his incarceration and, because he was considered a child abuser, not to be allowed to see his son upon his release.

The PT reviewed her notes with the prosecuting attorney (Fig. 1–1). The PT's notes were two to three lines at most, which was all that had been required by the home health-care agency at the time. The PTA's notes were fairly complete and appeared to follow the PT's plan of care (POC). However, the progress/daily notes (for the purposes of this textbook, progress and daily notes are interchangeable) certainly wouldn't meet the present criteria for third-party payers such as Medicaid or Medicare (discussed in Chapter 4). How were the PT and PTA going to respond to cross-examination by the opposing lawyers when their notes simply stated "pt. is improving" and "pt. tolerated treatment well"? These notes did not help either therapist recall the specifics of the patient's skilled physical therapy treatment sessions, about which they needed to testify. Both individuals wished their notes had been written more clearly and included more specific goals and outcomes.

The notes were reviewed, the information was recalled, and the PT and PTA were ready to testify. During their trips home, both the PT and PTA realized how necessary it was to provide quality documentation and found that the rule "if it isn't written, it didn't happen" took on more meaning. This court experience would have been so much easier for both therapists if the written notes had been in the same format currently required by third-party payers (see Chapters 4 to 6). To see the difference between the standards of care in 1998 and 2017, compare the note included in the court testimony (Fig. 1–1) with the example of how the session would have been documented today (Fig. 1–2). (Definitions of the abbreviations used in the notes are in Appendix A.)

EVOLUTION OF PT AND PTA RESPONSIBILITIES AND ROLE OF DOCUMENTATION

The event just described is an example of how documentation has evolved over time. This evolution has been a result of the changing responsibilities of the PT and PTA for treatment and documentation and the ever-changing requirements for reimbursement.

2-8-98: Pt. feeling better today. Pt. was seen for a 30 minute therapy visit.
  S: Mom told PTA that her son is cranky and stiff.
  O: Worked on sitting and rolling.
  A: Pt. able to sit by himself for short time periods.
  P: Continue PT sessions.

Figure 1—1 A note, written in 1998, from the medical chart containing the physical therapy progress notes for the patient.

2-8-98: Pt. has been seen at home for 10 physical therapy visits since hospital d/c on 1-5-1998. The physical therapy evaluation was on 1-8-98 and visits were set for 2x/week by the PTA and supervisory visits with the PT once a month. The session today was for 45 minutes. Pt. currently functions at a 6-7 month level in gross motor skills for his chronological age of 10.5 months. Mother reports central vision is still impaired as the pt. continues to turn his head and use his peripheral vision. The pt. will be seen for six more visits before re-evaluation and re-certification.

S: Mother stated the patient is not sleeping through the night and becomes quite agitated until she swaddles him and rocks him for several hours. Pt. continues to exhibit moderate hypertonicity overall with the right side more involved. Mother questions her son's development and is concerned about her husband who is unable to come home.

O: Patient can sit independently when placed in a sitting position, for over 1 minute. He can roll independently from prone to supine and supine to prone without using tone and with an appropriate flexor pattern. Patient can maintain an independent prone position on extended forearms for over 30 seconds and is beginning to pull his hips into flexion to approximate a four-point crawl position when in a prone position. Patient's PROM and AROM remain WNL and strength is 4/5 overall. Pt.'s alignment remains symmetrical and protective responses are present in all positions and all directions with a minimal delay noted on the right side. Independent manual muscle testing remains inappropriate due to the patient's young age. Exercises included positioning in independent sit, prone, and side sit with transitions in and out of each position. Transitions are accomplished with minimal assist.

A: Improvement in patient's gross motor skills continues with a good potential to meet the goal of independent sit with transition from the floor to sit within the next month. Hypertonicity has decreased from moderate to mild overall and patient is beginning to increase flexor patterns for improved sitting balance with an anterior pelvic tilt and beginning four-point crawl positioning. The home exercise program was reviewed with the mother and she correctly performed a return demonstration of all activities.

O:

P: Patient is scheduled 2x/week for 2 weeks with the PTA monitoring the home exercise program and gross motor progress and mother's handling skills. Programming will focus on increasing independent transition from floor to sit and independent four-point crawl position held for 30 seconds by the end of the next session. The PTA will set the supervisory visit with PT for 2-12-98.

—————————————————————————————— Kayla Therapist, LPTA
PT Lic. #123

Figure 1–2 An example of how the note from 1998 could be rewritten to meet the 2017 requirements for documentation.

Major Influences on PT and PTA Responsibilities

Three events have influenced the evolution of PT and PTA responsibilities and the role of documentation in patient care: (1) changes in referrals for physical therapy; (2) the establishment of Medicare, HMOs, PPOs, and additional third-party payers; and (3) the development of documentation classifications and models.

Changes in Referrals for Physical Therapy

The method by which physicians prescribe physical therapy has changed throughout the profession's short history. The changes have increased the PT's clinical decision-making power, led to the development of the physical therapy diagnosis, and offered the opportunity for autonomy in the practice of therapy.

THE PHYSICAL THERAPY PRESCRIPTION. Until the early 1960s, a patient commonly came to a PT with a referral from a physician in the form of a physical therapy prescription. That is, it read much like a medication prescription, as illustrated in Figure 1–3, or the instructions were more general, such as "ultrasound," "massage," or "exercise." The PT was required to follow the physician's orders and provide the treatment exactly as prescribed. If the PT did not agree with the treatment plan, he or she needed to discuss this with the physician in an attempt to agree on a more appropriate treatment plan. If the PT was not successful in convincing the physician to change the order, the physical therapy treatment provided may not have been as appropriate or effective as possible. The PT was practicing at the level of a technician, following precise directions from the physician and documenting briefly that the treatment was provided and whether the patient was improving. Autonomy in practice was not evident, nor was the PT expected to have much expertise.

P. T. Knowes, M.D.
123 Medical Building, Suite 1
Yourtown, NM 87405
(505) 111-222

Physical Therapy for Shelby Williams:

US at 1.5 w/cm^2 for 5 min. to the right deltoid insertion, followed by 10 min. of massage. AAROM 10 rep. for abduction (not to exceed 165°), flexion (not to exceed 170°), and external rotation (not to exceed 25°).

P. T. Knowes, MD

Figure 1—3   Illustration of a physician's order for physical therapy that tells the physical therapist exactly what to do. It resembles a medication prescription.

PTs ABLE TO EVALUATE AND TREAT.   In the early 1960s, PTs began convincing some physicians that a PT had the training and knowledge to evaluate a patient's neuromusculoskeletal system and determine the treatment appropriate for the patient's condition. A patient brought a physician's referral that provided the diagnosis and stated "evaluate and treat." The responsibilities of the PT expanded to include (1) determining the physical therapy diagnosis on the basis of medical diagnosis and evaluation results and (2) defining the interventions or treatment plan based on the physical therapy diagnosis and resulting dysfunction. The physical therapy problem was described in terms of the neuromusculoskeletal abnormality, and the treatment plan was directed toward correcting or minimizing this problem as it related to the patient's inability to function. The PT needed evaluation skills to identify physical therapy problems and to make clinical decisions regarding the treatment of those problems. Writing the initial, interim, and discharge evaluations became additional documentation responsibilities for every PT.

Because of the PT's evolving roles in physical therapy evaluation and treatment, the focus of a PT's education had to change, increasing the emphasis on scientific knowledge, evaluation skills, critical thinking, and research and decreasing the emphasis on treatment skills.

With PTs taking on more and more responsibilities in administration and the evaluation process, the role of the PTA was created to provide additional support in the treatment process and documentation. The first academic program for training PTAs was established in 1967. The PTA assumed the role of the technician, providing the physical therapy treatments under the direct guidance and supervision of the PT. Writing progress/daily notes was a documentation responsibility shared by the PT and PTA.

A PTA's training, although still focused on treatment skills, has expanded to emphasize the theories behind these treatment skills. This expansion provides the PTA with the knowledge to make clinical decisions within the parameters of the PT's treatment plan and the PTA's level of training and scope of practice. For these reasons, the PTA is held to the same professional standard for providing quality documentation related to the skilled treatment of patients and to provide a strong communication link with the supervising PT to ensure the prescribed POC is followed. For example, in home health settings, the PTA's responsibilities have evolved to allow the PTA to treat patients when the PT is not on the premises but is accessible through telecommunications. These parameters vary and are set by the individual state in which the PTA practices. In an acute setting, the PT is immediately available to the PTA to address multiple changes in patient status that might occur in this type of short-term treatment facility, as the patient is quickly progressed through to discharge.

DIRECT ACCESS TO PHYSICAL THERAPY.   Direct access allows a person access to the medical care system directly through a PT, without a physician's referral. The PT may evaluate the patient to determine whether the patient's condition is a disorder treatable by physical therapy. Nebraska, for example, has allowed direct access since 1957. California eliminated the need for a physician's referral in 1968, with a revision in 2013. Under the previous law, patients could be seen only for an evaluation, fitness and wellness services, and treatment for a condition that included a medical diagnosis. With the passing of Assembly Bill 1000, which went into effect on January 1, 2014, patient access to physical therapy services was expanded to include immediate treatment for up to 45 days or 12 visits, whichever came first.[2]

When Maryland's Physical Therapy Practice Act was amended in 1979 to allow direct access, many American Physical Therapy Association (APTA) state chapters launched their amendment campaigns. Today, all states have direct-access language in their state practice acts[2] that are either unlimited or provide provisions regarding its use. The following states have no restrictions to physical therapy, under direct access: Alaska, Arizona, Colorado, Hawaii, Idaho, Iowa, Kentucky, Maryland, Montana, Nebraska, Nevada, North Dakota, Oregon, South Dakota, Utah, Vermont, and West Virginia. The remainder of the states have either limited access or provisions toward direct access. For specific state guidelines, refer to the following website:[3] http://www.apta.org/uploadedFiles/APTAorg/Advocacy/State/Issues/Direct_Access/DirectAccessbyState.pd

Direct access gives the PT the opportunity for autonomy, but it also requires the PT to have the skills and knowledge to recognize conditions that are *not* problems that can be helped by physical therapy. The PT is responsible for referring a patient to a physician or other appropriate health-care provider when the patient exhibits signs and symptoms of a systemic disorder or a problem that is beyond the scope of practice or expertise of the PT. The PTA is responsible for reporting any signs, symptoms, or lack of progress that indicate a need for the PT to reevaluate the patient. For more information about direct access at the state level, visit: http://www.apta.org/StateIssues/DirectAccess

For those states that allow direct access and for those facilities in which reimbursement is possible under direct access, documentation becomes even more critical. It is incumbent upon the PT and the PTA to understand the ramifications of poor documentation related to skilled therapeutic intervention and to address those issues when providing documentation to third-party payers. Without such diligence, there is increased risk for nonreimbursement or delayed reimbursement of therapy services provided in any facility. From a legal standpoint, it is imperative that the supervising PT establish proper documentation and follow-up in order to ensure that the patient receives appropriate and skilled care for the physical therapy diagnosis and that such treatment remains within the scope of practice of that PT within the state in which the PT practices.

Establishment of Medicare

Before 1970, documentation in the medical chart was not always thorough or specific. Health-care providers knew documentation should be done well, but unfortunately, poor-quality documentation was easy to find. Typically, progress/daily notes were brief, consisting of one or two lines, and were subjective and/or judgmental in nature—for example, "Pt. feeling better today" (see Fig. 1–1). No standards for documentation existed, and those paying the health-care bills did not demand accountability for those bills.

This changed in the mid-1960s when the Health Insurance for the Aged and Disabled Act, known as Medicare, was enacted. With this act, the federal government began paying for medical care for the elderly. Within the Department of Health and Human Services, the Health Care Financing Administration (HCFA) issued standards for documentation to be followed for all patients receiving Medicare. Other insurance companies soon followed Medicare's example. Those paying the medical bills demanded that health-care providers be held accountable for the dollars spent. This accountability was determined through proper documentation that clearly identified the physical therapy problem, treatment goals and plans, and treatment results.[4] Consequently, the responsibilities for the supervising PT and the PTA evolved to include more specific parameters to demonstrate patient progression, and then treatment times were dictated for the medical diagnosis. Through the decades, Medicare has continued to make frequent revisions to the guidelines acceptable for patient care, and it is the responsibility of the PT and the PTA to remain abreast of such changes for each individual facility in which they are employed.

In addition to the establishment of Medicare, multiple changes have occurred in managed care and the use of private insurance companies. See Chapter 4 for further discussion of the different types of reimbursement and their effects on documentation and treatment.

Documentation Classifications and Models

Several taxonomies have evolved over the past four decades to aid in the documentation process for physical therapy services. The Nagi Disablement Model,[5] developed in 1969, was the first model used to provide a correlation between impairment and functional limitations. This model uses the patient's active pathology to help determine the relationship among the resulting impairment, functional limitation, and disability. In 1980, it was used as the groundwork to help revise the World Health Organization's International Classification of Impairments, Disabilities, and Handicaps[6] (ICIDH) and the International Classification of Functioning, Disability and Health[7] (ICF) in 2001. The ICF framework was groundbreaking because research using this framework was cross-cultural, involved more than 40 countries, and provided a common language to be used by all professionals treating patients in the rehabilitation setting. Because of its innovative design and vision, the APTA endorsed the use of ICF framework in 2010 and continues to disseminate this information to the public in all of the APTA documentation in their publications and on their website, as revisions occur (see Chapter 2 for additional details). Additionally, in 1992, the National Center for Medical Rehabilitation Research (NCMRR) provided support for specific definitions related to disability as referenced in research conducted by the National Institute on Disability and Rehabilitation Research (NIDRR).[8] Specifically, these classification methods helped provide a common language in the care of patients with disabilities. A summary of the classifications can be found in Table 1–1.

While the ICF framework has revised these taxonomies, it is important for the reader to understand the history of such models and their support for appropriate documentation in patient care. These taxonomies introduced a common definition for the following terms used in documentation:

- Impairment: A loss or abnormality of a physiological, psychological, or anatomical structure or function
- Functional limitation: A restriction of the ability to perform an activity or a task in an efficient, typically expected, or competent manner
- Disability: An inability to perform or a limitation in the performance of actions, tasks, and activities usually expected in specific social roles and physical environments

FUNCTION VERSUS IMPAIRMENT. For proper documentation to occur in the therapy field, *function* and *impairment* must be differentiated. According to the preceding classifications, impairment can lead to a functional problem, whereas a functional problem may not always cause impairment. A functional problem is usually patient-specific.

Physical Therapy Services Today

Our health-care system is now in a state of transition, and services provided to patients are being reduced because of limited financial resources. The physical therapy provider is placed in a position of competing for these limited funds. Physical therapy services will not be reimbursed when the treatments are not effective, efficient, and skilled. The patient or client seeks physical therapy because of problems resulting from a disease or injury that prevents

Table 1-1 Documentation Classification Methods		
Definition and Use of the ICIDH and ICF Classifications	**Definition and Use of the Nagi Disablement Model**	**National Center for Medical Rehabilitation Research Definition of Disabilities[7]**
ICIDH Classification: Provided a uniform standard of language for the description of health and health-related issues (1980).[5] ICF Classification: Updated the ICIDH classification to integrate the biomedical, psychological, and social aspects of diseases and their related disabilities, handicaps, and impairments (2001).[6]	Model of disablement to correlate impairment and functional limitations (1969).[4] This model provided a definitive summary of an active pathology and its relationship to the resulting impairment, functional limitation, and disability.	Provides a description of services to patients with impairments, functional limitations, and disabilities, or changes in these areas as a result of injury, disease, or other causes related to the pathology and societal limitations they might affect.

[Handwritten margin notes:]
Impairments: Pain, ↓'d ROM, ↓'d strength, ↓'d balance, ↓'d endurance
Fxnl limitations — unable to transfer, walk, stand, move a body part, — unable to jump, transition
Disability, social roles

the person from functioning in his or her environment. Therapeutic interventions are directed toward improving or restoring the patient's functional abilities by minimizing or resolving these problems in the most cost-effective manner.

Documentation that meets today's standards provides the basis for research to measure functional outcomes and identify the most effective and efficient treatment procedures. Documentation must describe what functional activities the patient has difficulty performing and must show how the interventions are effective in improving or restoring the patient's function. Documentation must be done properly if PTs and PTAs are to survive financially. Without proper documentation for the specific treatment given to a patient, reimbursement will not occur.

THE ROLE OF DOCUMENTATION IN PATIENT CARE

The term *quality care* as used in this text refers to medical care that is appropriate for and focused on the patient's problems relevant to the diagnosis. *Quality physical therapy care* is defined as care that follows the *Guide to Physical Therapist Practice*.[9] *The Guide to Physical Therapist Practice* is a publication by the American Physical Therapy Association and describes the following: (1) physical therapists and their roles in health care, (2) the generally accepted elements of physical therapy patient/client management, (3) the types of tests and measurements used by physical therapists, (4) the types of interventions physical therapists use, (5) the anticipated goals of the interventions, and (6) the expected outcomes of physical therapy patient/client management. Preferred practice patterns are descriptions about common physical therapy management strategies for specific diagnostic groups. The patterns serve as a guide for the physical therapist when planning comprehensive plans of care.[10]

To provide high-quality medical care, good communication among health-care professionals is absolutely essential. The PTA must accurately and consistently communicate with the supervising PT. The PTA may also share and coordinate information with other medical providers, including other PTs and PTAs who may fill in when the PTA is absent, occupational therapists and occupational therapy assistants, nurses and nursing assistants, physicians and physician assistants, speech pathologists, psychologists, social workers, and chaplains. The medical record is the avenue through which the medical team communicates regarding:

- Identification of the patient's problems
- Solutions for the patient's problems
- Plans for the patient's discharge
- Coordination of the continuum of care

This communication process helps ensure the patient receives a high quality of care from any provider.

The quality of care provided by the medical facility is determined by a review of the existing records. This review process is a way to monitor and influence the quality of health care provided by the facility. The information in the medical record is reviewed or audited for three purposes:

1. Quality assurance. Records are reviewed to determine whether the health care provided meets legal standards and appropriate health-care criteria (Box 1–1). This is done externally by agencies accrediting the facility and internally by a quality-assurance committee. Problem areas are identified and plans are made for correction and improvement. This is a continuous process; the quality-assurance committee usually meets on a regular basis, and accrediting agencies audit a facility every few years. PTAs are permitted to serve on the quality-assurance committee.
2. Research and education. Information in the medical record is used for research and for student instruction. Research helps validate treatment techniques and identify new and better ways to provide health care. The record is used for retrospective studies that measure outcomes to determine the most cost-effective treatment approach to patient care. Students are encouraged to question and challenge treatment procedures as part of their learning process.
3. Reimbursement. Third-party payers, such as Medicare, HMOs, PPOs, and insurance companies, decide how to reimburse providers for medical care by reading

---

Box 1–1   **Implications for the PTA: Legal Issues**

The medical record and all that is contained within it makes up a legal document and legal proof of the quality of care provided. The record protects the patient and the health-care providers should any questions arise in the future regarding the patient's care. Health-care providers work under the constant shadow of a possible malpractice lawsuit for each patient they come into contact with. Months or years after receiving treatment, a patient can become dissatisfied, leading to questions about the medical care received. Often these questions result in lawsuits, and many cases go to court because of the patient's claim that injury or illness was caused by an accident or negligence on the part of someone else. The PT, and possibly the PTA, may be called to testify in court about the therapy provided to the patient. Clear and accurate documentation is the best defense, demonstrating that safe and thorough patient care was provided.

---

the documentation in the medical record. The record must show that the patient's problems were identified and that treatment was directed toward solving those problems and discharging the patient while meeting his or her functional deficits as outlined in the POC (Box 1–2).

DOCUMENTATION STANDARDS AND CRITERIA

Documentation that ensures quality care follows the standards and criteria set by a variety of sources. Although the standards are similar, the PTA should be familiar with the criteria required by:

- The federal government
- State governments
- Professional associations
- Accrediting agencies
- Health-care facilities

Federal Government

As discussed previously, the federal government funds and administers Medicare. The PT and PTA must follow Medicare documentation requirements when treating a patient with this type of insurance. Because these requirements change frequently and can become complicated, both the PT and the PTA must stay informed and up-to-date in their knowledge of Medicare requirements. For more information, visit: http://www.cms.gov/center/provider.asp.[4]

State Governments

Although funded by the federal government, Medicaid, a government program providing health care to low-income individuals, is administered by the individual state governments. State governments also fund medical assistance and workers' compensation programs that have specific documentation criteria for patients with these types of insurance. The state may ask that specific data from the medical record be reported annually. Other documentation criteria, determined at the state level, may be influenced by the state's physical therapy legislation or practice act. The PT and PTA must be well informed about the rules, regulations, and guidelines of the Physical Therapy Practice Act in the state where they practice.

Box 1–2   **Implications for the PTA: Reimbursement Issues**

The insurance company or organization paying for the patient's medical services determines the reimbursement rate from the information recorded in the medical chart. Often payment is denied when the documentation does not clearly provide the rationale to support the medical care provided. With some insurance plans, the caregiver must provide effective patient care while containing the costs within a preset payment amount. The caregiver demonstrates accountability for these costs by thoroughly and properly documenting the care provided.

Professional Associations   Associations can recommend documentation standards, such as APTA's *Defensible Documentation,*[11] and those standards outlined in the *Guide to Physical Therapist Practice.*[10] These guidelines are the basis for the documentation instructions in this textbook and can be found on the APTA website at http://www.apta.org/Documentation/DefensibleDocumentation.

Accrediting Agencies   Accrediting agencies provide standards that health-care facilities must follow to meet accreditation criteria, including documentation requirements. Hospitals are accredited by The Joint Commission (formerly The Joint Commission on Accreditation of Healthcare Organizations [JCAHO]).[12] Rehabilitation facilities are accredited by the Commission on Accreditation of Rehabilitation Facilities (CARF).[13] PT and PTA educational programs also receive accreditation through the Commission on Accreditation in Physical Therapy Education (CAPTE).[14]

Health-Care Facilities   Each health-care facility has its own documentation criteria; most facilities incorporate federal, state, and professional standards into their own procedures. The PTA can follow all standards and criteria by remembering this good rule: Follow the policies and procedures at the facility where you work if they do not place you in a situation that is outside the scope of practice for your field or in a situation in which the therapeutic intervention is inappropriate or unethical.

SUMMARY   Documenting patient care in the medical record is one of the many responsibilities of the PT and the PTA. The medical record is a legal document that proves that medical care was given and holds the health-care providers accountable for the quality of that care. It is an avenue for constant communication among health-care providers that enables them to identify goals and monitor treatment progress. And insurance representatives read the medical record to determine whether or not to reimburse for the medical services provided.

Historically, the PT was a technician, providing physical therapy treatments that were prescribed, in detail, by the physician. Responsibilities have evolved such that the PT is now an evaluator, consultant, manager, and practitioner seeing patients (clients) without a physician's referral. The PTA provides treatment under the guidance and supervision of the PT.

Physical therapy services must be provided in an efficient and cost-effective manner because financial resources to fund health care are no longer as easily accessible. The outcomes must now focus on improving the client's functional abilities. With the introduction of the ICF framework and its endorsement by the APTA, more emphasis can now be placed on restoring the patient's functional level. Research must be done to measure the outcomes or results of physical therapy procedures and to define the most effective and efficient treatments for accomplishing the functional goals in order to demonstrate evidence-based practice as outlined in the APTA's *Guide to Physical Therapist Practice*. Proper documentation facilitates this research.

Providing up-to-date and valid physical therapy services is made possible by documentation that meets the standards and criteria set by federal and state governments, professional agencies, accrediting agencies, and individual clinical facilities. Although documentation formats differ from facility to facility, all incorporate the professional and legal standards and criteria. The PT and PTA should "follow the policies and procedures of [their] clinical facility" if specific rules and regulations are not otherwise addressed. The PT and PTA must maintain appropriate documentation to address patient treatments within their scope of practice. Documenting according to professional standards and legal guidelines will produce a medical record that protects the patient, the PT, and the PTA if the medical record is used in legal proceedings.

REFERENCES

1. Document and documentation. (2016). In *Merriam-Webster's online dictionary*. Retrieved from http://www.merriam-webster.com/dictionary
2. Signing of AB 1000 concludes busy legislative year for California chapter. (2013). *PT in Motion News.* Retrieved from http://www.apta.org/PTinMotion/NewsNow/2013/10/11/CA/
3. American Physical Therapy Association. (2016). *A summary of direct access language in state physical therapy acts.* Retrieved from http://www.apta.org/StateIssues/DirectAccess
4. Healthcare Finance Administration (HCFA), minimal data set (MDS), regulations, HCFA/AMA documentation guidelines, home health regulations. Retrieved from http://www.ncbi.nlm.nih.gov/pmc/articles/PMC2232246/
5. Nagi, S. Z. (1969). *Disability and rehabilitation.* Columbus: Ohio State University Press.
6. World Health Organization. (1980). *International classification of impairments, disabilities, and handicaps.* Geneva, Switzerland: Author.

7. World Health Organization. (2001). *International classification of functioning, disability and health.* Geneva, Switzerland: Author.

8. Center for an Accessible Society. (n.d.). *Research on definitions of disability from NIDRR.* Retrieved from http://www.accessiblesociety.org/topics/demographics-identity/nidrr-lrp-defs.htm

9. American Physical Therapy Association. (2014). Content, development and concepts. In *Guide to physical therapist practice* (3rd ed., Chapter 1). Alexandria, VA: Author.

10. American Physical Therapy Association. (2014). Standards of practice for physical therapy and the criteria. In *Guide to physical therapist practice* (3rd ed., Chapters 1 and 2). Alexandria, VA: Author.

11. American Physical Therapy Association. (2012). *Defensible documentation for patient/client management.* Retrieved from http://www.apta.org/Documentation/DefensibleDocumentation/

12. The Joint Commission on Accreditation of Healthcare Organizations. (1996). *Comprehensive accreditation manual for hospitals.* Oakbrook Terrace, IL: Author.

13. Commission on Accreditation for Rehabilitation Facilities. Retrieved from http://www.carf.org

14. Commission on Accreditation in Physical Therapy Education. Retrieved from http://www.capteonline.org/home.aspx

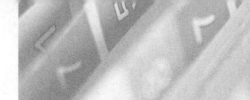

Review Exercises

1. Define **documentation.** Give an **example** of how it is used in physical therapy.

2. **Describe** what is meant by the following rule: "If it isn't written, it didn't happen."

3. **Describe** why the note in Figure 1–1 is **not** an appropriate record by today's documentation standards.

4. Identify the **three** major factors currently influencing the provision of health-care services and PT and PTA responsibilities.

5. **Describe** the changes in the process for obtaining a referral for physical therapy that have occurred since the early 1960s.

6. **Discuss** how changes in the process for obtaining a referral for physical therapy influenced the evolution of the responsibilities of the PT and the PTA.

7. Describe **three** purposes for which the medical record is reviewed or audited.

8. **Who** determines standards or criteria for documentation?

9. Explain **why** the PTA could use the rule "follow the policies and procedures at the facility where you work."

10. What is the **importance** of the ICF framework in documentation?

11. Explain the **differences** between the Nagi Disablement Model and the ICF framework.

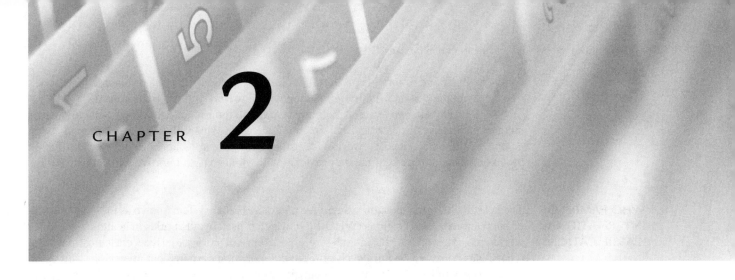

CHAPTER 2

The World Health Organization and the International Classification of Functioning, Disability and Health

LEARNING OBJECTIVES
INTRODUCTION
WHO FAMILY OF INTERNATIONAL
   CLASSIFICATIONS
THE ICF FRAMEWORK

SUMMARY
REFERENCES
REVIEW EXERCISES
PRACTICE EXERCISES

LEARNING OBJECTIVES

After studying this chapter, the student will be able to:

☐ Explain the importance of the World Health Organization (WHO) in the development of the International Classification of Functioning, Disability and Health (ICF)

☐ Describe the general role of the ICF in health care

☐ Understand the importance of the APTA's adoption of the ICF in patient treatment

☐ Explain the differences between the WHO reference, derived, and related classification systems

☐ Understand how to use the ICF and its application to functioning and disability

☐ Explain the difference between the Nagi Disablement Model and the ICF framework

☐ Identify the five domains of the ICF

INTRODUCTION

For decades, individuals dealing with medical issues related to patient care struggled to find a common means of communication to address treatment in various health-care settings. Because multiple agencies are involved in patient care, both in the United States and internationally, it was imperative that a common classification system, or language, be developed to identify specific health issues, pathologies, functional deficits, and physical limitations when addressing the treatment of patients in various health-care settings.

For that reason, the World Health Organization (WHO), the authority on health-care issues within the United Nations system and for global health matters, developed a family of classifications that may be used to compare health information internationally as well as nationally.[1] The International Classification of Diseases, Ninth Revision (ICD-9), along with the newly adopted ICD-10 (in the United States), is well known and used to classify diseases and other health problems. The International Classification of Functioning, Disability and Health (ICF), endorsed by WHO in 2001, provides additional information related to functioning and disability associated with health conditions. These two classification systems were developed to be complementary and to provide an overall picture of a person's disease or disorder and how it interacts with the person's ability to function within society and the environment.[2]

As a result, the two systems help provide a common language to be employed across cultures and borders as a critical link in communication. This link facilitates communication among health-care agencies worldwide, stimulates research, and provides rehabilitation professionals and other health-care providers with the means to improve clinical care for the patients they treat.

WHO FAMILY OF INTERNATIONAL CLASSIFICATIONS

The ICD and ICF classification systems are part of a broader system known as the WHO Family of International Classifications (WHO-FIC), which is used by all entities in health-care settings worldwide. The WHO-FIC includes reference classifications, derived classifications, and related classifications. Within each of these classification systems, parameters are addressed related to health issues (e.g., the ICD classification system and the ICF), diseases, and other issues not directly related to specific diseases or disabilities.

Reference classifications cover those parameters related to health-care issues affecting an individual's ability to function and include the following:

- The ICD coding system, introduced previously, which provides a numerical identification system for describing multiple diseases and health conditions that may have an impact on functioning that therapists may address (medical providers in the United States transitioned to the ICD-10 classification system as of October 1, 2015).
- The ICF, which provides a classification system that delineates how a health condition may have an impact on an individual's ability to function instead of focusing on the individual's specific health condition.
- The International Classification of Health Interventions (ICHI; with continued revisions at the time of this writing), which provides a common language for all health interventions.

Derived classifications provide more specialized classifications of diseases or disorders from the broader reference classifications (e.g., the International Classification of Diseases for Oncology, the ICF version for Children and Youth [ICF-CY], the Application of the ICF to Neurology).

Related classifications describe aspects of health not commonly addressed otherwise nor related to specific diseases or disabilities (e.g., the International Classification of Primary Care, Second Edition [ICPC-2]).[2]

THE ICF FRAMEWORK

Although both the ICD classification system and the ICF framework are important to therapists in the clinical setting, the ICF framework provides PTs and PTAs with the additional means to determine how a patient's function may be influenced by his or her disease. With the endorsement of the ICF framework in 2001, WHO provided a common language that could be used worldwide to describe health-related conditions and their interaction with function. WHO introduced this classification system following studies in more than 40 countries, making it a system free of cultural bias. It is based on both a medical model (specifically attributed to the individual with a disability or disease) and a social model (how that individual fits into society with environmental modifications made for that individual's disability or disease and the social acceptance of that individual).[2]

The ICF was not developed to take the place of another assessment method to treat individuals. It was developed to (1) provide a framework to help promote common terminology across disciplines, (2) provide a classification system independent of a specific disease or disorder, and (3) determine how a disability or disease might affect or limit an individual's ability to function and perform within society and/or his or her environment. This *universal* approach is more appropriate for treating the patient as an individual instead of using his or her specific disease or disability for identification.

The ICF belongs to the WHO family of international classifications, the best known member of which is the ICD-10 (the International Statistical Classification of Diseases and Related Health Problems). The ICD-10 gives users an etiological framework for the classification, by diagnosis, of diseases, disorders, and other health conditions. Therefore, the ICD-10 and ICF are complementary, and users are encouraged to use them together to create a broader and more meaningful picture of the experience of health of individuals and populations. Information on mortality (provided by the ICD-10) and information about health and health-related outcomes (provided by the ICF) can be combined in summary measures of population health. In short, the ICD-10 is used to classify causes of death, but the ICF classifies health.[2]

By using this ICF framework in the clinical setting, a therapist can classify a patient's functional status and outcomes, help set goals for treatment planning and monitoring, provide a comparison of interventions used for specific disabilities or disorders, and enhance electronic health records to assist in clinical decision-making.[2] In addition to being used to describe an individual's functioning, the ICF framework can also be used to organize data for research-based activities or in educational programs as an adjunct to clinical decision-making processes.

Prior to WHO's acceptance of the ICF framework, earlier models were developed and used to address disability and disease. As discussed in Chapter 1, the Nagi Disablement Model (1969) highlighted the individual's disability and impairment related to his or her pathology and functional limitations. With its revision in 2014, the APTA's *Guide to Physical Therapist Practice* reflects the newly endorsed ICF framework and its terminology in place of the Nagi model.

The American Physical Therapy Association's Endorsement of the ICF Framework

Following WHO's development of the ICF in 2001, it was adopted worldwide as an important tool to bring cultures, countries, and practitioners together and allow them to use a common language and further describe functioning. In keeping with this adoption practice, the APTA House of Delegates (HOD) unanimously voted to endorse the ICF framework during its June 2008 meeting in San Antonio, Texas. According to the APTA, the ICF provides a description/classification of the functioning of an individual and a standard language for function and disability for all agencies to utilize.[3]

As a result of the HOD vote, the language used in the ICF framework continues to be incorporated in all relevant American Physical Therapy Association documents and communication through a current review and revision cycle.[3] By developing this model and taking steps to develop a universal language to address health-related issues, the APTA has recognized the importance of a common language for all health-care professionals. This is especially true for PTs and PTAs, who promote the return to function following a disease, disorder, or injury. In addition to the support of the APTA for transition to the ICD-10 coding system for appropriate documentation, the World Confederation for Physical Therapy (WCPT) also recognizes the importance of developing and documenting agreed-upon standards for the practice of physical therapy worldwide. These standards include the following:

- Demonstrate to the public that physical therapists are concerned with the quality of the services provided and are willing to implement self-regulatory programs to maintain that quality.
- Guide the development of professional education.
- Guide practitioners in the conduct and evaluation of their practices.
- Provide governments, regulatory bodies, and other professional groups with background information about the professional nature of physical therapy.
- Effectively communicate with members of the profession, employers, other health professions, governments, and the public.

Not only does the WCPT encourage their members to follow such standards, they also set national practice standards in the areas of documentation, ethical behavior, quality assurance, and the like.[4]

For practicing PTs and PTAs, the ICF provides a common language that can be utilized across all nations and in all health-care settings and also offers an additional tool for identifying how a disease or disability can affect function for a patient in the clinical setting. In keeping with this framework, the acceptance of the ICD-10 coding system on October 1, 2015, provides increased specificity for diagnosis in treatment and lends support to the underlying components of the ICF model.

Components of the ICF Framework

WHO divided the ICF into two main components and their domains (see Table 2–1 for a description of each component and domain):

1. Part 1—Functioning and Disability
   - Body Functions
   - Body Structures
   - Activities and Participation
2. Part 2—Contextual Factors
   - Environmental Factors
   - Personal Factors

It is important to note that because of the variability of personal factors (e.g., race, sex, gender, age, educational level), such factors can be used in the ICF coding system but are not

Table 2–1	Descriptions of Each of the Five ICF Domains Within the Main Components of the ICF Framework
Domain	**Description**
FUNCTIONING AND DISABILITY	
Body Functions	Includes the physiological functions of body systems, such as: · Mental functions · Sensory functions and pain · Voice and speech functions · Functions of the cardiovascular, hematological, immunological, and respiratory systems · Functions of the digestive, metabolic, endocrine systems · Genitourinary and reproductive functions · Neuromusculoskeletal and movement-related functions · Functions of the skin and related structure
Body Structures	Anatomical parts of the body, such as organs, limbs, and their components, for example: · Structure of the nervous system · The eye, ear, and related structures · Structures involved in voice and speech · Structure of the cardiovascular, immunological, and respiratory systems · Structures related to the digestive, metabolic, and endocrine systems · Structures related to genitourinary and reproductive systems · Structures related to movement · Skin and related structures
Activity and Participation	*Activity* includes the execution of a task or action by an individual. *Participation* includes involvement in a life situation. Examples include the following: · Learning and applying knowledge · General tasks and demands · Communication · Mobility · Self-care · Domestic life · Interpersonal interactions and relationships · Major life areas · Community, social, and civic life
CONTEXTUAL FACTORS	
Environmental Factors	The physical, social and attitudinal environment in which people live and conduct their lives. These are either barriers to or facilitators of the person's functioning. Examples include the following: · Products and technology · Natural environment and human-made changes to environment · Support and relationships · Attitudes · Services, systems, and policies
Personal Factors	Those items related to age, ethnicity, occupation, etc.[6]

Source: Centers for Disease Control and Prevention. 2016. *The ICF model.* Retrieved from https://www.cdc.gov/nchs/data/icd/icfoverview_finalforwho10sept.pdf

utilized at this time within the framework. However, personal factors do have an impact on the patient's ability to function within the context of his or her health condition or disability (e.g., the WHO health conditions model in Fig. 2–1, discussed below).

Using the five domains outlined in Table 2–1, the ICF framework, along with the ICD-10 coding system, can be used to classify functioning and disability to provide a universal description of the disability and how the various domains interact and affect the ability of that individual to function appropriately. One of the initial methods to utilize the ICF framework is shown in Figure 2–1. This figure shows the basic ICF framework used to address a "health condition and the domains of the model."[5] This model can be used to provide more specific information regarding the interaction of the patient's health condition and his or her function as it relates to body functions, body structures, activity and participation, environmental factors, and personal factors. With the ICD-10 coding system, the therapist can now code for more specificity related to laterality of injury, activities that caused the injury, and the environment in which the injury occurred. While some of the information is not coded for medical treatment (e.g., personal factors), it does provide data for governmental and state health programs. Additionally, their interaction should be considered within the context of the patient's functioning. Again, because of the variability of the personal factors, they are listed but not classified, although they are very important, and their interaction should be considered within the context of the patient's functioning.

To support the ICF's importance and ease of use in assessing a person's function at a point in time in all types of settings, Figures 2–2 and 2–3 demonstrate how to use the ICF "Health

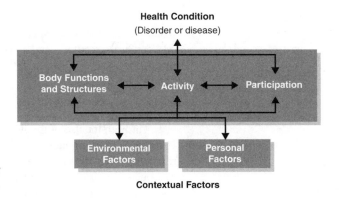

Figure 2–1 Universal assessment of disability using the ICF. *From:* World Health Organization. (2002). *Towards a common language for functioning, disability, and health: ICF.* Retrieved from http://www.who.int/classifications/icf/training/icfbeginnersguide.pdf, with permission.

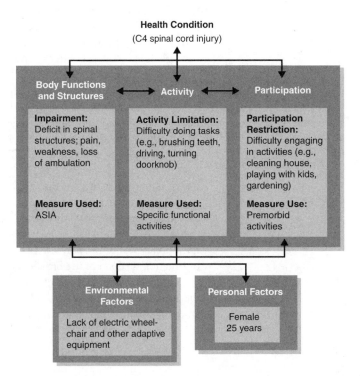

Figure 2–2 Use of the ICF to review a spinal cord injury (SCI).

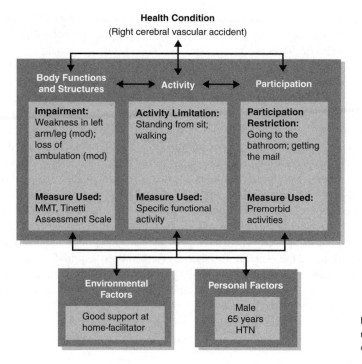

Figure 2—3 Use of the ICF to review a cerebral vascular accident (CVA).

Conditions" to assess a specific condition—in this case, a spinal cord injury (SCI; Fig. 2–2) or a cerebral vascular accident (CVA; Fig. 2–3). Through the use of the ICF framework as an informative tool of a patient with an SCI or a CVA, the patient's activity and participation levels can be considered. The ICF framework also helps describe a portion of the patient's physical health while providing an outcomes assessment to ensure comprehensive treatment of the individual patient.

Through the use of the ICF and ICD-10 systems, documentation plays an important role in defining the language used in the health-care setting. It also provides a means for proper reimbursement by third-party payers such as Medicare, Medicaid, HMOs, PPOs, and private insurance for those PTs and PTAs providing quality, skilled patient care. While these ICF codes and domains are not utilized in most clinics today, they provide a historical review of the ICF and help reiterate the importance of a coding system that is common among medical providers. Connected to the ICD-9 and ICD-10 coding systems, the universality of the providers to "speak the same language" when developing the interventions for the plan of care (POC) provides a better avenue to target functional outcomes appropriate for the patient.

SUMMARY   Based on reviews of the ICF in health care today, it was important to develop and utilize a common international language and to further define the differences between functioning and disabilities across cultures and borders. Through the use of the ICF and the necessity of developing clinical models to address function and outcomes in multiple settings, the importance of this framework was verified. APTA's endorsement of the ICF framework and the 2014 revision of the *Guide to Physical Therapist Practice* material provide additional support for the use of this framework and the ICD-10 coding system.

With the introduction of the ICF coding system, physical therapists and physical therapist assistants are able to follow the historical dynamics of the transition from the ICD-9 to the ICD-10 coding system for more focus on functionality and specificity of treatment. The initiation of the ICD-10 in 2015 increased the coding specificity for treatment related to issues of function, instead of the broader ICD-9 coding system that strictly identifies only the disease or diagnosis or for that system initially supported by the Nagi Disablement Model. Now, all therapists have a unified method to provide treatment across cultures, one that is easily understood by all clinicians and can be used in any type of setting.

REFERENCES

1. Madden, R., Sykes, C., & Bedirhan Ustun, T. (n.d.). *World Health Organization family of international classifications: Definition, scope and purpose*. Retrieved from http://www.who.int/classifications/en/FamilyDocument2007.pdf
2. World Health Organization. (n.d.). *International classification of functioning, disability, and health (ICF)*. Retrieved from http://www.who.int/classifications/icf/en
3. American Physical Therapy Association. (2008, July 10). APTA endorses World Health Organization ICF model. *Medical News Today*. Retrieved from http://www.medicalnewstoday.com/releases/114422.php
4. The World Conference for Physical Therapy (WCPT). 2015. *Policy statement: Standards of physical therapy practice*. Retrieved from http://www.wcpt.org/policy/ps-standards
5. World Health Organization. (2001). *International classification of functioning, disability, and health*. Geneva, Switzerland: Author.
6. Centers for Disease Control and Prevention. 2016. *The ICF model*. Retrieved from https://www.cdc.gov/nchs/data/icd/icfoverview_finalforwho10sept.pdf

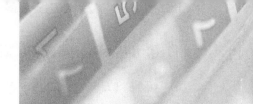

Review Exercises

1. **Explain** the importance of WHO's ICF conceptual framework in the health-care setting.

2. **Why** is it important for the APTA to endorse the ICF conceptual framework?

3. Explain the **use** of the ICF in determining the effect of a disease on a person's ability to function.

4. **Explain** how the ICD coding system **differs** from the ICF coding system.

5. **Describe** each of the five domains in the ICF framework.

6. Within the ICF framework, **which** parameters are included in Part 1?

7. Describe the **differences** between the Nagi Disablement Model and the ICF framework.

8. **When** was the ICD-10 coding system initiated in the United States?

9. **When** was the last revision of the *Guide to Physical Therapist Practice*?

PRACTICE EXERCISES

Identify which domain the following categories fall under by writing the corresponding letter in parentheses after each example:

- *body function (b)*

- *body structure (s)*

- *activities and participation (d)*

- *environmental factors (e)*

Example: *support (e)*

1. domestic life _____

2. technology _____

3. skin and related structures _____

4. attitudes _____

5. nervous system _____

6. learning _____

7. eyes and ears _____

8. self-care _____

9. relationships _____

10. speech _____

Identify which domain the following categories fall under by writing the corresponding letter in parentheses after each example

Example: *Difficulty with coordination activities due to a cerebellar stroke (body structure)*

1. Crawling across the room _____

2. Tightness in the IT band _____

3. Radiating pain down the left arm _____

4. Use of a front-wheeled walker (FWW) _____

5. Lifting and carrying objects with the arms _____

6. Difficulty judging width of door using wheelchair _____

7. Weakness in the diaphragm muscle _____

8. Use of a wheelchair to move about the house _____

9. Increased hypersensitivity to temperature changes _____

10. Difficulty following a one-step task _____

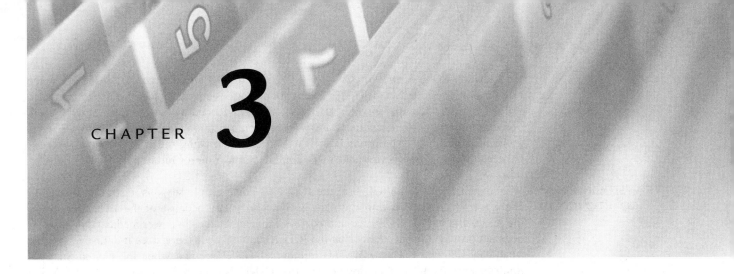

CHAPTER 3

Demystifying the ICD-10 Coding System

LEARNING OBJECTIVES

After studying this chapter, the student will be able to:

☐ Distinguish the difference between the ICD-9 and ICD-10 coding systems
☐ Understand the necessity for the ICD-10 coding system
☐ Differentiate between the initial, subsequent, and sequela encounters
☐ Understand the different characters in the ICD-10 coding system
☐ Describe the importance of functional limitation reporting in the billing process
☐ Identify functional outcomes in the plan of care
☐ Describe the importance of the PTA involvement in functional outcomes for the patient
☐ Understand the 8-minute rule for billing physical therapy services
☐ Describe the importance of the physician quality reporting system (PQRS) for reimbursement of services
☐ Explain the difference between functional limitation "G" codes and PQRS "G" codes

INTRODUCTION

Chapter 2 provided a historical review of WHO and the International Classification of Functioning, Disability and Health (ICF) that introduced a common language and coding system to better describe issues related to the provision of health care worldwide. With the inception of the ICF, the return to functional capabilities of the patient became paramount in the treatment, billing, and reimbursement process. Through the identification of the components of the ICF (body structure and function, activities and participation, and environmental and personal factors), now degrees of functioning and disability could be used to determine the interaction among these components as well as their impact on the ability of the patient to return to function and do so appropriately.

Through development of this universal language, a coding system was needed to delineate specific treatments for the patient based on his or her functional limitations compared with the patient's medical diagnosis. This new coding system also helped provide more information for billing to third-party payers and helped to ensure reimbursement for quality care.

This new coding system is the International Classification of Diseases (ICD), recently updated to the ICD-10 coding system, in the United States. The ICD-9 system has been used in the United States longer than in any other country in the world. The United States finally made the transition to the ICD-10 on October 1, 2015, following all other countries that had made this transition by 2008.[1] In the United States, for all entities covered under the Health Insurance Portability and Accountability Act (HIPAA), the ICD-10 coding system must now be used. Some automotive no-fault insurance and worker's compensation plans do not adhere to HIPAA guidelines, and it may be possible for them to continue using the ICD-9 coding system.[2] However, it would be wise to make this a complete transition for future purposes.

TRANSITION FROM ICD-9 TO ICD-10

Why transition from the ICD-9 to the ICD-10? For multiple reasons, as briefly discussed in the Introduction. This transition has become necessary because of the archaic nature of the ICD-9 and its inability to accommodate continued changes in newer medical diagnoses. It does not provide the specificity that the ICD-10 now provides, nor does it delineate specific functional outcomes, a necessity for reimbursement. Also, just when the United States is implementing the ICD-10 coding system, the ICD-11 is expected to launch in 2017.[3] Owing to changes in medical care, diagnoses, limitations with the ICD-9 coding system, the inability to add additional codes, and the necessity to become consistent with the rest of the world, the change to the ICD-10 coding system had to be made.

Differences Between the Two Coding Systems

Just what is the difference between the two coding systems? For a comparison, please refer to Table 3–1.

Table 3–1 Differences Between the ICD-9 and ICD-10 Coding Systems	
ICD-9	**ICD-10**
Uses approximately 17,000 diagnostic codes and 4,000 procedural codes	Uses approximately 69,000 diagnostic codes and 87,000 procedural codes
3–5 characters in length	3–7 characters in length
Digit 1 may be alpha or numeric	Digit 1 is alpha
Digits 2–5 are numeric	Digits 2–3 are numeric Digits 4–7 may be alpha or numeric
Limited spacing for adding new codes	Flexibility to accommodate new codes
Difficult to analyze data owing to multiple nonspecific codes that may share common meaning	Very specific
Does not support health data exchange with other countries	Supports health data exchange with other countries
Does not differentiate between traumatic and nontraumatic	Differentiates between traumatic and nontraumatic
Decimal occurs after third character	Decimal occurs after third character
No laterality of side affected	Laterality (right versus left side)
Does not distinguish dominant versus nondominant side	Distinguishes dominant versus nondominant side
Does not identify single versus bilateral condition	Identifies single versus bilateral condition
Does not identify the injury, place of occurrence, or activity in which the patient was involved that caused the injury	Identifies cause of traumatic injury, place of occurrence, and activity patient was performing when injury occurred
Does not differentiate between initial, subsequent or sequela encounters	Allows for differentiation between initial, subsequent, and sequela encounters
No placeholders used	May use placeholder (e.g., "X")

Here are some examples of the two codes:

	ICD-9	ICD-10
Lumbago:	742.2	M51.16
Pain in left hip:	719.45	M25.652
Cervicalgia	723.1	M25.611

This change from ICD-9 to ICD-10 involves a lot more coding for the physical therapist (PT) and the necessity for the physical therapist assistant (PTA) to understand what all the "fuss" is about. Since patients usually come to physical therapy because of injury or pain from injury, the supervising PT can begin coding the diagnosis and treatment codes using those two initial reasons for skilled physical therapy services. Chapter 4 outlines the differences between the medical and physical therapy diagnosis codes and the importance of identifying the exact deficit the patient has acquired based on the medical diagnosis and/or the physical therapy diagnosis. They may be the same codes, depending on the situation.

When using the ICD-10 coding system, it is critical for the evaluating PT to use as much specificity as possible in the coding process. This will help to ensure that all aspects of the diagnosis have been addressed and that third-party payers will provide reimbursement for such services. No longer can the treating therapist get by using the ICD-9 codes if working with a HIPAA-compliant payer. For those therapists seeing patients covered under workers' compensation and other private insurance companies, the ICD-9 may still be used. However, it is only a matter of time before the full conversion is adopted by all entities in the United States.

Alphabetical Versus Tabular List

To help therapists code medical diagnoses and injuries for the patients they treat, the Centers for Medicare & Medicaid (CMS) provide both alphabetical and tabular indices to best determine the code that meets the needs of the patient. Both of these indices are available in print or online through the CMS at https://www.cms.gov/medicare/coding/icd10/downloads/6_i10tab2010.pdf for the tabular list and at http://www.cdc.gov/nchs/data/dvs/2008Vol3.pdf for the alphabetical list.

Many electronic health record (EHR) programs have already made this transition, with the appropriate support for ICD-10, and provide similar access to printed and online versions of the two indices.

Both indices contain information important to the ICD-10 coding process and should be used in conjunction with each other. Some of the most common chapters used by an evaluating PT will be:

- Chapter 4: Endocrine, Nutritional, and Metabolic Diseases (E00-E89)
- Chapter 6: Diseases of the Nervous System (G00-G99)
- Chapter 13: Diseases of the Musculoskeletal System and Connective Tissue (M00-M99)
- Chapter 18: Symptoms, Signs, and Abnormal Clinical and Laboratory Findings, Not Elsewhere Classified (R00-R99)
- Chapter 19: Injury, Poisoning, and Certain Other Consequences of External Causes (S00-T88)
- Chapter 20: External Causes of Morbidity (V00-V99)

With the ICD-10 coding system, the first three placeholders are relegated to the category related to the injury, pain, and so on. The next three placeholders include the anatomical site, severity, and etiology, related to the category. The final placeholder is the extension or the time period when the patient accessed care for the injury. An example of an ICD-10 code is[4] **Injury of the Right Achilles Tendon—S86.011.D**, which can be translated as follows:

- **S86** denotes the <u>**category**</u> of the illness or injury
  - S specifically denotes injuries, poisonings, and certain other consequences of external causes related to a single body region.
  - S86 denotes an injury to muscle, fascia, and tendon at lower leg.

■ **011** denotes the etiology, anatomical site, severity, other vital details of the illness or injury.
  • S86.0 = **injury** of the Achilles tendon
  • S86.01 = **Strain** of the Achilles tendon
  • S86.011 = Strain of the **right** Achilles tendon
■ **D** denotes the extension for the code, which is used to document the episode of care for injuries and other conditions with external causes.
  • In this case, it is the subsequent encounter.
  • The letter "A" denotes the initial encounter.
  • The letter "S" indicates a sequela of the initial or subsequent encounters.[4]

While it is not the responsibility of the PTA to initially code the patient's diagnoses, it is important for the PTA to understand the basic coding process, the necessary specificity for billing, and the need for appropriate communication with the supervising PT to ensure quality care for the patient. One of the most important changes that occurred in the transition from the ICD-9 to the ICD-10 was the addition of the "7th" character. Its importance is discussed in the next section.

The 7th Character   The addition of the "7th" character in the ICD-10 coding system provides the treating therapist, medical record reviewers, and third-party payers with the ability to determine at what point the patient entered into the treatment process. The three primary codes that the evaluating PT will use for the 7th character are the characters for the initial (A) versus subsequent (D) versus sequela (S) encounters. This 7th character is used specifically for injuries and other types of deficits in the care of the patient. How the patient initially enters into treatment in the physical therapy facility helps determine the "encounter" code that will be used during his or her treatment.

Initial Encounter (A)   The initial encounter, identified by the letter "A," denotes the patient is receiving active care for an injury by a new medical professional. This could include a treatment provided by a surgeon, specialist, or general physician or in an emergency room setting, for example. In the case of a physical therapist, it would include a patient who walked into the clinic under direct access, without a referral from a physician, and prior to any other treatment from a medical professional. In most instances, it would be unusual for this code to be used by a physical therapist.

Subsequent Encounter (D)   The letter "D" identifies the subsequent encounter code and means the patient is receiving routine care for an injury during the healing or recovery phase. This is the most consistent code used for a physical therapy evaluation and treatment for patients referred for skilled physical therapy to treat injury/pain after having been seen already by another provider in the healthcare field.

The Sequela Encounter (S)   A sequela encounter is identified by the letter "S" and indicates that the initial injury has caused an additional deficit for which the patient may seek treatment. This would include a complication or a condition that might arise as a direct result from the initial injury. An example is the formation of scar tissue resulting from a burn. The burn may be the initial injury being treated, but treatment must also occur due to the resulting scar tissue, which resulted in loss of range of motion. The treatment for the scar tissue would be coded with the "S" extension, identifying the injury responsible for the sequela.[4] It is important to note that the CPT codes will remain unchanged under this new coding system and will continue to be used in the same manner as used under the ICD-9 coding system.

The Placeholder "X"   Because of the change in the number of spaces allocated with the transition to ICD-10, it was necessary to provide a placeholder, depending on the extent of alphanumeric options needed to provide the appropriate diagnosis code for a patient. For that reason, the letter "X" is used to denote that a code was not found for one of the specific placeholders but the extension is still necessary. Therefore, the letter "X" is used when there are less than six characters, but the

"7th" extension character is still required. An example is right knee contusion: S80.01X.D.[2] The following is an explanation of this new code:

- **S80** denotes the **<u>category</u>** of the illness or injury
  - S specifically denotes injuries, poisonings, and certain other consequences of external causes related to a single body region.
  - S80 denotes contusion of unspecified knee.
- **201X** denotes the etiology, anatomical site, severity, and other vital details of the illness or injury (in this case, there is no third number and "X" is used as a placeholder).
  - S80.01 = **contusion** of unspecified knee
  - S80.01X = contusion of the **right** knee
- **D** denotes the extension for the code, which is used to document the episode of care for injuries and other conditions with external causes. In this case, the letter "D" indicates the subsequent encounter.
  - The letter "A" denotes the initial encounter.
  - The letter "S" indicates a sequela of the initial or subsequent encounters.[4]

Activity Codes

The activity code is used to identify the type of activity the patient was engaged in when the injury occurred. Such codes can be found in the alphabetical or tabular indices, as needed. For example, Y93.012. indicates the following:

- **Y93** is the category code for activity.
  - 01 is the code for the activity walking, marching, and hiking.

Place of Occurrence Codes

In addition to the activity code, the place of occurrence is also used to identify where the injury happened (e.g., a soccer field), and those codes can also be found in the alphabetical or tabular indices, as needed. For example, Y92.0142 indicates the following:

- **Y92** is the category code for occurrence.
  - 014 is a private driveway to a single-family (private) house as the place of occurrence of the external cause.

Excludes Notes

In addition to this new coding information, it is important to note that, at times, certain conditions may be "excluded" in the billing process. This type of exclusion is used when similar diagnoses are being billed and must not be included together or need to be coded separately. There are two types of exclusions, Excludes type 1 and Excludes type 2.[5]

Excludes 1

A type 1 Excludes note is a pure excludes note. It means "NOT CODED HERE!" An Excludes 1 note indicates that the code excluded should never be used at the same time as the code above the Excludes 1 note. An Excludes 1 is used when two conditions cannot occur together, such as a congenital form versus an acquired form of the same condition.[5] In this case, only one of these codes may be used.

Excludes 2

A type 2 Excludes note represents "Not included here." An Excludes 2 note indicates that the condition excluded is not part of the condition represented by the code, but a patient may have both conditions at the same time. When an Excludes 2 note appears under a code, it is acceptable to use both the code and the excluded code together, for example, coding a pain in a joint and a pain in the leg.[5] In this case, both codes may be included, with only one condition being the one treated.

FUNCTIONAL OUTCOMES AND "G" CODES

With the inception of the ICD-10 coding system, it is much easier to determine the importance of the functional outcome for the patient receiving skilled physical therapy services. Use of the ICD-10 and functional limitation reporting (FLR) provides the evaluating PT with the means to code the initial or subsequent encounter of treatment in addition to the re-evaluation process through discharge. By using more functional codes, the PT can determine how well the functional outcomes were met and note any deterrents to progress and methods to better prepare the patient for discharge by meeting those functional goals, as outlined in the PT plan of care (POC). FLR using objective tools to track patient outcomes helps ensure quality care, progression through the PT POC, and provision of the necessary information for billing of PT services. Medicare, a government-subsidized insurance provided to those individuals aged 65 and over and those with certain life-threatening medical problems, requires therapists to use at least one outcome measurement tool to complete FLR and PQRS.[6] Examples include the Oswestry Low Back Pain Scale and the DASH. More information regarding Medicare and its coverage is discussed in Chapter 4.

It is the responsibility of the PTA to communicate any changes, progress, or regression to the supervising PT to ensure the patient receives the best skilled PT services to meet his or her needs for functional independence. Understanding the evaluation process and the new coding system allows both the PT and PTA to best determine progress and provide quality care to their patient. The processes of assessing progress toward the functional goals outlined in the PT POC have been set by CMS and are required for all patients receiving Medicare Part B. The following list delineates facilities that must provide FLR on their patients under Medicare:

Professionals: Therapists in Private Practice: Physical Therapists, Occupational Therapists, & Speech Language Pathologists

Physicians: Medical Doctors (MDs), Doctors of Osteopathy (DOs), Doctors of Podiatric Medicine (DPMs), & Doctors of Optometry (ODs)

Nurse Practitioners, Psychiatric (NPPs): Nurse Practitioners (NPs), Clinical Nurse Specialists (CNSs), & Physician Assistants (PAs)

Providers: Outpatients (OPs) and inpatients (IPs) receiving Part B therapy services, Rehabilitation Agencies, Home Health Agencies (HHAs), Comprehensive Outpatient Rehabilitation Facilities (CORFs), Outpatient Hospitals, including Emergency Departments, Critical Access Hospitals[6]

These functional outcomes along with the "G" codes are the PTA's way of documenting the patient's progression through the treatment process from the initial evaluation to discharge. The functional outcomes and resulting "G" codes are listed in Table 3–2.[6]

Along with the functional outcomes listed in Table 3–2, the PT must also use modifiers to report the severity of the functional limitation for the patient;[6] see Table 3–3.

These modifiers are reported based on the score from the outcome measurement tool used at the initial PT evaluation for each patient (e.g., Oswestry Low Back Pain Scale, Lower Extremity Functional Scale).

For every patient seen who has Medicare Part B, at least one of the "G" codes, with the accompanying modifier, must be used in the evaluation process to determine the best functional

Table 3–2 Functional Outcomes and "G" Codes

Functional Limitations Category/Type	Current	Goal	Discharge	Notes
Mobility: Walking and Moving Around	G8978	G8979	G8980	"A Current "G" code should be reported at
Changing and Maintaining Body Position	G8981	G8982	G8983	every reporting interval "except" discharge."
Carrying, Moving and Handling Objects	G8984	G8985	G8986	"A Goal "G" code should be reported at
Self-Care	G8987	G8988	G8989	every reporting interval."
Other PT/OT Primary Functional Limitation	G8990	G8991	G8992	"A Discharge "G" code should be reported at
Other PT/OT Secondary Functional Limitation	G8993	G8994	G8995	Discharge or at End of limitation."

Table 3-3	Modifiers to Report the Severity of Functional Limitation
Modifier	**Impairment Limitation Restrictions**
CH	0 percent impaired, limited or restricted
CI	At least 1 percent but less than 20 percent impaired, limited or restricted
CJ	At least 20 percent but less than 40 percent impaired, limited or restricted
CK	At least 40 percent but less than 60 percent impaired, limited or restricted
CL	At least 60 percent but less than 80 percent impaired, limited or restricted
CM	At least 80 percent but less than 100 percent impaired, limited or restricted
CN	100 percent impaired, limited or restricted

activity needed during the skilled physical therapy treatment sessions[6] to restore the patient to the highest functional level possible. Both the evaluating PT and the patient should decide which category best fits the needs of the patient based on the deficits that have occurred from the patient's injury, surgery, and so on at the initial evaluation and then again at each reassessment. While it is important to choose one primary functional outcome, more than one may be used, depending on the patient's deficits, to show progression of the patient's functional status throughout the rehabilitation process.

For example, a status post-shoulder may start out in the Self-Care category but then can progress to the Carrying, Moving, and Handling Objects category as he or she gains strength and AROM. It is important for the PTA to follow that POC to help determine the time for transition to another category based on the reassessment process. To best determine how the patient progresses from the initial evaluation through the reexamination process to discharge, the facility can use some of the basic functional outcome worksheets/questionnaires included here:

- Neck Disability Index
- Modified Oswestry Disability Scale
- Upper Extremity Functional Index (DASH or Quick DASH)
- Lower Extremity Functional Scale
- Tinetti Assessment of Gait and Balance
- Berg Balance Scale

These functional worksheets/questionnaires are required for the billing process in clinics and facilities, and without them such facilities may not be reimbursed for skilled physical therapy services.

PHYSICIAN QUALITY REPORTING CODING SYSTEM (PQRS)

Beginning July 1, 2013, CMS required all facilities treating patients with Medicare Part B insurance to identify specific quality measures when treating a patient in their clinic. Those measures are referred to as the Physician Quality Reporting System (PQRS). As of January 1, 2016, outpatient clinics were required to identify nine PQRS measures used throughout the treatment process for tracking purposes, if appropriate[8]; some facilities may not treat the type of patient for which a specific measure can be utilized (i.e., following a diabetic patient, if the clinic does not see those patients). Such measures are used to track patient care coordination, population health, safety, effective care, and crosscutting (APTA Learning Center).

Procedure and "G" Codes for Reporting Patient Data

The top reported PQRS coding measures for physical therapy are as follows[9]:

#128 Preventative Care and Screening: Body Mass Index (BMI) Screening and Follow-up

This is reported only at the initial evaluation and is expressed as weight/height (kg/m^2). The normal parameter for patients between the ages of 18 and 64 is a BMI greater than or equal to 18.5 but less than 25. For patients aged 65 and older, the BMI should be greater than or equal to 23 but less than 30. Here are the specific BMI codes:

G2480: Calculated BMI within normal parameters and documented at the initial evaluation

OR

G8417: BMI above normal, follow-up documented

OR

G8418: BMI below normal, follow-up documented

OR

G8422: Patient not eligible for BMI calculations (palliative care, pregnant, or refuses)

OR

G8938: BMI calculated, but patient not eligible for follow-up plan

OR

G8421: BMI not calculated, reason not given

OR

G8419: BMI outside normal parameters, __no__ follow-up plan documented

For billing and auditing purposes, it would never be advisable to show that any measure identified by a facility in the PQRS coding system was not documented or provided! While the codes for such instances are provided, they will raise a red flag in the documentation and billing processes, if used. The intent is for all information required to be provided.

#130 Documentation and Verification of Current Medications in the Medical Record

This measure is reported at the initial evaluation and documented when any changes occur throughout the treatment process. This list must include all prescriptions, over-the-counter medications, herbal remedies, and vitamin/mineral/dietary (nutritional) supplements and must contain the medication's name, dosage, frequency, and route of administration. Here are specific medication codes:

G8427: Current medications documented to the best of knowledge and ability

OR

G8430: Patient not eligible for medication documentation

OR

G8428: Current medications __not__ documented, reason not given

#131 Pain Assessment Prior to Initiation of Patient Treatment

This measure is reported at the initial evaluation and documented prior to and following every treatment session through discharge. For a clinical assessment of pain, a standardized tool should be used and should include the location, intensity, quality, and onset/duration of the reported pain. Tools could include a Verbal Rating Scale, Visual Analog Scale, Wong-Baker Faces Pain Rating Scale, Drawing Scale, and so on. Here are specific pain assessment codes:

G8730: Pain assessed with valid tool and follow-up plan documented

OR

G8731: Pain assessed as negative and no follow-up plan required

OR

G8732: Pain __not__ documented, reason not given

OR

G8509: Documentation of positive pain assessment; __no__ documentation of a follow-up plan, reason not given

#154 Falls: Risk Assessment

This is a two-part measure that is paired with Measure #155: Falls: Plan of Care. If the Falls Risk Assessment indicates the patient has documentation of two or more falls in the past year or any fall with an injury in the past year, then #155 should be reported also. Avenues to measure falls risk can include, but are not limited to, the following:

- Identification of fall history
- Assessment of gait, balance and mobility, and muscle weakness
- Assessment of osteoporosis risk
- Assessment of older person's perceived functional ability and fear related to falling
- Assessment of visual impairment
- Assessment of home hazards
- Assessment of cognitive impairment

Here are specific fall risk assessment codes:

3288F: Falls risk assessment documented

AND

1100F: Patient screened for future fall risk: documentation of two or more falls in the past year or any fall with injury in the past year

OR

3288F with 1P (modifier): documentation of medical reason(s) for not completing a risk assessment for falls (i.e., reduced mobility, immobile, confined to a chair)

AND

1100F: Patient screened for future fall risk: documentation of two or more falls in the past year or any fall with injury in the past year

OR

1101F: Patient screened for future fall risk: documentation of no falls in the past year or only one fall without injury in the past year

#155 Falls: Plan of Care

As discussed previously, this measure should be documented if the code 1100F is used. Specific codes for falls include the following:

0518F: Falls plan of care documented

OR

0518F with 1P: documentation of medical reason(s) for no plan of care for falls

OR

*0518F with 8P: Falls plan of care __not__ documented, reason not otherwise specified (**Avoid using the 8P, if possible**)*

Clinical recommendation statements that might support the plan of care for falls include the following:

- Gait training and advice on the appropriate use of assistive device(s) (AD[s])
- Review and modification of medication, especially psychotropic medication
- Exercise programs, with balance training as one of the components
- Treatment of postural hypotension
- Modification of environmental hazards
- Treatment for cardiovascular disorders

#182 Functional
Outcomes Assessment

Functional outcome assessments should be completed at the initial evaluation, on the 10th visit or 30th day (whichever comes first), and at discharge. For instance, if the patient is being seen only once a week, the re-evaluation would be on the 30th day. If the patient is being seen three times per week, then the re-evaluation would be on the 10th visit. Functional outcome assessments should be completed using standardized functional outcome assessment tools and documentation of a plan of care, based on the patient's deficiencies. Here are specific functional outcome codes:

> *G8539: Documentation of a functional outcome assessment using a standardized tool **and** documentation of a care plan based on identified deficiencies on the date of the functional outcome assessment.*

> **OR**

> *G8542: Documentation of a functional outcome assessment using a standardized tool: no functional deficiencies identified, care plan not required.*
> *G8942: Documented functional outcomes assessment and care plan within the previous 30 days.*

> **OR**

> *G8540: Documentation that the patient is not eligible for a functional outcome assessment using a standardized tool.*

> **OR**

> *G8541: Functional outcome assessment using a standardized tool not documented, reason not given.*

> **OR**

> *G8543: Documentation of a functional outcome assessment using a standardized tool: care plan **not** documented, reason not given.*

Through the use of these codes, the PT and PTA can effectively track these data for the patient and the third-party payer throughout the course of treatment.

8-Minute Rule for
Billing

CMS requires patients to be billed using specific time periods that can be divided up into units for consistency in treatment times and for billing purposes. For that reason, CMS developed the 8-minute rule, and some other third-party payers have followed with similar requirements. Medicare, along with other insurance companies, requires that patient care be divided into direct and nondirect care. For these purposes, the 8-minute rule is a specific component of the billing process. Patient treatment is based on the time that the patient is seen, both direct (time when the patient is physically being treated) and nondirect (time when the patient is receiving treatment unattended, such as ultrasound or hot packs). Treatment is based on the number of units for **direct** patient care only. Each unit of direct time ranges from 8 to 22 minutes. Untimed codes count only toward total treatment time, not direct time. It is important to remember that the units listed here apply only to **direct-timed code** units. Here is an illustration of the time allotted for the number of units that can be billed for skilled physical therapy care:[7]

> 0 units = 0–7 minutes
> 1 unit = 8–22 minutes
> 2 units = 23–37 minutes
> 3 units = 38–52 minutes
> 4 units = 53–67 minutes
> 5 units = 68–82 minutes
> 6 units = 83–97 minutes
> 7 units = 98–112 minutes
> 8 units = 113–127 minutes

Total Direct Minutes = the total time spent on **Direct-Timed Code** activities

Total Treatment Units is the name given to the total time spent on treating the patient. Total Treatment Units = **Total Direct Minutes +** minutes spent on **Untimed Codes (nondirect time).** For example, your patient with Medicare insurance is being billed for one unit of Gait Training, one unit of Therapeutic Exercise, and the Initial Examination or the use of cold packs. With two direct-timed coded units (1 unit of Gait Training + 1 unit of Therapeutic Exercise), you must choose a range between 23 and 37 minutes of Total Direct Minutes. The Total Treatment Minutes (the two direct-timed codes + the initial examination) is a combination of both Untimed and Direct-Timed Codes.[7]

PTA INVOLVEMENT

Although the PTA does not perform evaluations, he or she may assist the PT with the evaluation procedure. The PTA may take notes and help gather the subjective data. During the treatment process, the PTA may take measurements, perform some tests, and record the results as the patient makes progress through the POC. However, the PTA may not interpret the results. Performing the tests and recording the results constitute *data collection*. Interpreting the results involves making a judgment about their value. This is called *evaluating*. Examples of tests and measurements that make use of a PTA's data-collection skills include girth measurements, manual testing of muscle groups, and goniometry measurements to assess ROM. In addition, a PTA's skillset may include assessment of vital signs, falls, balance, and other functional outcomes using prescribed scales, indices, or other types of information that can be scored to provide an objective measurement of the patient's progress.

As part of their documentation responsibilities, PTAs must properly code each treatment session, the response from the patient to that treatment, and the progression made throughout the treatment process. Using the proper CPT codes (which remain unchanged with the initiation of the ICD-10 coding system) helps the supervising PT and the billing department ensure appropriate reimbursement for the skilled physical therapy services provided and provides necessary feedback for the supervising PT to code the reevaluation and discharge portion of the patient's POC.

Beginning January 1, 2017, CMS made changes to many of the common CPT codes for diagnosis and inpatient procedure codes previously in use. Both the PT and PTA need to be apprised of these changes as they occur and make adjustments to the treatment and billing processes. Codes for the physical therapy evaluation and re-evaluation will be discontinued, and the new physical therapy evaluation/re-evaluation codes will be based on a tiered system. This new system is based on the 2017 changes in the Physician Fee Schedule to delineate the different levels of complexity involved in the physical therapy evaluation. However, even though there will be a tiered level for PT evaluations, the fee schedule will not change. Here is a review of some of the proposed changes:

CPT Coding prior to January 2017	CPT Coding after January 2017
97001-PT Evaluation	97161-physical therapy evaluation: low complexity
97002-PT Re-evaluation	97162-physical therapy evaluation: moderate complexity
	97163-physical therapy evaluation: high complexity

To determine which of the new codes to select, the evaluating physical therapist will need to utilize the following four components:

1. Patient history and comorbidities
2. Examination and use of standardized tests and measures
3. Clinical presentation
4. Clinical decision-making

These components, along with the tiered level for physical therapy evaluations, will tie in with the different domains used within the ICF.[10]

During the course of a patient's treatment, the PTA is often expected to repeat the tests and measurements to record the patient's progress since the initial evaluation and re-evaluation. This objective data is more reliable when the same person performs the tests and measurements in a consistent manner throughout the course of the patient's treatment.

When writing progress/daily notes, the PTA refers to the problems, goals and outcomes, and treatment plans outlined in the initial and interim evaluation reports. Progress/daily notes should record the effectiveness of the treatment plan by comparing the patient's progress toward accomplishing the goals and outcomes with the status of the patient at the initial evaluation to ensure the appropriate "G" codes are used to track progress.

SUMMARY   From the transition of the ICD-9 to ICD-10, it is evident that many changes have occurred to which PTs and PTAs alike must continue to adjust. Even though PTAs are not directly responsible for the coding and billing process, they are responsible for assessing the functional outcomes of the patients under their care, communicating any changes in the plan of care to the supervising PT, and making recommendations to the PT for reassessment or possible discharge. Having an understanding related to the "G" codes used for reporting functional outcomes paired with following the PQRS measurement system helps the treating PTA grasp the complexity needed to assess the patient accurately from the initial evaluation through the discharge process and then precisely document the plan of care. With this understanding comes the ability to assist the evaluating PT with the entire process related to the patient's continuum of care and, it is hoped, a more positive functional outcome for that patient.

REFERENCES
1. Hansell, A. (2016). *Speaking in code: Documentation to support the ICD-10 code set.* Combined sections presentation, American Physical Therapy Association, Anaheim, California.
2. Gawenda, R. (2016). *The ABC's of ICD-10 for physical therapists.* Combined sections presentation, American Physical Therapy Association, Anaheim, California.
3. Healthcare IT News. (2010). Why move to ICD-10, if ICD-11 is on the horizon? Retrieved from http://www.icd10watch.com/headline/why-move-icd-10-if-icd-11-horizon
4. WebPT. (2015). *The physical therapist's crunch-time guide to ICD-10.* Retrieved from https://www.webpt.com/resources/download/the-physical-therapists-crunch-time-guide-to-icd-10
5. e-Meds Blog. (2015). ICD-9 vs ICD-10: Use of exclusions. Retrieved from http://www.e-mds.com/icd-9-vs-icd-10-use-exclusions
6. Medicare Learning Network. (2012). *Preparing for therapy required functional reporting implementation in CY 2013.* Retrieved from https://www.cms.gov/Outreach-and-Education/Outreach/NPC/Downloads/FunctionalReportingNPC.pdf
7. Medicare Quick Guide. (2014). *8-minute rule.* Retrieved from https://www.webpt.com/8-minute-rule
8. WebPT. (2016). PQRS 2016 FAQ [Web log post]. Retrieved from https://www.webpt.com/blog/post/pqrs-2016-faq
9. CMS. (2016). *2016 speciality measure sets.* Retrieved from https://www.cms.gov/Medicare/Quality-Initiatives-Patient-Assessment-Instruments/PQRS/MeasuresCodes.html
10. WebPT. (2016). *Understanding the new evaluation codes for 2017.* Rick Gawenda, PT, Author. Retrieved from https://www.webpt.com/ascend/files/handouts/Day%202_Understanding%20the%20New%20Evaluation%20Codes%20for%202017_handout.pdf?__hstc=194109170.e06eef88364d86cb0b0b60d28d2d97b6.1473811200109.1473811200111.1473811200112.2&__hssc=194109170.1.1473811200112&__hsfp=1773666937

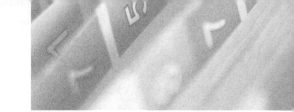

Review Exercises

1. List **four differences** between the ICD-9 and ICD-10 coding systems.

2. **What** is the 8-minute rule, and how is the time billed for two units?

3. What is the **purpose** of the "7th" character?

4. Explain the **difference** between the initial, subsequent, and sequela encounters.

5. What is the **difference** between a functional outcome code using FLR and a PQRS code?

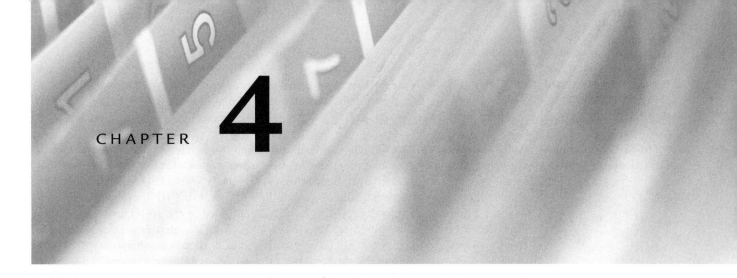

CHAPTER 4

Reimbursement Issues Related to Documentation

LEARNING OBJECTIVES	HEALTH-CARE REFORM LAW AND THE
INTRODUCTION	AFFORDABLE CARE ACT (ACA)
MANAGED CARE ORGANIZATIONS	HEALTH CARE AND POTENTIAL CHANGES
(MCOs)	TO DOCUMENTATION
MEDICARE	REIMBURSEMENT FOR PT VERSUS PTA
MEDICAID	STUDENT SERVICES
PROGRAM OF ALL-INCLUSIVE CARE FOR	SUMMARY
THE ELDERLY (PACE)	REFERENCES
WORKERS' COMPENSATION INSURANCE	REVIEW EXERCISES
OTHER MEDICAL INSURANCE OPTIONS	

LEARNING OBJECTIVES

After studying this chapter, the student will be able to:

☐ Differentiate between health maintenance organizations (HMOs), preferred provider organizations (PPOs), and other types of medical reimbursement

☐ Discuss the issues related to the declining use of HMOs and PPOs

☐ Understand Medicare (Parts A through D) and Medicaid reimbursement

☐ Identify the basic issues related to workers' compensation and private insurance coverage

☐ Understand options offered through health-care reform law and the Affordable Care Act

☐ Compare and contrast the documentation responsibilities of the PT and the PTA related to reimbursement in different health-care settings

☐ Differentiate between types of reimbursement for the PT and the PTA in specific health-care settings

☐ Discuss the reasons for nonreimbursement of services provided by a physical therapy aide in any clinical setting

INTRODUCTION

To more clearly understand the differences between the various resources that provide medical reimbursement and the importance of documentation, it is important to understand what each provider professes to cover for the individual, employer, employee, or company. This information helps such entities determine which provider they choose for reimbursement of medical services. Documentation and treatment can be very confusing to any individual trying to address the different requirements for managed care organizations (MCOs), Medicare, Medicaid, workers' compensation coverage, or private insurance. Without knowledge of services and scope of coverage, treating therapists will have difficulty determining what those parties require for appropriate patient treatment and documentation.

MANAGED CARE ORGANIZATIONS (MCOs)

It is helpful to review managed health care to obtain an understanding of services they provide. Such services are usually provided through health maintenance organizations (HMOs), preferred provider organizations (PPOs), and points of service (POS) organizations.

Health Maintenance Organizations (HMO)

An HMO is a type of MCO that provides health-care coverage through a limited number of physicians, hospitals, and other providers that have a contract with the HMO agency. An HMO covers only the care provided by those medical professionals who have agreed to treat patients within the confines of the guidelines and restrictions of that HMO. HMOs require individuals to select a primary care physician (PCP) from a list provided by the HMO network to follow the patient for all initial medical care. Then the PCP must provide referrals to other HMO agencies for all medical services that fall outside the scope of those that the PCP provides. HMOs monitor PCPs to ensure that the services they provide for each medical diagnosis are appropriate and not excessive in cost or type of treatment for the given diagnosis. In addition to medical care, HMOs provide preventive care, including such services as immunizations, well-care checkups, mammograms, and so forth that other types of insurance may not cover.[1] If a patient goes outside of an HMO's contract services, the individual will pay a higher rate for services received and, in some cases, may be responsible for the entire bill.

Preferred Provider Organizations (PPO)

A preferred provider organization (PPO) is a subscription-based MCO that gives members the option of choosing preferred providers from a list of contracted physicians or agencies that provide medical services through the PPO. A PCP is not required for coverage, and the patient does not need a referral for access to medical services. PPOs provide a substantial discount for their members. When patients belonging to a PPO network receive in-network medical care through their preferred providers, they are responsible only for paying their annual deductible and copays for their visits. If patients go "out of network" to get medical services, they will pay a higher rate directly to the physician or hospital and then can file a claim with their PPO to get reimbursed. PPOs earn money by charging access fees to the insurance company for the use of their network instead of charging premiums for medical services. PPOs also negotiate their fee schedules, handle disputes between the insurers and the providers, and can contract with each other to increase the strength of the relationship. Therefore, those insured by a PPO are billed at the reduced rate when they use the "preferred" provider. This increases the membership base for the company and continues to promote reduced rates for services; only members will be seen for such reduced rates. Additional services often used by PPOs include utilization reviews to review records and ensure appropriate services are being provided for the condition being treated, and precertification or prior approval requirements for nonemergency service, which help keep costs at a minimum.[1] Table 4–1 presents some of the differences between an HMO and a PPO,[1] but companies may also have different reimbursement procedures depending on their contracts.

Point of Service (POS) organizations

A point of service (POS) organization combines characteristics of an HMO and a PPO. POS organizations allow patients to either pick a PCP to manage their medical care within the network and provide referrals for other services or to use a provider outside of the network. If the patient chooses a provider outside of the network, however, he or she pays more for those medical services.[1] Even though MCOs are used throughout the country, the popularity of HMOs and PPOs began a serious decline in 2007.[2] This decline in popularity was due in part to decreased enrollment by individuals; an increase in the monthly premium fees required of individuals; and a decrease in the use of HMOs/PPOs by companies, due to escalating administrative costs.[2]

The Need for Something New

With the decrease in the use of HMOs and PPOs, other medical reimbursement companies have had to cover the gap by making improvements in procedures for negotiating with individual employees and the companies for which they work, reducing high-end administrative costs and ensuring the suitable coverage of employees and their dependents. There has been, and continues to be, inappropriate coverage of employees (or their dependents) who no longer require coverage, have passed the age of requiring coverage, or who simply do not meet the criteria for coverage as defined by the specific insurance company. For these reasons, the cost of medical reimbursements has escalated, and attempts are being made to ensure that inappropriate reimbursements

Table 4-1 Differences Between an HMO and a PPO

Type of Service	HMO	PPO
Can I choose my health-care providers?	You must choose a provider within the HMO network.	You may choose the provider from the list of contracted providers or you can go out of network (you may have to pay more for going out of network).
Do I need a PCP?	Yes. You cannot get services without a PCP and a referral.	No. You can see any provider you wish, but you will have to pay a higher rate for out-of-network providers.
Can I see a specialist (nonemergency)?	Yes, but your PCP must refer you to a specialist within the HMO network.	Yes. And you do not need a referral from your PCP, but you may have to pay more if the provider is out of network.
Do I file insurance claims?	No, all providers within the HMO network are required to file claims, and you do not receive a bill.	No. You do not have to file insurance claims if you are using the preferred provider. OR Yes. You do have to file insurance claims if you go to a provider who is out of network. Also you'll have to pay more, if not all, of the bill.

HMO = health maintenance organization; PCP = primary care physician; PPO = preferred provider organization

Source: Adapted from Bihari, M. (2010, April 15). HMOs vs. PPOs—What are the differences between HMOs and PPOs? About.com. Retrieved from https://www.verywell.com/what-are-the-differences-between-hmos-and-ppos-1739063

decline, ensuring more affordable and proper reimbursement for those individuals who do meet the criteria for coverage.[3]

Other options for health care have been researched and may lead to increased and better health care for individuals, decreased cost of health care, and increased interaction with the patient and the medical team through Patient-Centered Medical Home (PCMH) programs. With this type of health care, the individual is at the center of the medical process, while the "medical team" interacts and communicates to care for the patient. This reformed model of delivery system was crafted by the primary care professional organizations in 2007. The model has been endorsed by a broad coalition of health care stakeholders, including all of the major national health plans, most of the Fortune 500 companies, consumer organizations and labor unions, the American Medical Association, and a total of 17 specialty societies. At one point, 22 multistakeholder demonstration pilot projects were under way in 14 states, and the Centers for Medicare & Medicaid Services (CMS) conducted Medicare demonstration pilot projects in 400 practices in eight regional sites in 2009. Twenty bills promoting the PCMH concept have been introduced in 10 states.[4] It remains to be seen how the Affordable Care Act (ACA; discussed later in this chapter) will affect this type of health care and if it will continue to be as successful as it initially seems to have been.

MEDICARE

With the beginning of health-care coverage by Medicare (Title XVIII of the Social Security Act) in 1965, individuals aged 65 and older began to receive medical care subsidized by the federal government. In addition, since 1972 individuals younger than 65 who have permanent disabilities, end-stage renal disease, or Lou Gehrig's disease have also received Medicare coverage.[5] This coverage is independent of income or medical history (e.g., preexisting conditions) if an individual is 65 or older. Medicare is divided into four major parts—Part A, Part B, Part C, and Part D—for reimbursement in specific settings.

Medicare Part A (Original Medicare)

Medicare Part A coverage is available to individuals aged 65 or older, with the individual or his or her spouse being eligible for Social Security payments (they must have made payroll tax contributions for 10 years or more to qualify). Medicare Part A coverage provides insurance for treatment in hospitals and skilled nursing facilities and does not require premiums be paid by the individual. Individuals must enroll for Medicare Part A services during a 7-month period around the time they turn 65 (the period spanning the 3 months before their 65th birthday, the month they turn 65, and 3 months after their 65th birthday). Individuals should be aware that if they enroll during the last 4 months of their enrollment period, benefits could be delayed.[6] Individuals younger than age 65 can be eligible for Medicare coverage under specific conditions. Those with permanent disabilities, end-stage renal disease, or Lou Gehrig's disease are eligible for Medicare Part A after they first become eligible for Social Security Disability Insurance (SSDI). It can take up to 2 years before coverage under SSDI is granted, delaying qualification for Medicare benefits if the patient is younger than age 65. Usually enrollment in Medicare Part A is automatic, based on the individual's age and if the individual is receiving Social Security benefits. However, individuals aged 65 years and older who are still working and individuals diagnosed with end-stage renal disease are required to sign up for Medicare Part A by contacting Social Security.[6] If an individual fails to enroll in Medicare Part A during his or her enrollment period, he or she may enroll between January 1 and March 31 every year, and coverage will begin July 1 of that year. These individuals are required to pay a monthly penalty of 10% of the premiums for twice the period they were eligible to enroll but did not do so.[6] Individuals currently receiving coverage under an employer's insurance plan can wait until they retire from or leave their company to apply for Medicare coverage, and they will not pay higher premiums as long as they apply for Medicare within 8 months of retiring or leaving the company.

Medicare Part B   For Medicare Part B coverage, payment is voluntary and is made for physician visits, outpatient and therapy services outside of those provided in the hospital, and other medical services not paid for by Medicare Part A funds. The premiums for Medicare Part B coverage are usually paid by the individual in monthly premiums, most often through a deduction in the monthly Social Security payments to the individual. The same conditions are required for coverage as those required for Medicare Part A insurance, and the enrollment period is the same (the period spanning the 3 months before the individual's 65th birthday, the month he or she turns age 65, and the 3 months after his or her 65th birthday). Individuals who do not wish to receive benefits from Medicare Part B must notify Medicare so they don't get billed for them.[6] If an individual decides to enroll in Medicare Part B after the specified enrollment period, he or she will be responsible for additional penalties (as much as 10% of the Part B premiums) on a monthly basis for as long as he or she receives Part B coverage through Medicare.[6]

Individuals receiving coverage through TRICARE (coverage for active duty military personnel or retirees and their families) must have Part B coverage to maintain their TRICARE coverage.

Medicare Part C   Individuals are eligible for Medicare Part C coverage (Medicare Advantage Plan) if they live in the eligible service area, do not have end-stage renal disease, and are currently enrolled in Medicare Parts A and B. Medicare Part C coverage is provided through a private company, such as an HMO, PPO, or private fee-for-service plan provider. Medicare then pays hospitals, physicians, and other health-care providers for covered services by combining coverage for Parts A and B and prescription drug coverage. Copays tend to be lower with Part C coverage, and it provides coverage for additional benefits and services, such as Medicare Part D prescription drug coverage. Individuals who receive prescription drug coverage through a Medicare Advantage Plan [Part C] must be enrolled in both Part A and Part B portions of Medicare.[7]

Part C plans include the following:

- **Medicare Preferred Provider Organizations (PPOs):** Participants are able to see any doctor or specialist that they choose. If the doctor or specialist is not in the individual's PPO network, the participant's costs will increase. Individuals usually can see a specialist without a referral.
- **Medicare Health Maintenance Organizations (HMOs):** Participants are able to visit doctors in the HMO network only. In most cases, referrals are required to visit a specialist.
- **Medicare Private Fee-for-Service (PFFS):** Participants are able to see any doctor or specialist, but they must accept the PFFS's fees, terms, and conditions. Individuals do not have to have a referral to see a specialist.

- **Medicare Special Needs:** These plans are designed for people with certain chronic diseases or other special health needs. These plans must include Part A, Part B, and Part D coverage.
- **Medicare Medical Savings Account (MSA):** There are two parts to this plan:
  - A high-deductible plan under which coverage doesn't begin until the annual deductible is met
  - A savings account plan in which Medicare deposits money into an account for participants to use for health-care costs[8]

The criteria to enroll in a Medicare Advantage Plan are the same as for Medicare Part A and Part B. Similarly, individuals who choose to enroll after the designated enrollment period may be required to pay an additional penalty on top of the monthly premium.

Medicare Part D   Medicare Part D coverage (prescription drug coverage) is a new benefit that is also provided through private plans that contract with Medicare and that require the individual to pay a monthly premium.[2] Individuals must be enrolled in Part A or Part B to participate in a prescription drug plan under Medicare Part D. There are two types of Medicare Part D plans: Prescription Drug Plans (PDPs), which offer only prescription drug coverage and cover beneficiaries enrolled in Medicare Parts A and B, and Medicare Advantage with Prescription Drug Plans (MA-PDs), which offer both prescription drug coverage and medical coverage.[7]

Medicare Part D covers brand-name and generic prescription drugs at participating pharmacies. CMS approves the prescription drugs in the plan's formulary. As with all other Medicare plans, individuals who do not enroll in Medicare Part D during the designated enrollment period will be required to pay a penalty on any monthly premiums.

For additional information on reimbursed services under Medicare, please visit https://www.cms.gov/Medicare/Medicare-General-Information/MedicareGenInfo/index.html?redirect=/MedicareGenInfo/

Supplemental Insurance   Having Medicare coverage does not preclude an individual from carrying additional supplemental insurance (Medigap insurance) through agencies such as AARP, individual insurance companies such as Blue Cross/Blue Shield, or other types of insurance companies offered through an employer or the state. As with the various Medicare plans, individuals seeking supplemental Medigap insurance may choose to seek coverage through different plans, which can be very confusing. Consumers should discuss their options with the company from which they are seeking additional medical coverage.[9]

Medicare Reimbursement Issues   Because of the rising costs of medical care, the increasing burden on Medicare by the upcoming "baby boomers," the decrease in the number of workers compared with the number of beneficiaries, and the success of the new prescription drug benefit, Part A funds are projected to be exhausted by 2030.[2] Because of the financial challenges of providing adequate funding for Medicare services, individuals with chronic conditions and those from low-income families may not receive the types of services for which they are currently covered. For a fact sheet that addresses these continued challenges and possible solutions, please visit https://www.ssa.gov/oact/trsum/

Rising costs have also led CMS to impose more stringent requirements for Medicare reimbursement in different clinical settings. For example, on April 1, 2011, CMS's changes to the number of visits a PT must make in the home health setting went into effect. Previously, a physical therapist's review of therapy services provided by a PTA was required every 30 days, but now PTs are required to see a patient on the 13th and 19th therapy visits to provide a functional assessment and update the patient's plan of care (POC); these visits are in addition to the visit required every 30 days. The supervisory visit by the PT may be on any one of these visits but must be made within the 30-day time period. The PTA may not continue treating the patient until the PT attends the 13th and 19th visits and sees the patient on the 30th day. Again, all three visits must include a functional assessment to provide reasons for continued skilled physical therapy intervention in the home health setting.

With this new requirement, the PT may see the patient on the 13th or 19th visit, and this may also be the 30th day, depending on how the days are calculated. It might also mean the physical therapist sees the patient for the 13th or 19th visit one week and sees him or her again on the 30th day the next week. Consequently, the physical therapist may be seeing a home health patient for three visits within a 30-day time period, compared with one visit every 30 days prior to this change. Since these changes occurred, Medicare has made plans to cut reimbursements, putting additional burdens on home health agencies.[10] Additional changes and cuts will continue to occur as Medicare adapts to changes within the ACA.

It will be necessary for all therapists to check for continuing changes by frequently reviewing the following website: http://www.cms.gov/Manuals/IOM/list.asp#TopOfPage. Students and therapists may find the following two manuals to be most helpful when reviewing general information related to reimbursement, recent changes to reimbursement, and the services that Medicare covers:

- 100-01: Medicare General Information, Eligibility and Entitlement Manual[11]
- 100-02: Medicare Benefit Policy Manual[11]

For a summary of physical therapy services provided at different medical facilities that are covered in the annual Therapy Code List, please see the following website: https://www.cms.gov/Medicare/Billing/TherapyServices/AnnualTherapyUpdate.html

MEDICAID

Medicaid provides medical reimbursement to low-income working families and to some elderly and disabled individuals, depending on specific requirements. To qualify for Medicaid services, individuals must meet certain financial requirements for low-income status and other criteria determined by each state (e.g., age, pregnancy, disability, or blindness), in addition to being a U.S. citizen or a lawfully admitted immigrant with at least 5 years of legal residency. Families with children must meet specific requirements related to the federal poverty level (FPL), age of the individual, and disabilities. Medicaid faces the same challenges that Medicare does in trying to remain solvent while continuing to serve the populations for which it was created.[12]

PROGRAM OF ALL-INCLUSIVE CARE FOR THE ELDERLY (PACE)

The Program of All-Inclusive Care for the Elderly (PACE) is another option for health-care coverage for older individuals. PACE is an optional benefit—offered under both Medicare and Medicaid in some states and only under Medicaid in others—that provides comprehensive medical and social services in noninstitutional settings (e.g., patient's home, adult day care, inpatient facilities). A team of health-care professionals assesses the patient's needs, develops a POC, and delivers integrated services. Participants must meet certain eligibility requirements to qualify for such services.[13] For a listing of states that currently offer PACE services, visit https://www.cms.gov/medicare/health-plans/pace/downloads/pacefactsheet.pdf

WORKERS' COMPENSATION INSURANCE

Workers' compensation insurance is provided by an employer to cover an employee who is injured or becomes ill on the job, regardless of fault. Although workers' compensation benefits vary from company to company, workers' compensation laws require that all packages include the following six basic benefits:

- Medical care: Paid for by the employer to help the employee recover from an injury or illness caused by work
- Temporary disability benefits: Payments to an employee who loses wages because an injury prevents him or her from doing his or her usual job while recovering
- Permanent disability benefits: Payments to an employee who doesn't recover completely
- Supplemental job displacement benefits (if the date of injury is 2004 or later): Vouchers to help pay for retraining or skill enhancement if the employee doesn't recover completely and doesn't return to work
- Vocational rehabilitation (if the date of injury is before 2004): Job placement counseling and possibly retraining if the employee is unable to return to his or her previous job and the employer doesn't offer other work
- Death benefits: Payments to the employee's spouse, children, or other dependents if the employee dies as a result of a job-related injury or illness[14]

The employee, as a requirement of his or her employment, must notify the employer of a work-related injury or illness within the time period required by the company, or else the employee could forfeit his or her workers' compensation benefits.

Workers' compensation insurance also helps an employer monitor the progress of an employee who is disabled, providing employers with a mechanism for facilitating employees' return to work.[14] However, there is a cap for expenses related to the employee's recovery from the work-related injury or illness. For employees who cannot return to work because they are unable to continue in their current position, the company is required to provide alternative job training or permanent disability benefits. The employee does not have to prove employer negligence to claim benefits under workers' compensation. At this time, Texas is the only state that has an "elective" workers' compensation insurance provision, which means that employers may elect not to provide workers' compensation for their employees. All other states require employers to provide workers' compensation for their employees as no-fault liability insurance.[15]

What Does Workers' Compensation Insurance Cover?

An employee who suffers any injury or illness during his or her work-related employment is eligible for coverage under workers' compensation. The injury or illness may be related to a single incident or to multiple exposures in the workplace. However, the employer is protected from providing such coverage if the employee works while intoxicated or under the influence of drugs, or if he or she ignores the company's safety rules and regulations. Limits and types of coverage vary among states so it is important for employees to determine what their company will cover in the event such insurance is needed.

Because the employer provides workers' compensation insurance, an employee who receives workers' compensation benefits cannot sue the employer for personal injury or negligence on the job. In addition, benefits from this type of insurance are fixed, meaning that employees are compensated only up to a certain amount. This amount is based on a percentage of the employee's weekly salary received at the time of injury.

Because the employer provides workers' compensation insurance for the employee, the employer has the right to assign the employee to a physician with experience in workers' compensation injuries and illness and to follow the care and progress of that employee to ensure his or her return to work.

What Can the Employee Expect From Workers' Compensation Insurance?

Employees can expect the following from their workers' compensation insurance:[15]

- Workers' compensation systems do not require employees to share in the cost of medical services. Employees never pay a medical deductible or copayment for service.
- In all but seven states, workers' compensation laws require insurers to provide complete medical coverage without durational or monetary limitations. Special provisions limiting medical coverage apply in Arkansas, Florida, Hawaii, Montana, New Jersey, Ohio, and Tennessee.
- Workers' compensation benefits cover both permanent and temporary disabilities, which are further classified as either partial or total. For both temporary and permanent disabilities, workers' compensation pays between 66 ⅔% and 80% of lost wages, up to a set dollar maximum. Indemnity payments also are subject to time limits. Depending on the nature of the disability, payments are made for life, the "duration of disability," or a specified number of weeks. For example, in California, a worker who is determined to have a temporary total disability receives payments for the duration of his or her disability. An individual with a permanent total disability receives the state's temporary disability benefit—up to $490 per week—for life. Similarly, individuals with permanent partial disabilities, which allow employees to return to work in the same or a different function, receive lower benefits than do individuals with permanent total disabilities.
- Before paying temporary workers' compensation benefits, most states require employees to wait for a set period, usually between 3 and 7 days. If an employee can't work after the waiting period, he or she qualifies for disability payments. Temporary disability payments generally stop when an employee is able to return to work.

- Most states provide disfigurement benefits for serious injuries to the head, face, or neck (or any body part visible in the normal course of work) that "handicap employment" or hinder "earning capacity."
- Most workers' compensation laws require employers and insurers to pay for physical and vocation rehabilitation services. Employer responsibilities vary widely from state to state. Only North Carolina, Pennsylvania, and Wyoming do not have vocational rehabilitation provisions in their workers' compensation laws.
- Spouses of employees who are fatally injured receive workers' compensation death benefits, which include burial funds and vary by state (e.g., $3,000 in Alabama, $15,000 in Minnesota). Spouses with children receive greater workers' compensation benefits than do those without children. Children of employees who are fatally injured are generally paid benefits until they reach age 18, unless they are physically or mentally disabled, in which case they continue to receive benefits until they die or are no longer disabled. If the spouse of an employee who was fatally injured remarries, he or she is awarded a lump sum payment equal to 2 years of the benefits that he or she had been receiving.
- In every state, workers' compensation benefits are subject to offsets, or reductions, if the employee receives funds from other state or federal programs, such as a state unemployment agency or the U.S. Social Security Administration. Offsets can be as much as 50%.[1]

OTHER MEDICAL INSURANCE OPTIONS

Other options for medical coverage come in the form of private medical insurance companies that cover employees through an employer, with employees paying a certain percentage of the monthly premium and the employer covering the rest. Over the past 10 years, this percentage has increased for the employee, making this type of medical insurance difficult to maintain when salaries do not keep pace.[16]

Individuals who do not qualify for any type of medical coverage through employers or other avenues have minimal options, with the exception of the initiation of the Affordable Care Act (ACA) in 2012 (discussed in the next section). However, owing to the high cost of premiums under the ACA, many individuals have opted to pay the penalty for not having insurance, placing a greater burden on medical facilities, hospitals, physicians, and other health-care providers who treat such individuals on a cash-for-service basis.

In addition to the insurance options described previously, some individuals have the monetary means to self-insure by paying premiums to a private insurance company or to maintain a savings plan to cover medical expenses. In some states (e.g., New Mexico), a state insurance plan, in which individuals pay premiums based on the amount of the deductible that they choose, is available for those who are otherwise uninsurable. With this type of plan, state insurance companies underwrite the program while individuals pay monthly premiums.[18]

HEALTH-CARE REFORM LAW AND THE AFFORDABLE CARE ACT (ACA)

The Patient Protection and Affordable Care Act (PPACA, generally shortened to ACA) is another option for national health care. It was proposed in 2009, signed into law on March 23, 2010,[19] and, after much debate, was upheld as constitutional by the United States Supreme Court on June 28, 2012. The health-care reform package includes many changes to our health-care system, which began in 2010 with additional changes occurring over the next decade. For a review of these changes please visit the following websites:

- http://www.hhs.gov/healthcare/facts-and-features/key-features-of-aca-by-year/index.html
- https://www.healthcare.gov/
- http://www.apta.org/HealthCareReform/

Through these new health-care laws, individuals who are uninsured, those with preexisting conditions, and those who are self-employed will be able to receive coverage by purchasing insurance through federal or state exchange services.

- The uninsured and self-employed would be able to purchase insurance through state-based exchanges with subsidies available to individuals and families with income between 133 percent and 400 percent of the federal poverty level.

- Effective 2014, separate exchanges were created for small businesses to purchase coverage.
- Funding was made available to states to establish exchanges within 1 year of enactment and until January 1, 2015.[19]

At the time of this writing, what the new health-care reform law actually offers is still difficult to determine. The ACA will remain subject to additional changes over the next decade as some medical insurance providers struggle to remain financially viable. As of 2017, one of the largest medical insurance providers in the nation, United Healthcare, will no longer provide services through the ACA because of the small number of markets for these exchanges, the increased risk for the company over the short term, and the inability to serve such exchanges on an effective and sustainable basis.[17]

Individuals whose income is at or below the federal poverty level (FPL) will be able to receive subsidies for services purchased through an exchange as long as they do not receive benefits from any other source. In addition, insurance companies are no longer able to deny coverage to individuals with preexisting conditions. Children are covered through their parents' insurance until age 26 instead of 25, as previously allowed.[19] Actual provisions in this new health-care benefit package will be implemented over the next decade with final conversion slated for 2018, unless revised through legislative processes.

HEALTH CARE AND POTENTIAL CHANGES TO DOCUMENTATION

It remains to be seen how all of these proposed legislative changes and revisions, in addition to the development of new forms of coverage, will affect how documentation supports therapy services. However, without the PT and PTA providing proper documentation and appropriate services in various settings depending on the type of reimbursement venue, reimbursement will be difficult to obtain regardless of any outside factors. It is imperative that the treating therapist become knowledgeable about the requirements of individual payer sources and recognize what services can and will be reimbursed depending on the setting in which the patient receives treatment and on the therapist providing such treatment.

If the PT or PTA does not understand each individual payer's requirements for reimbursement and the settings for such reimbursement, it may result in fees being withheld for lengthy and costly review, fees remaining unpaid, or nonreimbursement for services provided. It takes quite the reimbursement detective to discover the requirements of each individual payer. Therefore, it is important to have a qualified billing expert in any setting to provide support for expected reimbursements for all types of patient care given in that setting.

REIMBURSEMENT FOR PT VERSUS PTA STUDENT SERVICES

With the ever-changing environment in reimbursement issues related to patient care provided by the student physical therapist in the clinical setting, it is difficult to determine which services will be reimbursed and which will not. For that reason, it is imperative that the Academic Coordinator of Clinical Education (ACCE) from the educational institution and the Center Coordinator of Clinical Education (CCCE) and the clinical instructor (CI) from the clinical site maintain frequent communication with each other. This communication needs to involve reviews of each state's physical therapy practice act and the policies and procedures of both APTA's Section on Health Policy and Administration (HPA) and CMS to ensure proper reimbursement for therapy services provided by student physical therapists in all types of health-care settings. Services provided by the student physical therapist used to be very limited in the billing process. With the involvement of educational institutions, clinics, APTA, and other organizations, such reimbursement issues have improved, and the number of services provided by students that will be reimbursed has increased.

However, in recent years, clinical facilities have found that reimbursement of student-provided services has become more limited within specific settings, and employers have found that certain types of services were not reimbursed at all. Such limitations prohibit student physical therapists from learning in all settings, in spite of their education and ability to provide quality therapeutic intervention in all settings. It is also important to reinforce that any type of intervention by a student physical therapist is always monitored or directly supervised by a CI, who is a physical therapist or physical therapist assistant for the clinical site, and that students need to be able to have multiple experiences in order to provide appropriate and skilled intervention in all types of health-care settings. Figure 4–1 outlines

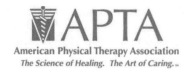

American Physical Therapy Association
The Science of Healing. The Art of Caring.

Last updated: 12/12/2011

Practice Setting	PT Student		PTA Student	
	Part A	Part B	Part A	Part B
Physical Therapist in Private Practice	N/A	X^1	N/A	X^1
Certified Rehabilitation Agency	N/A	X^1	N/A	X^1
Comprehensive Outpatient Rehabilitation Facility	N/A	X^1	N/A	X^1
Skilled Nursing Facility	Y^1	X^1	Y^2	X^1
Hospital	Y^3	X^1	Y^3	X^1
Home Health Agency	NAR	X^1	NAR	X^1
Inpatient Rehabilitation Facility	Y^4	N/A	Y^4	N/A

Contact: advocacy@apta.org

Key

Y: Reimbursable
X: Not Reimbursable
N/A: Not Applicable
NAR: Not Addressed in Regulation. Please defer to state law.

Y^1: Reimbursable: Therapy students are not required to be in line-of-sight of the professional supervising therapist/assistant (**Federal Register**, August 8, 2011). Within individual facilities, supervising therapists/assistants must make the determination as to whether or not a student is ready to treat patients without line-of-sight supervision. Additionally all state and professional practice guidelines for student supervision must be followed. Time may be coded on the MDS when the therapist provides skilled services and direction to a student who is participating in the provision of therapy. All time that the student spends with patients should be documented.

Medicare Part B—The following criteria must be met in order for services provided by a student to be billed by the long-term care facility:

- The qualified professional is present and in the room for the entire session. The student participates in the delivery of services when the qualified practitioner is directing the service, making the skilled judgment, and is responsible for the assessment and treatment.
- The practitioner is not engaged in treating another patient or doing other tasks at the same time.
- The qualified professional is the person responsible for the services and, as such, signs all documentation. (A student may, of course, also sign but it is not necessary because the Part B payment is for the clinician's service, not for the student's services.)

(RAI Version 3.0 Manual, October 2011).

Figure 4—1   Student supervision and Medicare. (Reprinted from http://www.apta.org/Payment/Medicare/Supervision, with permission of the American Physical Therapy Association. This material is copyrighted, and any further reproduction or distribution requires written permission from APTA.)

Individual Therapy:

When a therapy student is involved with the treatment of a resident, the minutes may be coded as individual therapy when only one resident is being treated by the therapy student and supervising therapist/assistant (Medicare A and Medicare B). The supervising therapist/assistant shall not be engaged in any other activity or treatment when the resident is receiving therapy under Medicare B. However, for those residents whose stay is covered under Medicare A, the supervising therapist/assistant shall not be treating or supervising other individuals **and** he/she is able to immediately intervene/assist the student as needed.

Example: A speech therapy graduate student treats Mr. A for 30 minutes. Mr. A.'s therapy is covered under the Medicare Part A benefit. The supervising speech-language pathologist is not treating any patients at this time but is not in the room with the student or Mr. A. Mr. A.'s therapy may be coded as 30 minutes of individual therapy on the MDS.

Concurrent Therapy:

When a therapy student is involved with the treatment, and one of the following occurs, the minutes may be coded as concurrent therapy:

- The therapy student is treating one resident and the supervising therapist/assistant is treating another resident, and both residents are in line of sight of the therapist/assistant or student providing their therapy; or
- The therapy student is treating 2 residents, <u>regardless of payer source,</u> both of whom are in line-of-sight of the therapy student, and the therapist is not treating any residents and not supervising other individuals; or
- The therapy student is not treating any residents and the supervising therapist/assistant is treating 2 residents at the same time, regardless of payer source, both of whom are in line-of-sight.

Medicare Part B: The treatment of two or more residents who may or may not be performing the same or similar activity, regardless of payer source, at the same time is documented as group treatment.

Example: An Occupational Therapist provides therapy to Mr. K. for 60 minutes. An occupational therapy graduate student, who is supervised by the occupational therapist, is treating Mr. R. at the same time for the same 60 minutes but Mr. K. and Mr. R. are not doing the same or similar activities. Both Mr. K. and Mr. R's stays are covered under the Medicare Part A benefit. Based on the information above, the therapist would code each individual's MDS for this day of treatment as follows:

Mr. K. received concurrent therapy for 60 minutes.

Mr. R. received concurrent therapy for 60 minutes.

Group Therapy:

When a therapy student is involved with group therapy treatment, and one of the following occurs, the minutes may be coded as group therapy:

- The therapy student is providing the group treatment and the supervising therapist/assistant is not treating any residents and is not supervising other individuals (students or residents); or
- The supervising therapist/assistant is providing the group treatment and the therapy student

Figure 4–1—cont'd

is not providing treatment to any resident. In this case, the student is simply assisting the supervising therapist.

Medicare Part B: The treatment of 2 or more individuals simultaneously, regardless of payer source, who may or may not be performing the same activity.

When a therapy student is involved with group therapy treatment, and one of the following occurs, the minutes may be coded as group therapy:
- The therapy student is providing group treatment and the supervising therapist/assistant is not engaged in any other activity or treatment; or
- The supervising therapist/assistant is providing group treatment and the therapy student is not providing treatment to any resident.

Documentation: APTA recommends that the physical therapist co-sign the note of the physical therapist student and state the level of supervision that the PT determined was appropriate for the student and how/if the therapist was involved in the patient's care.

$\mathbf{Y^2}$: Reimbursable: The minutes of student services count on the Minimum Data Set. Medicare no longer requires that the PT/PTA provide line-of-sight supervision of physical therapist assistant (PTA) student services. Rather, the supervising PT/PTA now has the authority to determine the appropriate level of supervision for the student, as appropriate within their state scope of practice. See $\mathbf{Y^1}$.

Documentation: APTA recommends that the physical therapist and assistant should co-sign the note of physical therapist assistant student and state the level of appropriate supervision used. Also, the documentation should reflect the requirements as indicated for individual therapy, concurrent therapy, and group therapy in $\mathbf{Y^1}$.

$\mathbf{Y^3}$: This is not specifically addressed in the regulations, therefore, please defer to state law and standards of professional practice. Additionally, the Part A hospital diagnosis related group (DRG) payment system is similar to that of a skilled nursing facility (SNF) and Medicare has indicated very limited and restrictive requirements for student services in the SNF setting.

Documentation: Please refer to documentation guidance provided under $\mathbf{Y^1}$

$\mathbf{Y^4}$: This is not specifically addressed in the regulations, therefore, please defer to state law and standards of professional practice. Additionally, the inpatient rehabilitation facility payment system is similar to that of a skilled nursing facility (SNF) and Medicare has indicated very limited and restrictive requirements for student services in the SNF setting.

$\mathbf{X^1}$: B. Therapy Students

1. General

Only the services of the therapist can be billed and paid under Medicare Part B. The services performed by a student are not reimbursed even if provided under "line of sight" supervision of the therapist; however, the presence of the student "in the room" does not make the service unbillable.

Figure 4–1—cont'd

EXAMPLES:

Therapists may bill and be paid for the provision of services in the following scenarios:

• The qualified practitioner is present and in the room for the entire session. The student participates in the delivery of services when the qualified practitioner is directing the service, making the skilled judgment, and is responsible for the assessment and treatment.

> • The qualified practitioner is present in the room guiding the student in service delivery when the therapy student and the therapy assistant student are participating in the provision of services, and the practitioner is not engaged in treating another patient or doing other tasks at the same time.

> • The qualified practitioner is responsible for the services and as such, signs all documentation. (A student may, of course, also sign but it is not necessary since the Part B payment is for the clinician's service, not for the student's services).

2. Therapy Assistants as Clinical Instructors

Physical therapist assistants and occupational therapy assistants are not precluded from serving as clinical instructors for therapy students, while providing services within their scope of work and performed under the direction and supervision of a licensed physical or occupational therapist to a Medicare beneficiary.

Documentation: APTA recommends that the physical therapist or physical therapist assistant complete documentation.

Figure 4—1—cont'd

the various reimbursements for services provided by a PT or PTA student in various settings as provided by Medicare.[20]

In addition, the Advocacy section of APTA further delineated the use of students in the clinical setting in their "Implementing MDS 3.0: Use of Therapy Students" policy update on October 8, 2010.[21] Again, through review of the information that APTA provides, educational institutions, clinical sites, therapists, and students can remain updated on the ever-changing revisions to these guidelines. Box 4–1 provides a summary of the Minimum Data Set Version 3.0 (MDS 3.0), on the involvement of therapy students in all aspects of treatment for the patient to receive Medicare reimbursement for therapy services. Additionally, the publication "Use of Students Under Medicare Part B" (Box 4–2) outlines the requirements for reimbursement in those settings that serve patients receiving Medicare Part B funds.

Reviewing the content from Box 4–1 and Box 4–2 should help the student physical therapist, the educational institution, and the clinical site better understand the types of services that Medicare can be billed for with regard to therapeutic intervention provided by the student in a specific setting.[21]

In addition to information regarding what types of student-provided services will be reimbursed and in which settings, APTA provides information to delineate the type of supervision necessary for the student physical therapist assistant in a specific setting (see Box 4–3).[20]

Use of Physical Therapy Aides   Historically, medical facilities have used physical therapy aides, not physical therapist assistants, to provide some patient preparation and care in treatment. The physical therapy aide is not licensed, does not complete any formal education in the physical therapy field, and is usually hired without any previous experience. They are trained within the facility for which they

(Text continued on page 60)

| Box 4-1 | Implementing MDS 3.0: Use of Therapy Students |

As facilities continue to change their current practices to implement the Minimum Data Set Version 3.0 (better known as MDS 3.0), one of the emerging issues is the manner in which they document and utilize therapy students. Under the new rules, in order to record the minutes as individual therapy when a therapy student is involved in the treatment of a resident, only one resident can be treated by the therapy student and the supervising therapist or assistant (for Medicare Part A and Part B). In addition, the supervising therapist or assistant cannot engage in any other activity or treatment when the resident is receiving treatment under Medicare Part B. However, for those residents whose stay is covered under Medicare Part A, the supervising therapist or assistant cannot be treating or supervising other individuals. Beginning on October 1, 2011, the student and resident no longer need to be within the line-of-sight supervision of the supervising therapist. CMS will allow the supervising therapist to determine the appropriate level of supervision for the student. The student is still treated as an extension of the therapist, and the time the student spends with the patient will continue to be billed as if the supervising therapist alone was providing the services.

Under Medicare Part A, when a therapy student is involved with the treatment, and one of the following occurs, the minutes may be coded as concurrent therapy:

· The therapy student is treating one resident and the supervising therapist or assistant is treating another resident, and the therapy student is supervised by the therapist at the appropriate level of supervision as determined by the supervising therapist; or
· The therapy student is treating two residents at the appropriate level of supervision as determined by the supervising therapist and the therapist is not treating any residents and not supervising other individuals; or
· The therapy student is not treating any residents and the supervising therapist or assistant is treating two residents at the same time, regardless of payer source.

The student would be precluded from treating the resident and recording the minutes as concurrent therapy under Medicare Part B.

Under Medicare Part A, when a therapy student is involved with group therapy treatment, and one of the following occurs, the minutes may be coded as group therapy:

· The therapy student is providing the group treatment at the appropriate level of supervision as determined by the supervising therapist and the supervising therapist or assistant is not treating any residents and is not supervising other individuals (students or residents); or
· The supervising therapist/assistant is providing the group treatment and the therapy student is not providing treatment to any resident.

Under Medicare Part B, when a therapy student is involved with group therapy treatment, and one of the following occurs, the minutes may be coded as group therapy:

· The therapy student is providing group treatment and the supervising therapist or assistant is present and in the room and is not engaged in any other activity or treatment; or
· The supervising therapist or assistant is providing group treatment and the therapy student is not providing treatment to any resident.

Recommended Skilled Nursing Facility Therapy Student Supervision Guidelines Submitted to CMS by the American Physical Therapy Association (APTA) During the Comment Period for the FY 2012 SNF PPS Final Rule

Please note: These suggested guidelines would be in addition to the student supervision guidelines outlined in the RAI MDS 3.0 Manual and all relevant Federal Regulations.

· The amount of supervision must be appropriate to the student's level of knowledge, experience, and competence.
· Students who have been approved by the supervising therapist or assistant to practice independently in selected patient/client situations can perform those selected patient/client services specified by the supervising therapist/assistant.

Box 4-1   Implementing MDS 3.0: Use of Therapy Students—cont'd

· The supervising therapist/assistant must be physically present in the facility and imme-diately available to provide observation, guidance, and feedback as needed when the student is providing services.
· When the supervising therapist/assistant has cleared the student to perform medically necessary patient/client services and the student provides the appropriate level of services, the services will be counted on the MDS as skilled therapy minutes.
· The supervising therapist/assistant is required to review and co-sign all students' patient/client documentation for all levels of clinical experience and retains full respon-sibility for the care of the patient/client.
· Therapist assistants can provide instruction and supervision to therapy assistant students so long as the therapist assistant is properly supervised by the therapist.

   These changes as well as other changes regarding MDS 3.0 took effect October 1, 2011. If you have questions regarding this provision or other provisions within MDS 3.0, please contact the APTA at advocacy@apta.org or at 800.999.2782 ext. 8533.

Box 4-2   Use of Students Under Medicare Part B

The purpose of this document is to provide clarification on the circumstances under which physical therapy students may participate in the provision of outpatient therapy services to Medicare patients, and whether or not such services are billable under Medicare Part B. Specifically, this document addresses student participation in the provision of services in the following settings: private practice physical therapy offices, rehabilitation agencies, comprehensive outpatient rehabilitation facilities (CORFs), skilled nursing facilities (SNFs) (Part B), outpatient hospital departments, and home health agencies (Part B).

Background
CMS issued a program memorandum (AB-01-56) on the provision of outpatient therapy services by therapy students on April 11, 2001. In this program memorandum (http://www.cms.hhs.gov/Transmittals/downloads/AB0156.pdf), CMS provided an-swers to frequently asked questions regarding payment for the services of therapy students under Part B of the Medicare program.

   In response to inquiries from the American Speech Language Hearing Association (ASHA), CMS issued a follow-up letter dated November 9, 2001, to ASHA in which they further clarified the policy on payment of student services that they outlined in the Q and A program memorandum. On January 10, 2002, CMS also issued a similar letter to AOTA on the subject. The follow-up letters to ASHA and AOTA were not intended to signify a change in the policy issued in the program memorandum; they were merely intended to provide further clarification.

   Specifically, in the program memorandum (AB-01-56), CMS stated, in part, that "services performed by a student are not reimbursed under Medicare Part B. Medicare pays for services of physicians and practitioners (e.g., licensed physical therapists) authorized by statute. Students do not meet the definition of practitioners listed in the statute." Regarding whether services provided by the student with the supervising ther-apist "in the room" can be reimbursed, CMS stated that "Only the services of the ther-apist can be billed to Medicare and be paid. However, the fact that the student is 'in the room' would not make the service unbillable. Medicare would pay for the services

Continued

Box 4-2   Use of Students Under Medicare Part B—cont'd

of the therapist." In response to another question, CMS stated that "the therapist can bill for the direct services he/she provides to patients under Medicare Part B. Services performed by the therapy student are not payable under Medicare Part B."

In the letter to ASHA, CMS once again restated, in order to be paid, Medicare Part B services must be provided by practitioners who are acting within the scope of their state licensure. CMS further described circumstances, under which they consider the service as being essentially provided directly by the qualified practitioner, even though the student has some involvement. Such services would be billable. Specifically, CMS states:

"The qualified practitioner is recognized by the Medicare Part B beneficiary as the responsible professional within any session when services are delivered."

"The qualified practitioner is present and in the room for the entire session. The student participates in the delivery of services when the qualified practitioner is directing the service, making the skilled judgment, and is responsible for the assessment and treatment."

"The qualified practitioner is present in the room guiding the student in service delivery when the student is participating in the provision of services, and the practitioner is not engaged in treating another patient or doing other tasks at the same time."

"The qualified practitioner is responsible for the services and as such, signs all documentation (A student may, of course, also sign but it is not necessary since the Part B payment is for the clinician's services, not for the student's services)."

In response to a request from AOTA, CMS issued a summary of their understanding of the typical scenario involving students for which occupational therapists seek payment. The information provided in this letter mirrors what was stated in the letter provided to ASHA.

Acceptable Billing Practices

Based on the information provided by CMS and MedPAC, it is possible for a physical therapist to bill for services only when the services are furnished jointly by the physical therapist and student. APTA recommends that physical therapists consider the following factors in determining whether or not a physical therapist may bill Medicare Part B for a service when the therapy student is participating in the provision of the service.

· Physical therapists should use their professional judgment on whether or not a service is billable, keeping in mind the importance of integrity when billing for services.

· Physical therapists should distinguish between the ability of a student to provide services to a patient/client from the ability to bill for student services provided to Medicare Part B patients. A student may provide services to any patient/client provided it is allowable by state law. This does not mean, however, that the services provided by the student are billable to Medicare, Medicaid, or other private insurance companies.

· As CMS states, only services provided by the licensed physical therapist can be billed to Medicare for payment. Physical therapists should consider whether the service is being essentially provided directly by the physical therapist, even though the student has some involvement in providing the care. In making this determination, the therapist should consider how closely involved he or she is involved in providing the patient's care when a student is participating. The therapist should be completely and actively engaged in providing the care of the patient. As CMS states in their letter, "the qualified practitioner is present in the room guiding the student in service delivery when the student is participating the provision of services, and the practitioner is not engaged in treating another patient or doing other tasks at the same time." The therapist should direct the service, make the skilled judgment, and be responsible for the assessment and treatment. There should be checks and balances provided by the physical therapist throughout the entire time the patient/client is being managed.

· The physical therapist should ask him- or herself whether the billing would be the same whether or not there is a student involved. The therapist should not bill beyond what

---

Box 4-2   Use of Students Under Medicare Part B—cont'd

they would normally bill in the course of managing that patient's care. The individual therapist or the employer should not benefit financially from having the student involved in the clinical experience in the practice or facility.

Conclusion
It is crucial that physical therapists be aware of and comply with Medicare regulations governing the circumstances in which physical therapy students may participate in the provision of physical therapy services. CMS has clearly stated its policy that student services under Part B are not billable, and that only services provided to Medicare beneficiaries by the PT may be billed. APTA will continue to work to ensure that physical therapy students receive the clinical training they need in order to provide valuable, high-quality physical therapy services to patients/clients.

Reprinted from http://www.apta.org/Payment/Medicare/Supervision/PartB/, with permission of the American Physical Therapy Association. This material is copyrighted, and any further reproduction or distribution requires written permission from APTA.

Box 4-3   Use of PTAs Under Medicare

Please note that physical therapists are licensed providers in all states and physical therapist assistants are licensed providers in the majority of states. As licensed providers, the state practice act governs supervision requirements. Some state practice acts mandate more stringent supervision standards than Medicare laws and regulations. In those cases, the physical therapist and physical therapist assistant must comply with their state practice act. For example, in a skilled nursing facility in New Jersey, a physical therapist must be on the premises when services are furnished by a physical therapist assistant, despite the fact that Medicare requires general supervision. New Jersey's state practice act requires direct supervision rather than general supervision, and therefore, the physical therapist and physical therapist assistant would have to comply with this requirement.

Certified Rehabilitation Agency (CRA)
CRAs are required to have qualified personnel provide initial direction and periodic observation of the actual performance of the function and/or activity. If the person providing services does not meet the assistant-level practitioner qualifications in 485.705, then the physical therapist must be on the premises.

Comprehensive Outpatient Rehabilitation Facility (CORF)
The services must be furnished by qualified personnel. If the personnel do not meet the qualifications in 485.705, then the qualified staff must be on the premises and must instruct these personnel in appropriate patient-care service, techniques, and retain responsibility for their activities. A qualified professional representing each service made available at the facility must be either on the premises of the facility or must be available through direct telecommunications for consultation and assistance during the facility's operating hours.

Home Health Agencies (HHA)
Physical therapy services must be performed safely and/or effectively only by or under the **general** supervision of a skilled therapist. General supervision has been traditionally described in Health Care Financing Administration manuals as "requiring the initial direction and periodic inspection of the actual activity." However, the supervisor need not always be physically present or on the premises when the assistant is performing services.

Continued

Box 4–3   Use of PTAs Under Medicare—cont'd

Inpatient Hospital Services

Physical therapy services must be those services that can be safely and effectively performed only by or under the supervision of a qualified physical therapist. Because the regulations do not specifically delineate the type of direction required, the provider must defer to his or her physical therapy state practice act.

Outpatient Hospital Services

Physical therapy services must be those services that can be safely and effectively performed only by or under the supervision of a qualified physical therapist. Because the regulations do not specifically delineate the type of direction required, the provider must defer to his or her physical therapy state practice act.

Private Practice

Physical therapy services must be provided by or under the *direct* supervision of the physical therapist in private practice. CMS has generally defined direct supervision to mean that the supervising private practice therapist must be present in the office suite at the time the service is performed.

Physician's Office

Services must be provided under the *direct* supervision of a physical therapist who is enrolled as a provider under Medicare. A physician cannot bill for the services provided by a PTA. The services must be billed under the provider number of the supervising physical therapist. CMS has generally defined direct supervision to mean that the physical therapist must be in the office suite when an individual procedure is performed by supportive personnel.

Skilled Nursing Facility (SNF)

Skilled rehabilitation services must be provided directly or under the *general* supervision of skilled rehabilitation personnel. "General supervision" is further defined in the manual as requiring the initial direction and periodic inspection of the actual activity. However, the supervisor need not always be physically present or on the premises when the assistant is performing services.

---

were hired and have no formal training in patient care. Conversely, the physical therapist assistant has formal training from an accredited physical therapist assistant program in an educational setting, completes clinical training following a didactic program, and sits for a national licensing examination (in most states) to be licensed to practice as a physical therapist assistant. APTA has provided current information regarding the type of supervision needed for physical therapy aides and the guidelines related to reimbursement for services they provide in all settings. Physical therapy aides are not considered adequately trained to deliver any type of patient-centered treatment and can only assist the PT or PTA who is providing appropriate care to a patient. For clarification of the role of the physical therapy aide in all treatment settings, refer to Box 4–4.

Box 4–4   Use of Physical Therapy Aides Under Medicare

Certified Rehabilitation Agency (CRA)

In order for services to be reimbursed under Medicare Part B benefit, they may not be provided by a physical therapy aide regardless of level of supervision.

CMS's policy is that the therapy aide may assist the professional therapist or therapist assistant to perform a specific therapy service. The aide should never be the provider of the service.

Comprehensive Outpatient Rehabilitation Facility (CORF)

In order for services to be reimbursed under Medicare Part B benefit, they may not be provided by a physical therapy aide, regardless of level of supervision.

CMS's policy is that the therapy aide may assist the professional therapist or therapist assistant to perform a specific therapy service. The aide should never be the provider of the service.

Home Health Agencies (HHA)

Under Medicare Part A regulations, all therapy services offered by the HHA, either directly or under arrangements, must be provided by a qualified therapist or a qualified therapist assistant under the therapist's supervision and in accordance with the plan of care. The qualified therapist assists the physician in evaluating level of function, helps develop the plan of care (revising as necessary), prepares clinical and progress notes, advises and consults with the family and other agency personnel, and participates in in-service programs. (42 CFR §484.32)

An HHA that wishes to furnish outpatient physical therapy or speech pathology services must meet all the pertinent conditions of this part and also meet the additional health and safety requirements set forth in subpart H of part 485 of this chapter to implement section 1861(p) of the Act. (42 CFR 484.38)

Inpatient Hospital Services

Physical therapy services must be those services that can be safely and effectively performed only by or under the supervision of a qualified physical therapist. According to 42 CFR Section 482.56 of the Medicare hospital conditions of participation, "physical therapy, if provided, must be provided by staff who meet the qualifications specified by medical staff, consistent with state law." Because the regulations do not specifically delineate the type of direction required, the provider must defer to his or her physical therapy state practice act.

Outpatient Hospital Services

In order for services to be reimbursed under Medicare Part B benefit, they may not be provided by a physical therapy aide regardless of level of supervision.

CMS's policy is that the therapy aide may assist the professional therapist or therapist assistant to perform a specific therapy service. The aide should never be the provider of the service.

Physical Therapist in Private Practice

In order for services to be reimbursed under Medicare Part B benefit, they may not be provided by a physical therapy aide, regardless of level of supervision.

CMS's policy is that the therapy aide may assist the professional therapist or therapist assistant to perform a specific therapy service. The aide should never be the provider of the service, however, and employees must be personally supervised by the physical therapist.

Continued

Box 4-4   Use of Physical Therapy Aides Under Medicare—cont'd

Physician's Office/"Incident to" Billing

Effective July 25, 2005, in order for services to be reimbursed under Medicare Part B benefit, they may not be provided by a physical therapy aide, regardless of level of supervision.

Skilled Nursing Facilities

Effective July 30, 1999, "the therapy assistant cannot supervise a therapy aide. It is up to the professional therapist to ensure that the assistant is capable of performing therapy services without the more stringent 'line-of-sight' level of supervision required by therapy aides. A therapy aide must be supervised personally by the professional therapist in such a way that the therapist has visual contact with the aide at all times. Therapy aides are not to perform any services without 'line-of-sight' supervision. Similarly, a therapy aide must never be responsible for provision of group therapy services, as this is well beyond the scope of services that they are qualified to provide."

Additionally, the rule states that set-up time, as well as time under the therapist's direct supervision, counts as reportable therapy minutes on the MDS.

Use of Aides in the Delivery of Skilled Services

Per the RAI manual instructions released on November 9, 2009, aides cannot be used to deliver skilled services. Aides should be used to provide support services and those services cannot be counted towards the minutes on the MDS. This policy is further detailed in the 2010 SNF PPS Final Rule.

From August 2003 through October 1, 2009, the following policy regarding the use of aides in SNFs was in effect. As of October 1, 2009, this policy is no longer effective.

Supervision (Medicare A only): Aides cannot independently provide a skilled service. The services of aides performing therapy treatments may only be coded when the services are performed under line-of-sight supervision by a licensed therapist when allowed by state law. This type of coordination between the licensed therapist and therapy aide under the direct, personal (e.g., line-of-sight) supervision of the therapist is considered individual therapy for counting minutes. When the therapist starts the session and delegates the performance of the therapy treatment to a therapy aide while maintaining direct line-of-sight supervision, the total number of minutes of the therapy session may be coded as therapy minutes.

SUMMARY   Changes continue to occur regarding what types of therapy services are reimbursed, the level of therapy that is reimbursed, the percentage of reimbursement fees that is paid, and the types of settings for which reimbursement occurs. These changes continue to make a difficult situation much worse for those providing medical services to patients in various health-care settings. Because of the ever-changing requirements of MCOs, Medicare, Medicaid, private insurance providers, workers' compensation insurance providers, and other agencies, the therapist, student, clinical site, and educational institution must remain diligent in their oversight of regulations and activities related to documentation and reimbursement.

Without such diligence in the clinical setting, various therapeutic interventions may not be reimbursed, the facility could lose necessary reimbursement, and students may be unable to complete their education in a supervisory setting with a valued and experienced supervising therapist.

REFERENCES

1. Bihari, M. (2016, April 21). HMOs vs. PPOs—What are the differences between HMOs and PPOs? About.com. Retrieved from https://www.verywell.com/what-are-the-differences-between-hmos-and-ppos-1739063

2. Rural Assistance Center. (n.d.). Medicare frequently asked questions: Who is covered by Medicare? Retrieved from https://www.ruralhealthinfo.org/topics/medicare#faqs

3. Bihari, M. (2014, June 19). Health reform and the doctor shortage in the U.S.: Availability of primary care physicians—the Massachusetts experience. Retrieved from http://healthinsurance.about.com/od/reform/a/PCP_shortage.htm

4. Rittenhouse, D. R., & Shortell, S. M. (2009). The patient-centered medical home: Will it stand the test of health reform? *JAMA, 301*(19), 2038–2040 Retrieved from http://jama.jamanetwork.com/article.aspx?articleid=183908

5. Centers for Medicare & Medicaid Services. (n.d.). Regulations, guidance, and standards. Retrieved from https://www.cms.gov/home/regsguidance.asp

6. Medicare. (2011). Understanding Medicare enrollment periods: How do I get Medicare Part A and Part B? Retrieved from http://www.medicare.gov/Publications/Pubs/pdf/11219.pdf

7. Centers for Medicare & Medicaid Services. (n.d.). Medicare program—general information. Retrieved from http://www.cms.gov/MedicareGenInfo/

8. Medicare Consumer Guide. (2012). Medicare advantage plans—Part C. Retrieved from http://www.medicareconsumerguide.com/medicare-part-c.html

9. AARP. (2016). Medicare supplemental insurance plans. Retrieved from https://www.aarpmedicaresupplement.com/

10. Centers for Medicare & Medicaid Services. (2011, May 6). Pub 100-02 Medicare benefit policy: Home health therapy services. Retrieved from http://www.cms.gov/transmittals/downloads/R144BP.pdf

11. Centers for Medicare & Medicaid Services. (2012, April 5). Manuals. Retrieved from http://www.cms.gov/Manuals/IOM/list.asp#TopOfPage

12. Who is covered by Medicaid? (n.d.). Retrieved from http://www.medicaidwebsites.com/whoiscoveredbmedicaid.php

13. Program of all-inclusive care for the elderly (PACE). (n.d.). Retrieved from https://www.cms.gov/Medicare/Health-Plans/pace/Overview.html

14. California Department of Industrial Relations. (n.d.). Division of workers' compensation—Answers to frequently asked questions about workers' compensation for employees. Retrieved from http://www.dir.ca.gov/dwc/WCFaqIW.html

15. United States Department of Labor. (2016). Workers' compensation. Retrieved from https://www.dol.gov/general/topic/workcomp

16. Drummond-Dye, R., Elliott, C., & Lee, G. R. (2010, February). *Emerging issues in Medicare, Medicaid, and private insurance.* Presented at the Health Policy & Administration Combined Sections Meeting, San Diego, CA.

17. La Monica, P. R. (2016, April 19). Unitedhealthcare to exit most Obamacare exchanges. *CNNMoney.* http://money.cnn.com/2016/04/19/investing/unitedhealthcare-obamacare-exchanges-aca/

18. New Mexico Medical Insurance Pool. (n.d.). Retrieved from http://www.nmmip.org

19. Jackson, J., & Nolen, J. (2010, March 21). Health care reform bill summary: A look at what's in the bill. CBSNews.com. Retrieved from http://www.cbsnews.com/8301-503544_162-20000846-503544.html

20. American Physical Therapy Association. (n.d.). Use of physical therapist assistants (PTAs) under Medicare. Retrieved from http://www.apta.org/Payment/Medicare/Supervision/UseofPTAs/

21. American Physical Therapy Association. (2011). Implementing MDS 3.0: Use of therapy students. Retrieved from http://www.apta.org/search.aspx?q=implementing%20MDS%203.0

Review Exercises

1. What are the **three** reasons noted in the chapter for the declining use of HMOs and PPOs?

2. Explain the **difference** between using a PCP in an HMO and using a PCP in a PPO.

3. For **which** individuals will Medicare provide insurance coverage?

4. **What** do Medicare Part A and Medicare Part B **cover?**

5. **Who** qualifies for Medicaid?

6. What is **PACE?**

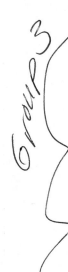

7. What is **workers' compensation insurance**?

8. Is it **true** that all employers must provide workers' compensation insurance for their employees? Explain **why** or **why not.**

9. Does the **employee** pay premiums for workers' compensation insurance?

10. Are there any circumstances in which an employer does **not** have to provide workers' compensation insurance?

11. What **type** of coverage can the employee expect the employer to provide through a workers' compensation claim?

12. What can an individual do for medical insurance coverage if the individual does **not qualify** for a program where he or she is employed, works privately, or simply does not qualify for coverage?

13. What is the **purpose** of the Affordable Care Act?

14. Why is proper documentation **important** for reimbursement for services in health care?

15. Are Medicare Part A therapy services that are provided by a PT or PTA student in an outpatient setting **reimbursed?**

16. Are Medicare Part A therapy services that are provided by a PT or PTA student in an inpatient rehabilitation setting reimbursed?

17. Can a PTA be a clinical instructor for a PTA student in **any** setting?

18. Under Medicare Part A, what **conditions** may be coded as concurrent therapy for a student therapist?

19. In a home health setting, what is the ruling for the **type** of supervision the PTA must treat under?

20. What **interventions** can a physical therapy aide provide, and which ones will Medicare reimburse the facility bill for?

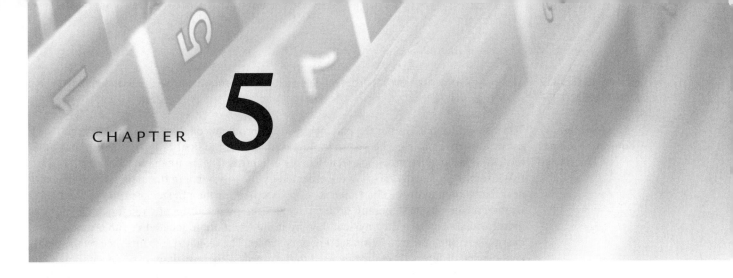

Documentation Content and Organization

LEARNING OBJECTIVES

After studying this chapter, the student will be able to:

☐ Identify the six categories of documentation content

☐ Briefly describe the content to be documented in each category

☐ Differentiate between the medical diagnosis and the physical therapy diagnosis

☐ Locate information in the medical record, based on an understanding of how medical record content is organized

☐ Organize the information to be documented in a physical therapy note into a logical sequence

☐ Present documentation content in at least three different formats

INTRODUCTION

The medical record is the written account of a patient's medical care. The medical record documents the medical care provided from a patient's admission through discharge.

The content within the medical record can be grouped into six categories:

1. The problem(s) requiring medical treatment
2. Data relevant to the patient's medical or physical therapy diagnosis
3. Treatment plan or action(s) to address the problem(s)
4. Goals or outcomes of the treatment plan
5. Record of administration of the treatment plan
6. Treatment effectiveness or results of the treatment plan

This information can be documented in many different ways (e.g., written evaluations, daily/progress notes, specialized reports) and in various types of medical records.

This chapter begins by briefly describing the six categories of content typically documented in the medical record. (In-depth explorations of these categories for physical therapy documentation are discussed in Chapters 9 through 13.) The chapter then discusses how to document this information by describing the various types of medical records, the various ways to organize the content in the medical record, and the various ways to record the information to be included in the medical record.

WHAT IS BEING DOCUMENTED?

This section describes the six different categories of information typically found in the medical record.

The Problem(s) Requiring Medical Treatment

The medical team identifies the patient's medical problems on the basis of the data collected by various disciplines. The physician determines the medical diagnosis (Dx), and other professionals identify problems related to the diagnosis that are treatable within their respective disciplines. The diagnosis is documented by the physician in the medical chart, usually near the beginning of the chart, in a section specified for the physician's report. The identification of the physical therapy problem, called the physical therapy diagnosis (PT Dx), is usually documented in the physical therapy initial evaluation, located in either the physical therapy section or the evaluation section of the chart. The diagnosis documented by the physician may be different from the one used in the physical therapy diagnosis, depending on the patient's medical history. For example, the medical diagnosis may be identified as a fracture of the right femur, but the physical therapy diagnosis would be loss of strength and range of motion to the right hip and knee due to the fracture of the right femur. With the launch of the ICD-10 coding system on October 1, 2015, the ability to differentiate between the two diagnoses has become easier. In addition, due to the increased specificity required, with the use of the ICD-10, therapists will be able to provide more clarification related to the diagnoses and increased reimbursement for skilled PT services. The PTA would be cognizant of the cause of the loss of function (i.e., the fracture of the right femur) but only would be responsible for treating the loss of function. Other problems are discussed in other health-care providers' evaluations.

In the example of the student in the motorcycle accident in Table 5–1, possible problems identified by the physicians, nurses, and social workers may include the following:

1. Compound fracture of the shaft of the right femur
2. Lacerations into the right quadriceps muscles
3. Infected open wound on the right anterior thigh
4. Edema of the right foot
5. Suspected chemical dependency
6. Fever
7. Elevated blood pressure

The PTA treats the loss of function related to the medical diagnosis, as outlined in the plan of care (POC) developed by the supervising PT. The supervising PT might evaluate how all seven medical diagnoses listed above affect the patient's function within the developed POC and might include all diagnoses as they relate to the physical therapy treatment sessions. For example, the treating therapist would need to monitor the open wound to determine whether it is healing properly. The PT would also monitor the fever, elevated blood pressure, and edema of the right foot to ensure that none of these issues is worsening, which could adversely affect the patient's progress regarding physical therapy goals and interventions. With the increased use of the ICF framework, additional skilled therapy services may be needed to address the loss of function that the patient has experienced because of a specific disability or disease.

Data Relevant to the Patient's Medical or Physical Therapy Diagnosis

It is important to understand the differences between the medical diagnosis and the physical therapy diagnosis in order to ensure the PTA's proper documentation of patient treatment and to delineate why skilled physical therapy services are necessary.

Medical Diagnosis

The medical diagnosis is the description of a systemic disease or disorder that is determined by the physician's evaluation and diagnostic tests. "Diagnosis is the recognition of disease. It is the determination of the cause and nature of pathologic conditions."[1] The medical diagnosis is equivalent to the pathology in the APTA and the Nagi frameworks. In the example of the student in the motorcycle accident (see Table 5–1), the medical diagnosis was "a fractured femur and infected lacerations."

Table 5–1	Examples of Data Gathered by Various Services for a Patient in a Motorcycle Accident
Discipline/Service	**Data**
Admitting clerk	Past admission to the hospital
	Insurance information
	Nearest relative
	General information about the accident
Physician	Medical history
	Detailed information about the accident
	Physical examination results
	Orthopedic examination results from orthopedic surgeon
	Diagnostic and laboratory test results, such as x-rays
Nurse	Vital signs
	Bowel and bladder function
	Skin condition
	General nutritional status
	General ability for self-care, communication, and decision-making
Physical therapist	Flexibility or joint range of motion
	Muscle strength
	Sensation
	Posture
	Ability to move about in environment
	Functional level (pre- and postaccident)
Occupational therapist	Specific ability for self-care in activities of daily living
	Vocational abilities
	Homemaking abilities
	General vision, hearing, and communication abilities
Social worker	Home environment and lifestyle
	More specific financial concerns
	General emotional development
	Family support and adjustment

Physical Therapy Diagnosis

The physical therapy diagnosis is not a medical diagnosis. According to Sahrmann,[2] the physical therapy diagnosis is the identification of pathokinesiologic (i.e., having to do with the study of movements related to a given disorder) problems associated with faulty biomechanical or neuromuscular action. In Sahrmann's definition, faulty biomechanical or neuromuscular action is termed *impairment,* and pathokinesiologic problems are called *functional limitations.*

In APTA's original model, the physical therapy diagnosis consisted of the patient's impairments and functional limitations, whereas in the ICF framework, the physical therapy diagnosis consists of the patient's impairments and disabilities affecting his or her ability to function. In both models, the physical therapy treatment objectives are to eliminate or minimize the impairments and functional limitations or disabilities. The desired outcome of the physical therapy treatment is preventing or minimizing the severity of the disability on that function. Since June 2008, APTA has embraced WHO's definitions and use of the specific terms as outlined in the ICF framework (see Chapter 2).

Impairments

Impairments are abnormalities or dysfunctions of the bones, joints, ligaments, muscles, tendons, nerves, or skin, or problems with movement resulting from an injury to or abnormality of the brain, spinal cord, or pulmonary or cardiovascular systems. A few common examples of dysfunctions treatable by physical therapy include muscle weakness; tendon inflammation; connective tissue tightness with limited range of motion (ROM) in the joints; muscle spasms; edema; and difficulties moving in bed, moving from sitting to standing, and walking. Impairments in the physical therapy diagnosis may be the same as in the medical diagnosis, such as "a rotated L5 vertebra" with muscle spasms and pain limiting a truck driver's sitting tolerance to 5 minutes. The physician, after determining through x-rays and evaluation that the L5 vertebra is rotated, may indicate this as the medical diagnosis. If the patient went to see the PT first, the PT, after performing the evaluation, may identify the rotated vertebra. This, plus the muscle spasms, is the musculoskeletal dysfunction part of the physical therapy diagnosis. A patient may have a medical diagnosis with a physical therapy diagnosis, such as "rheumatoid arthritis with adhesive capsulitis of the anterior capsule limiting shoulder ROM and interfering with the patient's ability to put on a shirt and sweater." In this case, "rheumatoid arthritis" is the medical diagnosis, and "adhesive capsulitis limiting shoulder ROM" is part of the physical therapy diagnosis.

Functional limitations

The physical therapy diagnosis must include the patient's functional abilities or inabilities. The patient comes to physical therapy because of an inability to function adequately in his or her environment. In the examples cited previously, the patient with the fractured femur cannot bear weight on the fractured leg during ambulation, the truck driver with the rotated L5 vertebra cannot sit longer than 5 minutes, and the patient with rheumatoid arthritis cannot put on a shirt and sweater. These functional problems become the basis for determining the outcomes toward which the physical therapy treatments are directed, and the rate of progress toward accomplishing the goals and outcomes determines the duration of the physical therapy services.[1] As previously discussed in Chapter 2, the use of the ICF framework for coding the patient's functional capabilities, in conjunction with the use of the ICD codes, provides a more unified method of treatment to address how that disease or disability affects the individual's ability to function.

Differentiation Between the Medical Diagnosis and Physical Therapy Diagnosis

The PTA should distinguish between the medical diagnosis and the physical therapy diagnosis when treating and documenting. Examples of medical diagnoses include the following (with ICD-9/ICD-10 codes included in parentheses):

1. Multiple sclerosis (340/G35)
2. Rheumatoid arthritis (714.0/M06.9)
3. Fractured right femur (821.1/S72.90XB)
4. Cerebral vascular accident secondary to thrombosis (434.01/I63.30)
5. Compression fracture of T12 vertebra with compression of spinal cord (839.21/S23.101A)

Physical therapy diagnoses that may be associated with the first two medical diagnoses listed previously are discussed in Box 5–1. With the initiation of the ICD-10, it has become imperative for the physician and PT to provide more specific information related to the patient's diagnosis affecting his or her functional capabilities based on information related to laterality, traumatic versus nontraumatic, dominant versus nondominant side, and so on. This provides the treating therapist and third-party payers a much better avenue to distinguish progress over the course of treatment from skilled physical therapy services.

Treatment Plans or Actions to Address the Problem(s)

The list of the patient's medical problems is used to plan the patient's medical treatment. Appropriate strategies for resolving or minimizing the problems are outlined by professionals in the various disciplines involved. These strategies are the treatment plans. In the case of the student who was in a motorcycle accident (see Table 5–1), the physician would design a treatment plan for medication to stop the infection and then for surgery to pin and stabilize the fractured femur. The nurse may design a treatment plan for positioning the right foot to reduce the edema, providing wound care, and monitoring blood pressure. The social worker may design a treatment plan to help the patient address his suspected chemical dependency. Later, the PT may design a treatment plan to teach the patient to walk with crutches. In the example with the truck driver, the PT may design a treatment plan that includes applying a physical agent to relax muscle spasms, performing mobilization techniques to derotate the L5 vertebra, and educating the driver about sitting support, proper posture, and appropriate lifting techniques. These treatment plans, described in the medical record, would include the frequency and duration of the treatment procedures.

| Box 5–1 | Physical Therapy Versus Medical Diagnosis |

Physical Therapy Diagnosis
Ataxia of lower extremities with inability to ambulate independently.

Discussion
A patient with the medical diagnosis of multiple sclerosis may have the physical therapy diagnosis of ataxia (the impairment) and the functional problem of inability to ambulate (the functional limitation). In the past, the result of the treatment was documented by a description of the improvement in impairment (e.g., "pt.'s coordination improved as pt. able to place Ⓡ heel on Ⓛ knee"). Today, treatment effectiveness is documented by a description of a decrease in the functional limitation, such as improvement in the ability or quality of the patient's ambulation (e.g., "pt. able to walk to mailbox [approximately 75 ft] without assistive device but needs standby assist because of occasional loss of balance").

Physical Therapy Diagnosis
ROM deficits in right shoulder limiting the ability to put on shirt and sweater.

Discussion
The patient with the medical diagnosis of rheumatoid arthritis may have the physical therapy diagnosis consisting of the impairment, ROM deficits, and the functional limitation of difficulty in dressing. In the past, it was acceptable to document treatment effectiveness in degrees of increased ROM (e.g., "shoulder flexion 0°–100°, an improvement of 20° since initial evaluation"). Today, a description of the patient's ability to put on his or her shirt or sweater, along with the improvement in degrees of ROM, documents the treatment effectiveness (e.g., "patient able to put on loose-fitting pullover sweater without assistance") and adds meaning to the ROM degrees related to a functional activity.

Informed Consent to the Treatment Plan

All aspects of the treatment plan, including the purposes, procedures, expected results, and any possible risks or side effects of treatment, must be explained to the patient and family. In some cases, the patient may participate in designing the plan. The patient or a representative for the patient should agree to the treatment plan and procedures. His or her decision to consent to the treatment (informed consent) is based on the information provided about the treatment. In many medical facilities, a formal informed consent form or document must be signed before treatment is initiated. When a patient is receiving physical therapy, the PT designs the treatment plan and reviews the plan with the patient. Thus, the appropriate person to obtain the informed consent signature is the PT, not the PTA. Once signed, this form is placed in the patient's medical record.[3] For electronic medical records (EMRs), the PT or PTA will electronically sign the note in the patient's medical record. It would be in the best interest of the PTA to ensure that informed consent has been obtained prior to the PTA continuing any additional services. Obtaining informed consent provides the patient with the opportunity to decline the treatment or decline the therapist providing the treatment if the patient is uncomfortable with either the procedure or the therapist.

Goals or Outcomes of the Treatment Plan

All health-care providers identify the goals or outcomes to be accomplished by their treatment plans. In the case of the student involved in the motorcycle accident (see Table 5–1), the physician's goals may be to treat the infection and stabilize the fractured femur so healing can occur. The nurse's goals may be to monitor the patient and prevent any other problems as a result of the patient's injury and temporary inactivity. The social worker's goal may be to help the patient find the most appropriate resources and help for his chemical dependency.

The functional outcomes toward which the PT's treatment plan are directed should include the patient's expectations (i.e., what is meaningful to the patient) for eliminating or minimizing the patient's functional limitations. The physical therapy goals are directed toward eliminating or minimizing the patient's impairments.

Therefore, the physical therapy goals and outcomes are planned with collaboration between the patient and the PT. The goals for the truck driver, for example, are to decrease his low back pain (M54.5) and improve his trunk ROM (F0115ZZ), whereas his functional outcome is to be able to sit for at least 2 hours so he can return to work.

The functional outcome for the student in the motorcycle accident is to learn how to use crutches so that he can return to college. The goals and outcomes give the PTA direction for planning the treatment sessions, progressing the patient within the POC, and recommending the termination of treatment. The PT and the PTA need to stay focused on the purpose of the treatment plan, gearing everything during a treatment session toward improving or resolving the functional problem that brought the client to physical therapy initially. Likewise, all documentation should be focused on the treatment appropriate for the goals and outcomes and on the progress toward accomplishing the functional outcomes. As discussed in Chapter 2, for patients receiving physical therapy under Medicare, therapists must also follow strict guidelines to track progress through the treatment process. This is done through the use of functional codes specific to the patient's deficits, utilizing the three types of "G" codes for the initial exam, re-evaluation, and discharge period of treatment.

Record of Administration of the Treatment Plan

The medical record contains proof that the treatment plan is being carried out. Recording the administration of the treatment procedures can range from simply checking off items listed in a flow chart or checklist to writing a narration or report about the treatment in daily, weekly, or monthly therapy notes. Whether notes are handwritten or an EHR system is utilized, such treatment plans should be followed and properly documented to ensure appropriate and timely medical care for the patient.

Progress/Daily Note

The progress/daily note (for the purposes of consistency, the term "daily" notes will be used from this point forward in this text) is a record of the treatment provided for each problem, the patient's reaction to the treatment procedures, progress toward goals and outcomes, and any changes in the patient's condition. Although both the PT and the PTA write daily notes, this text is directed toward the skills that the PTA needs to write quality notes or to enter information in the EMR to support progress within the prescribed POC, which was developed by the supervising PT.

Daily notes ensure that communication is occurring between the supervising PT and the PTA to determine whether the patient is meeting the short-term and long-term goals that have been set and to ensure that frequent assessment and re-evaluation are occurring and include plans for discharge. Daily notes also provide a written record for third-party payers (e.g., Medicare, Medicaid, private insurance) to determine whether the patient is making progress under the prescribed POC and whether continued skilled therapy services are still warranted.

Treatment Effectiveness or Results of the Treatment Plan

The content related to treatment effectiveness contains an interpretation of the patient's response to the treatment. It is the most important content in the medical record and is considered the "bottom line" of the health-care business. The therapist notes whether or not goals were met, thus documenting the effectiveness of the treatment plan and if expected progression within the prescribed POC has occurred. This information tells the reader about the quality of the medical care provided. The researcher uses this content to measure outcomes and determine the efficacy of treatment procedures. The third-party payer reads this information to determine whether the medical care met the requirements for reimbursement and the necessity for skilled intervention.

TYPES OF MEDICAL RECORDS

Once familiar with the different categories of information typically found in the medical record, it is important to become familiar with the various types of medical records that heath-care workers may encounter.

Until the 1970s, hospitals typically used source-oriented medical records (SOMRs). In the 1970s, the problem-oriented medical record (POMR) was introduced, offering another way to organize information. The PTA who works in several different clinical facilities may see both types of records. More commonly, however, facilities use variations and combinations of SOMRs and POMRs. Today, the PTA may also use functional outcome reports (FORs), which are organized according to the functional abilities of the patient.

Source-Oriented Medical Records (SOMRs)

The SOMR is organized according to the medical services offered by the clinical facility, such as in a hospital or rehabilitation facility. A section in the chart is labeled with a tab marker or color-coded for each discipline. For example, the SOMR might be organized with the physician's section first, followed by sections for nursing, physical therapy, occupational therapy, and then test results. Caregivers in each discipline document their content (e.g., data, problems, treatment plans, goals, daily notes, and treatment effectiveness) in the section designated for their discipline. The sections must be clearly marked for easy identification so that the reader can locate the information. Source-oriented organization is criticized because the time required to read through each section for information makes the record difficult to audit for reimbursement and quality control.

Each professional on the medical team is responsible for reading the chart frequently, communicating with other medical professionals, and staying informed about the patient's latest treatments and condition. Otherwise, professionals in one discipline might identify a patient's problem and begin treatment while professionals in the other disciplines may not be aware that the problem exists. For example, a nurse discovers high blood pressure and obtains medication orders from the physician. The nurse records this information in the section for nursing notes. The patient experiences side effects from the new medication that affect his or her ability to fully understand the PTA's exercise instructions. If the PTA has not taken the time to read the nursing section of the patient's chart and, therefore, is unaware of the additional medication, the PTA may incorrectly assume and document in the physical therapy section that the patient is being uncooperative. To ensure communication and coordination among the health-care providers, regular meetings are necessary so that medical personnel can discuss the patient's problems and progress. A written record of these meetings that includes a list of attendees should be placed in the patient's chart.

Problem-Oriented Medical Records (POMRs)

In the 1970s, Dr. Lawrence Weed introduced the POMR in an attempt to eliminate the disadvantages associated with the SOMR. Content in the POMR is organized around the identification and treatment of the patient's problems. The components or sections of the POMR are organized in the following sequence, thus ordering information about the patient's medical care from admission to discharge:

1. Database
2. Problem list
3. Treatment plans
4. Daily notes
5. Discharge notes

Each section contains the appropriate information from each discipline. For example, the data gathered by the physician, PT, and occupational therapist (OT) are recorded in the database section. For each of these disciplines, the problems identified are listed in the problem list section, the treatment plans in the treatment plan section, and the daily notes in the daily note section. Each caregiver may record on the same page within each section. Alternatively, subsections may be designated for each discipline within the main sections of the POMR.

Communication among disciplines is enhanced with the POMR because all of the problems identified and treated by each discipline are in one place. This form of organization also allows specific information, such as treatment results, to be found easily should the record be audited.

Functional Outcome Reports (FORs)

Swanson[4] proposed the use of the FOR, a structured approach for reporting functional assessment and outcomes (Box 5–2). The sequence of the information in the FOR is as follows:

1. Reason for referral
2. Functional limitations
3. Physical therapy assessment
4. Therapy problems
5. Functional outcome goals
6. Treatment plan and rationale

The "reason for referral" section includes the medical diagnosis, medical history, and subjective data. The "functional limitations" and "physical therapy assessment" sections contain

> ### Box 5-2   Example of an Initial Functional Outcome Report (FOR)
>
> **Reason for Referral**
>
> Patient post-meniscectomy of left knee reports pain (8/10), stiffness, and difficulty with walking and other upright mobility activities.
>
> **Functional Limitations**
>
> | Activity | Current Status |
> |---|---|
> | Sit-to-stand transfer | Independent |
> | Standing balance | Performs independently, with cane, WB on Ⓛ knee 50% |
> | Flat terrain ambulation (speed) | Performs with cane for more than 18 sec for 20 ft |
> | Flat terrain ambulation (endurance) | Tolerates less than 5 min |
> | Ambulation on uneven terrain | Unable without LOB |
> | Stair climbing | Ascends two steps, descends two steps with railing and minimum assistance |
>
> **PT Assessment**
>
> Medical diagnosis status post-meniscectomy is further defined to include residual left knee joint inflammation.
>
> Positive test findings: Positive fluctuation test; limited strength; quadriceps 3/5 and hamstring 4/5, indicative of synovial effusion.
>
> **Therapy Problems**
>
> 1. Pain on compression maneuvers of the left knee: sit to stand, periodically during gait cycle, during all phases of stair climbing.
> 2. Difficulty in coordinating gait cycle with use of cane to reduce stress to left knee with normal stance phase on Ⓛ side due to pain level of 8/10.
>
> **Functional Outcome Goals**
>
> | Activity | Performance | Due Date |
> |---|---|---|
> | Flat terrain ambulation (speed) | Independent without device; 20 ft in 9 sec | Within 14 days |
> | Flat terrain ambulation (endurance) | Tolerates unassisted walking for 30 min | Within 21 days |
> | Uneven terrain ambulation | Tolerates for a minimum of 15 min | Within 14 days |
> | Stair climbing | Ascends and descends 15 steps with reciprocal gait | Within 21 days |
>
> **Treatment Plan With Rationale**
>
> Application of anti-inflammatory modalities with instruction for follow-up home program to minimize post-activity edema.
>
> Lower extremity strength training with instruction in progressive home exercise program. Patient instructed in activity limits and restrictions during the course of care.
>
> *Source:* Swanson, G. (1993). Functional outcome report: The next generation in physical therapy reporting. In D. Stewart & H. Abeln (Eds.), *Documenting functional outcomes in physical therapy.* St. Louis, MO: Mosby Yearbook.

objective data. The physical problems are identified based on the data. The functional goals are listed, and the report concludes with the treatment plan and how it relates to accomplishing the functional goals. This type of documentation format more closely follows the requirements of the ICD-10 coding system, in conjunction with the SOAP format, discussed under organizational models.

LOGICAL SEQUENCING OF CONTENT IN THE MEDICAL RECORD

The content provided in medical records can be organized using several different models. Most content organization models use a problem-solving approach to sequence the information. First, the data are gathered. Second, the data are interpreted and a judgment is made to identify the physical therapy diagnosis. Next, goals and outcomes are determined to direct the focus of physical therapy interventions. Finally, a treatment plan is designed to accomplish the goals and outcomes.

Organization Models

Five content models are used to teach PTAs how to organize and present the information describing the medical treatment and how to determine what information is necessary. Medical facilities determine which of the following models they use on an individual basis:

1. SOAP (subjective, objective, assessment, and plan)
2. PSP (problem, status, plan)
3. PSPG (problem, status, plan, goals)
4. DEP (data, evaluation, performance)
5. Paragraph or narrative

Table 5–2 compares the organization models and their methods of incorporating documentation content. Examples of the PSP, PSPG, and paragraph models are given in Figures 5–1, 5–2, and 5–3, respectively.

SOAP Model

SOAP notes are perhaps the most widely used type of documentation and the documentation most commonly used in the 1970s and 1980s before the widespread use of computers and EMRs. This type of documentation provides the new therapist and the student with an outline to document what happens during the patient treatment session. It also provides a means of chronicling the patient's progress and recommendations for continuing care. This type of format provides beginning therapists with an organized method to outline what they hear from

Table 5–2 Comparing Organization Models				
Documentation Content	**SOAP**	**PSP**	**PSPG**	**DEP**
Problem	Pr	P	P	D
Subjective data	S	P	S	D
Objective data	O	S	S	D
Treatment effectiveness	A	S	S	E
Goals/outcomes	A	S	G	P
Plan	P	P	P	E

Pr = Problem; P = Plan in SOAP and Performance in DEP; D = Data; S = Subjective Data in SOAP and Status in PSPG; O = Objective data; A = Assessment; E = Evaluation; G = Goals

---

ABC Physical Therapy Clinic, Anytown, USA

June 1, 2017

P: 47 YOM, college math professor, Dx: chronic LBP syndrome; mild Ⓛ spine DJD; probable lumbar extension dysfunction; r/o HNP.

S: Pt. states, "I feel 50% better. The pain in my Ⓡ leg is gone now. I can sit for over an hour w/o any pain." Pt. attended back school on May 15, 2017. Exam: GMT/AROM WNL, ⒷLE, FAROM, Ⓛspine, w/o any c/o Sx. Neg. spasm, TTP, deformity. Neg. SLR to 85° Ⓑ, neg. Fabere. Gait, posture, SLR WNL. Performs extension exercises w/o difficulty or Sx.

P: Cont w/MH PRN, tid extension exercises, 10–15 reps. F/U w/ Dr. Brown scheduled for tomorrow. PT F/U 2–3 weeks or PRN. Pt. understands home program; pt. questions about exercise techniques answered. _____

——————————————————————————————— Aaron Therapist, PT

Figure 5—1 A note written using the PSP model. (Adapted from Scott, R. W. [1994]. *Legal aspects of documenting patient care* [p. 79]. Gaithersburg, MD: Aspen, with permission.)

Therapy Clinic, USA

June 1, 2017

P: 47 YOM, college math professor, Dx: chronic LBP syndrome; mild Ⓛ spine DJD; probable Lumbar extension dysfunction; r/o HNP.

S: Pt. was discharged as inpatient on May 5, 2017, and placed on OP home PT program of MH PRN and active extension exercises, tid X 10-15 reps. Today pt. states "I feel 50% better. The pain in my Ⓡ leg is gone now.
I can sit for over an hour w/o any pain." Pt. attended back school on May 15, 2017. Exam: GMT/AROM WNL, BLE, FAROM, Ⓛ spine, w/o any c/o Sx. Neg. spasm, TTP deformity. Neg. SLR to 85° Ⓑ, neg. Fabere. Gait, posture, SLT WNL. Performs extension exercises w/o difficulty or Sx.

P: Cont. w/MH PRN, tid extension exercise, 10-15 reps F/U w/ Dr. Brown scheduled for tomorrow. PT F/U 2-3 weeks or PRN. Pt. understands home program; pt. questions about exercise techniques answered.

G: Decrease residual Sx 50% X 2-3 wks; I pain-free ADL; prevent recurrence through good body mechanics.

Aaron Therapist, PT

Figure 5—2 A note written using the PSPG model. This is a physical therapist's 4-week outpatient reevaluation form. (Adapted from Scott, R. W. [1994]. *Legal aspects of documenting patient care* [p. 79]. Gaithersburg, MD: Aspen, with permission.)

6-27-17: Dx: Status post pinned fractured R femur, dependent ambulation because of NWB on R leg.

Patient states he feels dizzy when he sits up but is eager to start walking on crutches and go home. Pt. c/o dizziness first time standing during treatment. BP before treatment 120/70 mmHg, first time up in // bars 108/65 mmHg, second standing trial 118/70 mmHg, after treatment 128/72 mmHg. Pt. responded to gait training with axillary crutches/minimal assist for sense of security and vc for posture and heel contact/NWB on Ⓡ/swing through gait 100 ft 2 X in hall, bed↔bathroom, and on carpet. Able to Ⓘ sit↔stand with crutches from bed/lounge chair/toilet. Pt.'s progress toward functional outcome of community ambulation with crutches 50%. BP adjusting to upright position. Will teach stairs, ambulation on grass and car transfers tomorrow AM. Will notify PT discharge evaluation scheduled for tomorrow PM.

Jesus Therapist,
PTA Lic. #7890

Figure 5—3 Note written in a paragraph or narrative model.

the patient, to provide measurable goals, to analyze the treatment session, and to plan for continued treatment and referral to other health-care providers. See Box 5–3 for an example of each section of the SOAP note. It is one of the simplest documentation methods used and will be discussed in detail in Chapters 10 through 13.

PSP and PSPG Models

A model used more typically for daily notes or interim evaluation reports is one that describes the problem, status, and plan (PSP) for the patient treatment, a variation of the SOAP note. The patient's physical therapy problem and diagnosis and medical diagnosis are stated under the first P (problem) section. Subjective and objective data about the patient's condition at the time of the interim evaluation are documented under the S (status) section. The second P (plan) section contains the modified treatment plan indicated by the clinical findings. The PSPG model adds a G section for functional goals. Review Figures 5–1 and 5–2 for examples of notes in PSP and PSPG models.[3]

DEP (Data, Evaluation, Performance goals) Model

DEP is a performance-based documentation model designed by El-Din and Smith.[5] The subjective and objective data (D) are combined into one section. In the evaluation section (E), data are interpreted and physical therapy diagnoses are identified; the treatment plan is also included in this section. The performance goals (P) section contains the functional goals for treatment and the expected time frame for meeting these goals.

Paragraph or Narrative Model

A paragraph or narrative reporting format describes treatment sessions in a more descriptive manner and does not provide the type of structure that you might find in other models. This type of reporting is used to describe short treatment sessions with a patient or any type of interaction with other health-care personnel responsible for the patient's care. This type of note

> **Box 5–3**   **SOAP Note Format**
>
> S: This section includes subjective types of information—reported by the patient, family, caretakers, or other health-care providers—that are related to the patient's treatment and response to the treatment.
>
> O: This section includes all the objective types of information, including specific measurements, range of motion, strength ratings, functional levels, tone, therapeutic exercises, number of repetitions and sets of exercises, and any other measurable treatment protocols.
>
> A: This section contains assessment information related to the patient's response to the treatment session, a summary of how the session was conducted and completed, and the introduction of a home program with a review of and changes in patient status.
>
> P: This section contains the continued plan for treatment, communication with the supervising PT, recommendations from the supervisory visit, and recommendations for any necessary referrals or plans for discharge to another facility or to the patient's home.

can review a simple treatment session, document a brief discussion with another health-care worker regarding the patient's treatment session or progress, or provide a simple discussion of the patient's progress. Because this type of note is less structured, however, important information may be omitted.

Regardless of the type of organization model used, it is the PT's responsibility to evaluate the patient and set the POC, and it is the PTA's responsibility to treat the patient within that POC and provide frequent assessments of how the patient is meeting the goals set within the POC. The PTA never sets the short- and long-term goals, but he or she may have input into those goals through communication with the supervising PT. If the patient is not progressing within the prescribed POC set by the supervising PT, it is the responsibility of the PTA to communicate this information to the PT so that the PT can re-evaluate the patient and amend the POC.

Guidelines for Adapting to the Organization Models

The PTA can easily adapt to any organization model for the medical record by using the following problem-solving approach to sequence the information:

1. Introduce the daily note with a list or statement that tells the reader the physical therapy diagnoses for which the note is written.
2. Place the subjective and objective data first. Compare them with or relate them to the data in the initial or interim examination report.
3. Discuss the meaning of the data as they relate to treatment effectiveness and progress toward accomplishing the goals and functional outcomes listed in the initial or interim evaluation report.
4. Discuss the plan for future treatment sessions and involvement of the PT.

Figures 5–1, 5–2, and 5–3 illustrate different content organizations for daily notes. See Figure 1–2 in Chapter 1 for an example of a SOAP note.

FORMATS FOR RECORDING CONTENT

Information can be recorded using a variety of formats. For example, evaluations and daily notes may be either handwritten or typed. The daily notes may be narrative (i.e., written in paragraph form) or written in an outline format, such as the SOAP note. How the information in the medical record is organized depends on the preference of the medical facility. Each facility determines the format to use for recording data. The PTA must be familiar with the facility's charting procedures and must always follow the facility's policies, procedures, and format.

Computerized Documentation

According to the Office of the National Coordinator for Health Information Technology, "An electronic health record (EHR) is a digital version of a patient's paper chart. EHRs are real-time, patient-centered records that make information available instantly and securely to authorized users. While an EHR does contain the medical and treatment histories of patients, an EHR system is built to go beyond standard clinical data collected in a provider's office and can be inclusive of a broader view of a patient's care."[6]

Currently EHRs are designed for completing evaluations and daily notes on the computer. Many facilities have one or more computers in the department for staff members to use when completing documentation, or the practice may provide individual tablets for employees. A few facilities have a computer terminal in every hospital room or in every treatment area of a physical therapy department. This allows the therapist to enter information in the patient's chart immediately following the treatment session. Physical therapy documentation software often is advertised in publications such as *Physical Therapy* and *PT in Motion.* There are several kinds available on the Web, such as WebPT (www.webpt.com),[7] ReDoc (www.rehabdocumentation. com),[8] Therapy Charts (www.therapycharts.com),[9] Clinicient (www.clinicient.com),[10] and HealthWyse (www.healthwyse.com).[11] While the PTA may not be responsible for procuring such programs, he or she may be asked for input into such programs when the clinic may be looking at a transition into EHRs.

A word of warning is necessary about computerized documentation. This chapter discusses how the content of the daily note must be individualized to each patient to clearly demonstrate how each patient is responding to the physical therapy treatment plan. Computerized documentation programs typically have preprogrammed statements or phrases that can be selected and combined to quickly compose the content of the daily note. The PTA must be careful that the selection of these phrases clearly distinguishes this patient from other patients and that the content clearly describes the necessity for providing skilled physical therapy services. The software should allow the writer to type in his or her own words and phrases to individualize the note for specific patient treatments. In addition, EHRs can be difficult to use, time consuming, and challenging to edit once information has been entered. On the positive side, EHRs can:

- Make notes easier to read
- Result in fewer errors and less waste
- Contribute to a decrease in unwarranted variations in practice
- Provide cost savings and faster reimbursement
- Provide consistency in information among patients
- Allow therapists to enter information as they treat the patient
- Provide timely updates for coding
- Help with updates related to changes in Medicare requirements
- Help identify problems within the documentation process related to inappropriate billing issues

APTA provides education and assistance in assessing and implementing EHRs.[12] Its Health Information Technology's (HIT) Advisory Group developed the EHR adoption toolkit in 2012 and then revised it through 2016. This toolkit provides PTs with a meaningful guide to understand and adopt EHRs into their practices. The toolkit was researched and adopted in response to Medicare's Meaningful Use Program initiatives, which penalize providers who do not meet the requirements for their documentation. The EHR toolkit provides four parts to help clinicians decide whether adopting EHRs will be advantageous for their practice:

- Part 1: Background information on why there is a push to adopt EHRs and a brief introduction to the federal issues that impact physical therapist practice
- Part 2: Basic information on what PTAs need to understand for the successful adoption of an EHR system; this includes what constitutes an EHR and suggestions to help the PTA consider his or her current environment and workflow
- Part 3: Expands the PTA's knowledge about the available types of EHR software and hardware; this section also provides considerations for choosing the right technology partner
- Part 4: Successful implementation makes a smooth transition when adopting an EHR; this section describes an organized approach and clear communication with all members of the facility's staff and provides suggestions for implementation[13]

Flow Charts and Checklists   Much of the data, such as the patient's vital signs and functional status and the physical therapy interventions provided, can be recorded on flow charts, fill-in-the-blank forms, and checklists for day-to-day treatment sessions. By using these formats, the medical professional can easily scan the form to gather information and quickly record information in the chart. Hospitals, long-term care facilities, and rehabilitation centers are facilities where the PTA will find narrative or outlined (commonly SOAP) notes, checklists, and flow charts. Figure 5–4 is an example of a flow chart for recording physical therapy treatments. Figure 5–5 illustrates two daily note forms combining a checklist or a flow chart with brief statements or a narration. A fill-in-the-blank form is depicted in Figure 5–6.

DATE:

Orientation/Mood					
UE Strength/EX - bicep/tricep					
- W/C push up/rowing					
- shld flex/abd/horz abd/add					
TRANSPORT:					
- Transport to dept W/C/cart/amb					
Abductor pillow/knee immobilizer/prothesis/tilt tbl.					
- standing table					
GAIT: DEVICE:					
//bars; walker; crutches; cane; Qcane; none					
wt. bearing; NWB; TTWB; PWB; FWB; WBAT					
pattern: 2pt./3pt./4pt.					
distance/endurance					
Balance - sit/stand/walk					
Balance Act: lat/post/braid/line/sit/ball					
Stairs: rail/without rail/gait sequence					
TF's bed mobility					
toilet/raised seat/reg/commode bedside					
slidingboard transfer					
shower seat/car transfer					
supine → sit; sit → supine/sit to stand					
EX isometric quads, glut, HS, abd/ball squeeze					
ankle pump/circle/ DF/PF/Ev/Inv					
hip flexion supine/sit/stand					
SLR flexion supine/stand					
SLR extension prone/stand/side lie					
SLR abduction supine/side lie/stand					
TKE supine/sit/SAQ/LAQ					
Bridging 1 leg/both					
knee AAROM sit/prone/supine					
PROM hip/knee/UE/ankle					
AAROM hip/knee/UE/ankle					
Stretching LE/UE					
Positional ROM/prone/long sit					
CPM					
Modalities H.P./ice/US/whirlpool					
Neuromusc. Re-Educ. Biofeed/CVA rehab					
HHA/Family instruction in:					
TF's-bed/toilet/shower/chair					
positioning/EX program					
walking program					
Written home program provided					
CHARGE - abbreviation for treatment					
THERAPIST					

SPC 337022   **REHABILITATION PHYSICAL THERAPY**

Restraints: NA/pelvic/vest

DNR Y/N

Precautions: _____

Figure 5—4   Flow-chart form for recording physical therapy treatment.

Letters   Physical therapists in private practice may communicate information about a patient to other medical professionals by letter. The data are recorded in the office through any of the models already mentioned, but they are periodically summarized in letter format (Fig. 5–7). This type of format is commonly used when the patient's progress is being reported to a physician.

Cardex   Within the physical therapy department, the patient's treatment goals and current intervention plan may be recorded in a cardex format. This 4- by-6-inch card is kept in a folder designed to hold many cards for quick access. Some clinics may use a larger form (8½ by 11 inches) for similar purposes: to help track exercise programs for their patients. The information is written in pencil so it can be updated easily. For example, in the morning the card may read that the patient ambulates from his bedroom to the nursing station and ambulates on the carpet in the lounge area. However, during the treatment session later in the afternoon, the patient ambulated past the station and to the stairs. The patient also managed three stairs for the first time. Now the information needs to be erased, and the new ambulation distance and the stair-climbing must be described. However, the treating therapist must ensure that the information regarding the patient's progress has been included in the chart for review by medical personnel and

HOME CARE/HOSPICE SERVICES

Patient's Name:	Last	First	Age	Date	Time	Visit Frequency	Date Next Visit

Mood	Orientation	Cooperation	Communication	Pain	Rx Tolerance

		TREATMENTS			**COMMENTS**
	Modalities	**WB Status**	**Ambulation**	**Exercise:**	
	Bed mobility	Non wt. bearing	Distance		
	Elec. stim.	Partial	Assist.		
	Ex. active	Toe touch	Balance		
	Ex ROM	Full	Coord.		
	Ex back	Non amb.	Pattern		
	Ex breathing		Stairs		
	Ex coord.				
	Ex isometric	**Equipment**	**Transfers**	**Problems/Progess:**	
	Ex man. resist	Walker	Bed		
	Ex mm re-ed.	Crutches	Toilet		
	Ex PRE	Cane	Tub		
	Ex gait trng.		Chair		
	Massage		Car		
	Packs	**ROM**			
	Stump wrap				
	Transfers		Other		
	Tx				
	Ultrasound				
	Evaluation				
	MD contact				
	Instruction		**Follow-through/Response:**		
	Patient				
	Support Person				
	HHA				

THERAPIST SIGNATURE

Figure 5—5A   Physical therapy progress/daily note forms that combine presentation styles. This form combines a checklist with brief statements.

Physical Therapy Daily Progress Notes						
MODALITIES:	DATE/Initials	DATE/Initials	DATE/Initials	DATE/Initials	DATE/Initials	DATE/Initials
Hot Pack/Cold Packs						
Massage/Ice Massage						
Electrical Stimulation						
Traction						
Ultrasound						
Kinetic Activity						
Therapeutic Exercise						
Neuromuscular Re-ed						
Functional Activities						
Training in ADLs						
Serial Casting						
Gait Training						
Orthotics/Prosthetics Train.						
Wound Care						
Whirlpool Therapy						
Conference						
Consultation						
Other						

Date	Comments:

Assessment:

Goals:

Plan:

(Name)	Date
(Name)	Date
(Name)	Date

Treatment Diagnosis:

Figure 5—5B   Physical therapy progress/daily note forms that combine presentation styles. This form combines a flow chart with narration.

Level of Independence	Without Help	Uses Device	Help of Another	Device and Help	Dependent/ Does Not Do	Not Determined
Feeding						
Hygiene/Grooming						
Transfers						
Homemaking						
Bath/Shower						
Dressing						
Bed Mobility						
Home Mgt.						

Physical Environment: _____

_____

Psychosocial: _____

Safety Measures: _____

_____

Equipment in Home: _____

Emergency No: _____ *Nutritional Req: _____ Allergies: _____

Unusual Home/Social Environment: _____

*Known Medical Reason Pt. leaves home: _____

Other Services Involved: _____ Prognosis: _____

Vulnerable Adult Assessment: _____ Low Risk _____ High Risk _____

Caregiver Status: _____

Pulse: _____   BP: _____

Current Medications: _____   _____

                        _____   _____

                        _____   _____

Patient's Prior Status: _____

_____

Scheduled MD Follow-up Appt(s): _____

_____

Name: _____

Rx#: _____

Figure 5—6 Form with a fill-in-the-blank format.

August 2, 2017
RE: Mr. Isaiah Morris
Dx: Femur Fx

Update on Progress:

Mr. Morris is making good progress recovering from the fracture of the (L) femur. Patient is now able to ambulate 100 feet with a quad cane and SBA, 4x/day. Pt. has full AROM in (L) LE and strength is 4/5 in all muscles. Recommend continued therapy 2x/week with continuation of daily home program.

Figure 5—7 Example of a letter format.

third-party payers. When the PTA is treating a patient, he or she refers to the cardex information. Updating the information on a regular basis is essential to ensure the patient is progressing toward accomplishing the treatment goals outlined in the POC. This cardex is used within the physical therapy department; it is not a part of the patient's medical record. An intervention plan outlined on a cardex is depicted in Figure 5–8.

Templates Templates are forms developed by a medical facility to shorten the patient documentation time and to ensure a more orderly and complete reporting process for all employees. These forms

DX: R CVA with hemiplegia **INITIAL DATE:** 3-24-17

PRECAUTIONS: Broca's Aphasia, feeding tube **UPDATE:** 4-20-17

Exercise	Set	Rep	Equipment	Assist	Goals
PROM/AAROM (L) UE & LE, prone	1	10		muscle belly	1. (I) bed mobility
Knee flexion	1	10	1# cuff weight	tapping	2. (I) unsupported sit
TKE long sit	1	10	2# cuff weight	verbal cues	3. (I) w/c mobility
	1	as many as he can; goal of 10 reps			4. Standing pivot transfer with min assist of 1
	2	10	2# cuff weight	verbal cues	
	2	10	2# cuff weight		**TDD:**
Standing 10 min; work on eye tracking and lip closure	2	10	1# cuff weight	Standing table	**TDP:**

Patient's Name	Age	Sex	MD	PT	RM#	Unit
Marquis W.	**71**	**M**	**Sanchez**	**Jiminez**	**E123**	**12**

Transfers	Method	Assist	Other
bed↔w/c, w/c↔mat, w/c↔toilet w/c↔straight chair	Stand pivot to (R) side	Max. x 1	Practice squat pivot transfer w/c ↔ mat moving toward (L).

Pregait/Gait

Stand in//bars-max assist x 1 – midline with mirror and wt. shifting to (L). Watch (L) knee – no hyperextension.

Sitting balance in w/c with arms removed and in armless straight chair. Min assist x 2. Work on head movement, eye tracking, wt. shifting, and trunk rot.

W/c mobility – room to bathroom, room to dining room, to PT, OT and Speech departments. Check seating/cushion, (L) scapula protracted, and arm on tray.

Figure 5—8 A treatment plan outlined on a cardex, commonly used in physical therapy departments to keep treatment procedures current.

can be developed in an EHR or on paper. Various companies now provide these types of documentation materials, and many of the larger facilities tend to use them. When using this type of format, several problems develop related to the inability of the therapist to provide any detailed narrative that may ensure quality patient care. This format also makes it difficult for students and new therapists to develop the skills necessary for quality reporting of patient care because it may not allow for delineation of specific treatment techniques to address individual patient goals. This format does not allow new PTAs to learn how to organize their thought processes to address the POC in an outline fashion and may make it difficult for the PTA to remember to address all aspects of the POC in his or her documentation.

Standardized Forms Used in Documentation

The PTA also may need to fill out various standardized forms, surveys, or scales to provide appropriate documentation in patient care. Common forms include those used to treat children in the educational setting using individualized education programs (IEPs) and various Medicare forms that have been developed for specific medical facilities.

Individualized Education Programs (IEPs)

In public schools, physical therapy, occupational therapy, speech therapy, and psychological services provided to a student are planned and recorded in a format called an individualized education program (IEP). This format is in accordance with several laws passed by Congress relating to the provision of services to facilitate the education of students with disabilities. Professionals providing these services (e.g., teacher, OT, PT, school psychologist, speech pathologist) are included on the IEP team. The team records educational goals and objectives to be accomplished during the school year and holds meetings periodically to review the goals and objectives. The team also meets with parents a minimum of once every 6 months to make any needed changes. Box 5–4 lists the components of an IEP. These components are essentially the same as those of a physical therapy evaluation and daily note. Figure 5–9 provides an example of the PT's contribution to the annual long-term goals and instructional objectives in an IEP written for a student. The PTA does not write the physical therapy goals and objectives for the IEP but plays an important role by providing input for their planning. The PTA working in the school environment documents the progress being made toward accomplishing the physical therapy goals.[13]

Medicare Forms

Standardized Medicare forms are used to chart the medical care given to patients covered by Medicare. The Health Care Financing Administration (HCFA) specifies the format and timelines for recording and submitting data. The Medicare Plan of Treatment for Outpatient Rehabilitation (Form CMS-700; see Fig. 5–10) and the Updated Plan of Progress for Outpatient

---

Box 5-4   Components of an IEP

1. A statement of the student's current levels of educational performance
2. A statement of annual goals, including short-term instructional objectives
3. A statement of the specific special-education and related services to be provided to the student and the extent to which the child will be able to participate in regular education programs
4. The projected dates for initiation of services and the anticipated duration of the services
5. Appropriate objective criteria, evaluation procedures, and schedules for determining, on at least an annual basis, whether the short-term instructional objectives are being achieved (34CFR 300.334)

Source: Martin, K. D. (1990). Individualized educational program and individualized family service plan. In American Physical Therapy Association, *Physical therapy practice in educational environments: Policies and guidelines* (p. 61). Alexandria, VA: Author.

Learner's Name:	
Annual Goals, Short-term Instructional Objectives	
Thoroughly state the goal. List objectives for the goal, including attainment criteria for each objective.	Goal #_____ of _____ Goals

Goal:

The student will independently move about the school building and within the classroom using a wheelchair to participate in all daily school activities, and the student will independently transfer from wheelchair to desk seat, to floor for participation and position change in 6 months.

Short-term Instructional Objectives

1. The student will independently open doors to the gymnasium and maneuver the wheelchair through the entrance to the gym 1/3 trials in 3 months.
2. The student will independently transfer from wheelchair to floor and back into the chair 1/3 trials in 3 months.
3. The student will safely and independently maneuver the wheelchair around the tables in the cafeteria 1/3 trials in 3 months.

IEP Periodic Review

Date Reviewed: _____
Progress made toward this goal and objective

The learner's IEP

☐ Meets learner's current needs and will be continued without changes.

☐ Does not meet learner's current needs and the modifications (not significant) listed below will be made without an IEP meeting unless you contact us.

☐ Does not meet learner's current needs and the significant changes listed below require a revised IEP. We will be in contact soon to schedule a meeting.

Note to Parent(s): You are entitled to request a meeting to discuss the results of this review.

Figure 5–9 An example of the PT's contribution to the goals and instructional objectives on an IEP written for a child in school.

Rehabilitation forms (Form CMS-701, see Fig. 5–11) are intended to be evaluation forms. These forms should not be completed by a PTA.[14]

The approval for physical therapy services is renewed or recertified periodically (at present, every 30 days in most states). Recent changes in some types of settings may require more frequent reviews (e.g., services provided through Medicare in a home health setting now require a reassessment by the supervising physical therapist made on the 13th visit, on the 19th visit, and on the 30th day). In an outpatient setting, Medicare requires a review following the 10th visit or 30th day (whichever comes first) after the initial PT evaluation. When the PT completes an updated functional evaluation and recommends that skilled physical therapy services continue for the patient to meet the goals, these forms become an interim evaluation and are necessary to track those changes. If the patient has reached the maximum benefit or has met the goals, these forms serve as a discharge evaluation. The PTA can provide the PT with information about the status of the patient, but the PT completes the evaluation and discharge forms.

DEPARTMENT OF HEALTH AND HUMAN SERVICES
CENTERS FOR MEDICARE & MEDICAID SERVICES

PLAN OF TREATMENT FOR OUTPATIENT REHABILITATION
(COMPLETE FOR INITIAL CLAIMS ONLY)

1. PATIENT'S LAST NAME	FIRST NAME	M.I.	2. PROVIDER NO.	3. HICN

4. PROVIDER NAME	5. MEDICAL RECORD NO. *(Optional)*	6. ONSET DATE	7. SOC. DATE

8. TYPE	9. PRIMARY DIAGNOSIS *(Pertinent Medical D.X.)*	10.TREATMENT DIAGNOSIS	11. VISITS FROM SOC.
☐ PT ☐ OT ☐ SLP ☐ CR ☐ RT ☐ PS ☐ SN ☐ SW			

12. PLAN OF TREATMENT FUNCTIONAL GOALS | PLAN

GOALS *(Short Term)*

OUTCOME *(Long Term)*

13. SIGNATURE *(professional establishing POC including prof. designation)* | 14. FREQ/DURATION *(e.g., 3/Wk. x 4 Wk.)*

I CERTIFY THE NEED FOR THESE SERVICES FURNISHED UNDER THIS PLAN OF TREATMENT AND WHILE UNDER MY CARE ☐ N/A

17. CERTIFICATION

15. PHYSICIAN SIGNATURE | 16. DATE

FROM   THROUGH   N/A

18. ON FILE *(Print/type physician's name)*
☐

20. INITIAL ASSESSMENT *(History, medical complications, level of function at start of care. Reason for referral.)*

19. PRIOR HOSPITALIZATION

FROM   TO   N/A

21. FUNCTIONAL LEVEL *(End of billing period)* PROGRESS REPORT   ☐ CONTINUE SERVICES **OR**   ☐ DC SERVICES

22. SERVICE DATES
FROM   THROUGH

Form CMS-700-(11-91)

Figure 5—10   Medicare Plan of Treatment for Outpatient Rehabilitation, Form CMS-700.

DEPARTMENT OF HEALTH AND HUMAN SERVICES
CENTERS FOR MEDICARE & MEDICAID SERVICES

UPDATED PLAN OF PROGRESS FOR OUTPATIENT REHABILITATION
(Complete for Interim to Discharge Claims. Photocopy of CMS-700 or 701 is required.)

1. PATIENT'S LAST NAME	FIRST NAME	M.I.	2. PROVIDER NO.	3. HICN

4. PROVIDER NAME	5. MEDICAL RECORD NO. *(Optional)*	6. ONSET DATE	7. SOC. DATE

8. TYPE
☐ PT ☐ OT ☐ SLP ☐ CR

☐ RT ☐ PS ☐ SN ☐ SW

9. PRIMARY DIAGNOSIS *(Pertinent Medical D.X.)*   10. TREATMENT DIAGNOSIS   11. VISITS FROM SOC.

12. FREQ/DURATION *(e.g., 3/Wk. x 4 Wk.)*

13. CURRENT PLAN UPDATE, FUNCTIONAL GOALS *(Specify changes to goals and plan.)*

GOALS *(Short Term)*   PLAN

OUTCOME *(Long Term)*

I HAVE REVIEWED THIS PLAN OF TREATMENT AND RECERTIFY A CONTINUING NEED FOR SERVICES.   ☐ N/A   ☐ DC

14. RECERTIFICATION
FROM   THROUGH   N/A

15. PHYSICIAN'S SIGNATURE

16. DATE

17. ON FILE *(Print/type physician's name)*
☐

18. REASON(S) FOR CONTINUING TREATMENT THIS BILLING PERIOD *(Clarify goals and necessity for continued skilled care.)*

19. SIGNATURE *(or name of professional, including prof. designation)*

20. DATE

21.
☐ CONTINUE SERVICES **OR**   ☐ DC SERVICES

22. FUNCTIONAL LEVEL *(At end of billing period — Relate your documentation to functional outcomes and list problems still present.)*

22. SERVICE DATES
FROM   THROUGH

Form CMS-701(11-91)

Figure 5—11 Medicare Updated Plan of Progress for Outpatient Rehabilitation, Form CMS-701.

SUMMARY   This chapter has provided an overview of the multiple methods that can be used to document the patient's evaluation, POC, and discharge process in different types of clinical settings. In addition, the reader was introduced to several different types of forms that can be used to document treatment sessions for patients under their care. It is important to note that PTs and PTAs must be able to distinguish between a medical diagnosis and a physical therapy diagnosis to determine how the treatment plan will best meet the needs of the patient. It is also important to note that the sequencing of information related to the patient and his or her POC is organized and easy for all interested stakeholders to access for continued care, reimbursement, and quality assurance. For such purposes, the information documented in the medical record should consist of the following:

1. The problem(s) requiring medical treatment
2. Data relevant to the patient's medical and physical therapy diagnoses
3. Treatment plan or action(s) to address the problem(s)
4. Goals or outcomes of the treatment plan
5. Record of administration of the treatment plan
6. Treatment effectiveness or results of the treatment plan

The documentation content describes the medical care from the moment the patient is first seen by a medical professional. The information on the effectiveness of the treatment is used to determine the quality of the care provided, measure outcomes, research the most effective treatment procedures, and determine reimbursement.

When documenting patient data, it is important for the PTA to understand the difference between the medical diagnosis and the physical therapy diagnosis. The physical therapy diagnosis is the identification of the abnormalities and dysfunctions (impairments) causing a functional limitation. The functional limitation is the primary reason the patient seeks physical therapy, and improvement of this limitation is the goal of physical therapy treatment.

Information about treatment procedures (e.g., their purposes, expected results, and any possible risks or side effects) must be explained to the patient or a representative of the patient. The patient or his or her representative must agree to the treatment plan before it is started. This agreement, called informed consent, is often made official by the patient's signing an informed consent form, which is placed in the medical record.

In addition to following a POC set forth by a supervising PT, the PTA must be cognizant of standardized forms that can be used to determine the POC for the patient. Such forms include those used in the school setting to address the annual goals for a student receiving therapy services in the IEP and forms developed and required by Medicare in specific clinical settings (e.g., Forms CMS-700 and CMS-701). Through a thorough review of this type of information, the PTA will have a better understanding of the documentation requirements in the facilities in which they may be employed.

REFERENCES

1. American Physical Therapy Association. (2003). *Guide to physical therapist practice* (2nd ed.). Alexandria, VA: Author.
2. Sahrmann, S. A. (1988). Diagnosis by physical therapist—a prerequisite for treatment. A special communication. *Physical Therapy, 68*, 1703–1786.
3. Scott, R. W. (1994). *Legal aspects of documenting patient care.* Gaithersburg, MD: Aspen.
4. Swanson, G. (1995, December). *Essentials for the future of physical therapy, every therapist's concern. A continuing education course.* Duluth: American Physical Therapy Association, Minnesota Chapter.
5. El-Din, D., & Smith, G. J. (1995, February). *Performance-based documentation: A tool for functional documentation.* Reno, NV: American Physical Therapy Association.
6. HealthIt.gov. (2016). What is an electronic health record? Retrieved from https://www.healthit.gov/providers-professionals/faqs/what-electronic-health-record-ehr
7. WebPT. (n.d.). Retrieved from http://www.webpt.com
8. ReDoc. (n.d.). Retrieved from http://www.rehabdocumentation.com
9. Therapy charts. (n.d.). Retrieved from http://www.therapycharts.com
10. Clinicient. (n.d.). Retrieved from http://www.clinicient.com
11. HealthWyse. (n.d.). Retrieved from http://www.healthwyse.com
12. American Physical Therapy Association. (2016, May 8). Electronic health records: Guide to understanding and adopting electronic health records. Retrieved from http://www.apta.org/EHR/Guide/Decision/
13. Martin, K. D. (1990). Individualized educational program and individualized family service plan. In American Physical Therapy Association, *Physical therapy practice in educational environments: Policies and guidelines* (p. 61). Alexandria, VA: Author.
14. Centers for Medicare & Medicaid Services. (n.d.). Hospital center. Retrieved from http://www.cms.hhs.gov/center/hospital.asp

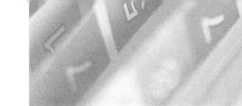

Review Exercises

1. List the **six categories** of documentation content and describe the content of each category.

2. Compare and contrast the **medical** diagnosis and the **physical therapy** diagnosis.

3. What is **impairment?** Give **three** examples.

4. **Define** a functional limitation.

5. **Explain** the **difference** between a source-oriented and a problem-oriented medical record.

6. Provide the **definition** for the following acronyms: SOAP, PSPG, and DEP.

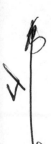

7. List **three** formats in which documentation content may be presented and identify the **types** of physical therapy facilities most likely to use each format.

8. What is an **IEP** and in **which** clinical setting is it used?

PRACTICE EXERCISES

Practice Exercise 1 ➤   *You read in the PT's initial evaluation that your patient has a fractured right femur that has healed. He is left with 2/5 strength (normal strength is 5/5) in the quadriceps and is unable to transfer independently in and out of bed or a chair.*

What is the medical diagnosis (pathology)? _____

What is the impairment of the musculoskeletal system? _____

What is the functional limitation? _____

Practice Exercise 2 ➤   *You read in the PT's evaluation that your patient has had a cerebral vascular accident (i.e., stroke) and now has difficulty moving his left arm and leg. The PT states that the patient has weakness and extensor hypertonicity in his left lower extremity with inability to ambulate stairs independently.*

What is the medical diagnosis (pathology)? _____

What is the impairment of the neuromuscular system? _____

What is the functional limitation? _____

Practice Exercise 3 ➤   *You read in the PT's evaluation that your patient has an incomplete spinal cord injury causing lower extremity paraparesis and an inability to stand.*

What is the medical diagnosis (pathology)? _____

What is the impairment? _____

What is the functional limitation? _____

Practice Exercise 4 ➤   *Identify the medical diagnosis (pathology), impairment, functional limitation, and disability after each patient description.*

1. Mr. Cruz, a professional football player, will never be able to play football again because he fractured a vertebra and severed his spinal cord. His legs are paralyzed and he cannot stand or walk.

   Medical diagnosis (pathology) _____

   Impairment _____

   Functional limitation _____

   Disability _____

2. Sable received third-degree burns on both hands, and the scar tissue causes limited ROM in her fingers and wrists. She is unable to pick up or manipulate small objects, so she is unable to return to any work that requires fine hand manipulation.

Medical diagnosis (pathology) _____

Impairment _____

Functional limitation _____

Disability _____

3. Mrs. Cohen has rheumatoid arthritis with limited ROM in both knees and hips. She is unable to climb stairs or steps, so she must live and function in an environment that has no stairs or steps.

Medical diagnosis (pathology) _____

Impairment _____

Functional limitation _____

Disability _____

4. Mr. Liu's left leg was crushed in a motor vehicle accident. His leg was amputated just above his knee. He does not have the muscle strength to walk with his prosthesis (artificial leg) without the help of a cane. He will not be able to return to his job as a railroad brakeman.

Medical diagnosis (pathology) _____

Impairment _____

Functional limitation _____

Disability _____

5. Jarett received a head injury in a snowmobile accident. He now has difficulty maintaining his balance when walking and frequently feels dizzy. He walks with a wheeled walker and always needs someone nearby, in case he feels dizzy while walking.

Medical diagnosis (pathology) _____

Impairment _____

Functional limitation _____

Disability _____

6. A little girl in the third grade has spina bifida, which has caused her legs to be very weak. She can walk independently with crutches, but she cannot maintain her balance when she tries to open doors.

Medical diagnosis (pathology) _____

Impairment _____

Functional limitation _____

Disability _____

Practice Exercise 5 ➤

You are a PTA working on the orthopedic floor at the local hospital. You are treating Earl, a 62-year-old farmer, who has just had surgery for a ® total knee arthroplasty. The PT saw him on day one (12-5-16, 0930), post-operation. The discharge goals are (1) independent ambulation on tile, carpet, ascending and descending stairs, and walking up inclines using the least restrictive and most appropriate assistive device; and (2) independent transfers. Active knee ROM should be 90° at discharge. Treatments to include CPM, 1 hr on/1 hr off until 90° is reached; isometric exercises for quads, glutes, and hamstrings; ankle pumps; TKE; SLR; and active knee flexion. Gait training is to start on day one in the a.m. on tile surface using standard walker and mod A. A cold/ice pack may be used on the knee as needed to reduce swelling. BP 135/85 mm Hg, pulse at 85 BPM in sit.

Document all of the treatment sessions on the flow sheet that follows.

Day 2 (12-6-16, 0915): *All isometric exercises independent with good coordination. CPM increased to 50°. Active knee motion while supine –10° of extension to 40° flexion. BP 140/85 mm Hg, pulse 90 BPM. Bed mobility transfers (supine to sit) mod. assist of one to support knee. Unable to do SLR independently, needing min A. In sitting, still requires support to ® knee as pain (10/10) too severe for initiation of ROM exercises. Ice pack to knee almost continuous. Drain in place for a.m. session; removed by p.m. session. Able to stand at side of bed, WBAT ® LE using standard walker. Did not attempt ambulation because of pain (10/10).*

Day 3 (12-7-16, 1030): *All bed mobility activities are Ⓘ and all transfers are min A. Able to sit at side of bed, Ⓘ, with AROM to 65° flex in am and 70° flex in p.m., with pain 8/10. Active knee motion while supine –5° of extension to 60° flexion. AROM knee flexion to 65° with TKE to 0°. BP 140/85 mm Hg, pulse at 72 BPM before standing. Stood at side of bed with mod. assist of one, WBAT to approx. 50% of body weight on ® LE, using standard walker. Took four steps to chair, then sat, with SBA. Uses standing pivot transfer with standard walker. BP 145/88 mm Hg, pulse 100 BPM. Independent with all exercises. CPM increased to 65° flex in a.m. and 70° in p.m. Able to ambulate 50 ft 1X with FWW walker, WBAT at 50% body weight. Continues to keep ice pack on knee for swelling and pain control.*

Day 4 (12-8-16, 1030): *Ambulated 50 ft 2X with FWW walker on level surface, tile, and carpet with min A. Used stairs, marking time, with Ⓑ hand rails, 6 steps up and 6 steps down x2. BP 140/80 mm HG, pulse 82. Sitting AROM 75° with pain 6/10, CPM increased to 80° with pain 6/10. Supine AROM 0°–75° flexion. Ⓘ with SLR. p.m.: Ambulated 50 ft 2X with walker, SBA. Ambulated 60 ft 1X with crutches on level, min. assist of one. Remains PWB with up to 75% body weight. AROM sitting to 75°, supine 0°–70°. SBA for supine to sit transfer, independent transfer sit to stand. Independent with SLR. Ice pack discontinued this am.*

Day 5 (12-9-16, 0900): *Independent with all exercises and all standing pivot transfers. CPM discontinued last night by nursing. BP 140/85 mm Hg, pulse 85, pain was 5/10. Ambulates independently 125 ft with crutches, 3-point step through gait on tile and carpeting. Ⓘ on stairs and inclines. Knee AROM sitting from 0° ext. 90° flex., supine 0°–85°. PT to see patient in p.m. for re-evaluation and discharge planning on 12-10-16.*

TOTAL KNEE ARTHROPLASTY

	Date		Date		Date		Date		Date	
	am	pm	am	pm	am	pm	am	pm	am	pm
CPM Degrees										
CPM Time										
Pain Levels at Treatment										
Knee ROM AA = Active Assist A = Active Supine										
Sitting										
Exercises: Isometrics Quads/Gluts/HS										
Ankle Pumps										
TKE										
SLR										
Active Knee Flex										
Transfers: Bed Mobility										
Toilet/Commode										
Shower Seat										
Car Transfer										
Standing Pivot										
Sliding Board										
Supine <- -> Sit										
Sit <- -> Stand										
Balance: Sitting										
Standing										
Ambulation: Device										
Weight Bearing										
Pattern										
Distance										
Surface										
Assist										
Stairs										
Blood Pressure										
Pulse										
Modalities										
THERAPIST										

PHYSICAL THERAPY PROGRESS

PRECAUTIONS:

NAME:

Practice Exercise 6 ➤   *Write "MD" by the medical diagnoses, "IMP" by the impairments, and "FL" by the functional limitations.*

_____   1. Diabetes

_____   2. Rhomboid strength 3/5

_____   3. Instability

_____   4. Unable to reach top of head

_____   5. Multiple sclerosis

_____   6. Fractured neck of the femur

_____   7. Inability to walk one block

_____   8. Cannot sleep more than 3 hours

_____   9. Frequent falling with ambulation

_____   10. T10 paraplegia

_____   11. Severed ulnar nerve

_____   12. 10°–90° knee flexion

_____   13. Cerebral palsy

_____   14. Hypermobility

_____   15. Unable to sit unsupported

_____   16. Circumducted gait pattern

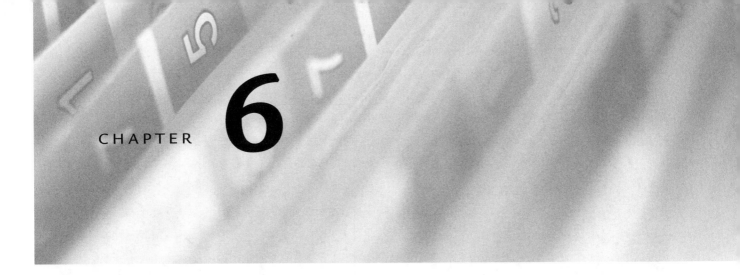

CHAPTER 6

Physical Therapy Patient Management and Documentation Responsibilities

LEARNING OBJECTIVES
INTRODUCTION
FIVE ELEMENTS OF PHYSICAL THERAPY
   PATIENT MANAGEMENT
TYPES AND CONTENT OF EXAMINATIONS
   AND EVALUATIONS

DOCUMENTATION SPECIFICS
SUMMARY
REFERENCES
REVIEW EXERCISES
PRACTICE EXERCISES

LEARNING OBJECTIVES

After studying this chapter, the student will be able to:

☐ Identify the five elements of physical therapy patient management
☐ Distinguish between the examination and the evaluation
☐ Explain the elements of the documentation process
☐ Understand the necessity for reexamination and re-evaluation
☐ Explain the difference between examination, evaluation, and discharge
☐ Identify the basic information included in the summation of care
☐ Compare and contrast documentation responsibilities between the PT and the PTA
☐ Use "person-first" terminology

INTRODUCTION

Chapter 5 reviewed the different types of documentation models, discussed terms used to delineate how patient treatment can be documented, and provided some examples of documentation formats. This, however, is only the beginning of the documentation process. It is also important for the PTA to understand the examination and evaluation process that occurs between the patient and the PT. In addition, the relationship between the supervising PT and the PTA is very important, and appropriate documentation and communication for continued skilled patient care is imperative. Consequently, having an understanding of the examination and evaluation process, completed by the supervising PT, is very helpful in understanding a patient's overall plan of care (POC) that the PTA will follow when treating patients.

FIVE ELEMENTS OF PHYSICAL THERAPY PATIENT MANAGEMENT

According to APTA's *Guide to Physical Therapist Practice,* "The physical therapist integrates five elements of patient/client management—examination, evaluation, diagnosis, prognosis, and intervention—in a manner designed to maximize outcomes."[1] While the PT is responsible for the main management duties that are the foundation for generating the POC, there are implications for the PTA that must also be considered (Fig. 6–1).

PTA Prognosis Implications

The final determination for the level of improvement attained through PT intervention remains the responsibility of the supervising PT. The PTA is responsible for communicating any changes in the patient's ability to complete the plan of care, as ordered or if it needs to be changed by the supervising PT. The PTA may make changes in timing and frequency if they remain within the plan of care provided by their supervising PT.

Prognosis (Including Plan of Care)

Determination of the level of optimal improvement that may be attained through intervention and the amount of time required to reach that level. The plan of care specifies the interventions to be used and their timing and frequency.

Intervention

Purposeful and skilled interaction of the physical therapist with the patient/client and, if appropriate, with other individuals involved with the care of the patient/client, using various physical therapy procedures and techniques to produce changes in the condition that are consistent with the diagnosis and prognosis. The physical therapist conducts a reexamination to determine changes in patient/client status and to modify or redirect intervention. The decision to reexamine may be based on new clinical findings or on lack of patient/client progress. The process of reexamination also may identify the need for consultation with or referral to another provider.

PTA Intervention Implications

This is the purposeful and skilled interaction of the PTA with the patient/client and, if appropriate, with other individuals involved in the care of the patient/client, using various physical therapy procedures and techniques to produce changes in the condition that are consistent with the diagnosis and prognosis. The PTA will re-assess the patient/client's status to determine if the current plan of care meets the needs of the patient or if the PT needs to re-evaluate the patient/client and develop a new plan of care.

PTA Diagnosis Implications

This section is determined by the referring physician and the evaluating physical therapist. This is beyond the scope of practice for the PTA. However, if the diagnosis the patient is being treated for changes in any manner, it is the responsibility of the PTA to communicate this to the supervising PT to have the PT determine if a change in the plan of care is necessary.

Diagnosis

Both the process and the end result of evaluating examination data, which the physical therapist organizes into defined clusters, syndromes, or categories to help determine the prognosis (including the plan of care) and the most appropriate intervention strategies.

Outcomes

Results of patient/client management, which include the impact of physical therapy interventions in the following domains: pathology/ pathophysiology (disease, disorder, or condition); impairments, functional limitations, and disabilities; risk reduction/prevention; health, wellness, and fitness; societal resources; and patient/client satisfaction.

PTA Outcomes Implications

These would include the results of patient/client management, which include the impact of physical therapy interventions in the following domains: pathology/ pathophysiology (disease, disorder, or condition); impairments, functional limitations, and disabilities; risk reduction; prevention; health, wellness, and fitness; societal resources; and patient/client satisfaction. The ultimate short- and long-term goals to achieve these outcomes remain the responsibility of the supervising PT.

PTA Evaluation Implications

This is not a skill that lies within the scope of practice of a PTA and must be performed by the supervising PT. The PTA may be present for the evaluation.

Evaluation

A dynamic process in which the physical therapist makes clinical judgments based on data gathered during the examination. This process also may identify possible problems that require consultation with or referral to another provider.

Examination

The process of obtaining a history, performing a systems review, and selecting and administering tests and meaures to gather data about the patient/client. The initial examination is a comprehensive screening and specific testing process that leads to a diagnostic classification. The examination process also may identify possible problems that require consultation with or referral to another provider.

PTA Examination Implications

The initial process of obtaining the history, performing a systems review, and selecting and administering tests and measures to gather data about the patient/client is the responsibility of the supervising PT. Once this information has been gathered and documented, the PTA may then perform tests and measurements within their scope of practice to determine if the patient is meeting the PT's goals outlined within the plan of care.

Figure 6—1 Treatment responsibilities of the PT versus the PTA. (Adapted from American Physical Therapy Association. [2014]. *Guide to physical therapist practice* [3rd ed.], with permission.)

The *examination* is the process for gathering subjective and objective data about the patient and includes three areas:

- Patient/client history
- Systems review
- Test and measurements[2]

The *evaluation* is the clinical judgment the therapist makes based on the examination. The evaluation results in the determination of the diagnosis, prognosis, and interventions. The *diagnosis* is both the process and the end result of evaluating the examination data. The *prognosis* is a judgment about the optimal level of improvement the patient may attain and the amount of time needed to reach that level. *Interventions* are the skilled techniques and activities that make up the treatment plan.[2]

TYPES AND CONTENT OF EXAMINATIONS AND EVALUATIONS

The PT should always perform an initial examination and evaluation and a discharge examination and evaluation of the patient and may perform one or more interim evaluations, depending on the length of time the patient is receiving physical therapy care and the requirements of the third-party payer. The PT follows APTA's "Defensible Documentation" elements[3] outlining the recommended documentation format for reporting the examination and evaluation process. These guidelines are included in Appendix B and are a valuable resource for the treating PT and PTA.

The categories for content of the medical record that should be addressed in the PT documentation include (see Appendix B for details)[3]:

- Initial examination and evaluation
- History
- Systems review
- Tests and measures
- Evaluation
- Diagnosis
- Prognosis
- Plan of care
- Reexamination and re-evaluation
- Visit/encounter notes
- Discharge summary

After the supervising PT completes the evaluation and develops the POC, but prior to greeting the patient for the first treatment, the PTA should review this information. When reviewing this important information, the PTA should be cognizant of the diagnosis for which the patient is being treated and the PT's recommendation for meeting the functional deficits that the diagnosis has generated and that prevent the patient from fully functioning in his or her environment. It is also important for the PTA to communicate any inconsistencies or questions he or she might have related to the POC to the supervising PT in advance of the first meeting with the patient. This communication link is imperative in providing appropriate, skilled patient care while working toward the discharge process.

The specific clinical setting in which the PT and PTA provide patient care often determines the type of documentation that must be gathered. APTA's *Guide to Physical Therapist* Practice[1] provides templates for documentation review of medical records to check for appropriate documentation specifics.

DOCUMENTATION SPECIFICS

In addition to the basic sections of a SOAP note, other identifying information should be included in the medical record of a patient receiving physical therapy services (see Appendix B). This includes the information gathered in the PT's evaluation, which is completed in the first session with the patient. The evaluation includes the patient's POC. Using the updated ICD-10, the supervising PT must also appropriately identify the complete diagnosis and delineate the impact on the patient's ability to function. Following this designation, the PTA begins and continues to follow the initial POC, assesses the patient's progress, and reports to the PT. Through this reporting process, the PTA should communicate the need for a change in the POC because the patient goals have or have not been met, the need to progress the patient, or the need to develop a discharge plan. The PTA is not responsible for determining when to discharge the patient but is responsible for communicating the patient's progression toward being ready for discharge. Again, without the communication link between the PT and the PTA, there is little evidence that the patient received skilled therapy intervention or progressed within the prescribed POC.

Initial Examination and Evaluation

The initial examination and evaluation are performed the first time the PT meets with the patient. This written report contains the following information:

1. History, observations, and identification of risk factors: General statistics about the patient are obtained before the evaluation is performed. Some of this information may be found elsewhere in the chart, such as in the notes from admissions, the emergency room, or the physician. Examples include name, age, sex, medical diagnosis, date of birth, physician, complications, and precautions. All these data are required in the medical record, but they may not all need to be in the PT's evaluation if they are already located elsewhere in the chart.

2. Component identification: Components of an evaluation should include information about the following:
   a. Strength (Evaluate the patient's muscle strength on a scale from 0 to 5, with 5 representing expected normal functional strength, comparing both sides, when appropriate)
   b. Active and passive range of motion (ROM) (What is the normal range for the joint being tested? Is it functional or within normal range? Does it impair function? Are there any restrictions due to soft tissue deficits or pain? How does the ROM of the joint being tested compare with that of the joint on the other side of the body (when applicable)?
   c. Functional abilities (What activities can the patient perform appropriately, and what can he or she no longer do because of the diagnosis or disease? It is also important to ask the patient what activities he or she would like to be able to do that the disease or diagnosis has limited or prevented and whether he or she is independent in any activities of daily living [ADLs]).
   d. Pain level (The patient's pain level should always be addressed during treatment to determine whether the intervention decreases or increases pain. The patient should use a visual analog scale—0 to 10, with 10 being the worst pain the patient has ever felt—to determine what his or her pain level is and report that to the treating therapist both prior to and following the treatment session. In addition, it is essential to ask the patient to report where the pain is located.)
   e. Presence of abnormal muscle tone (Is the tone decreased or increased, and does it affect the patient's level of function? Where is it located? Which side? What increases or decreases the tone?)
   f. Ability to communicate and understand simple commands (What are the patient's receptive and expressive language skills? Can the patient use other methods of communication, such as writing, when he or she cannot speak?)
   g. Need for adaptive equipment (What equipment is necessary to increase appropriate and safe function and mobility for the patient? Has the patient been measured properly to use the assistive device? Has the patient been trained to use the device correctly?)
   h. Presence of automatic reactions (Does the patient demonstrate the ability to catch him- or herself following loss of balance? In which direction can the patient catch him- or herself? Does the patient know he or she is losing balance? Can he or she accept challenges to static versus dynamic balance? Are any of the reactions delayed but present?)
   i. Presence of any abnormal reflex patterns (Are there any abnormal reflex patterns present that interfere with the patient's ability to function, e.g., asymmetrical

tonic neck reflex [ATNR], plantar grasp reflex, Babinski reflex? Are they primitive, pathological, or obligatory? Are they symmetrical or asymmetrical?)

j. Level of independence in daily care (At what level can the patient function in his or her day-to-day life, and does he or she need assistance during any ADLs? How much assistance does the patient need, and when does he or she need it?)

k. Alignment (What is the patient's alignment like? Can the patient sit erect, or does he or she lean to one side, forward, or backward? To which side does the patient lean? Does the patient realize he or she is not upright, and can the patient move into upright and midline orientations upon request?)

l. Quality of movement (Can the patient move in a smooth, coordinated manner as he or she transitions in and out of different positions and on and off of different types of furniture in a sit-to-stand motion?)

m. Cognitive abilities (Is the patient oriented to person, place, or thing? Can he or she understand simple and/or complex commands? Does the patient have good body schematics? Can he or she understand basic activities, such as sit-to-stand, etc.?)

Providing this type of information in a PT evaluation gives both the patient and the treating PTA a better idea of just where the deficits lie for this patient and what interventions should be included in the POC to increase or restore the patient's functional level. The treating PT and PTA should be aware of the activities that re necessary to help restore the patient to the highest functional level possible within the treatment protocol outlined by the third-party payer.

3. Subjective data: Information obtained directly from the patient during the interview with the PT or PTA. Examples include the onset of injury/disease/pain, chief complaint, location of complaints, functional limitations, home situation, lifestyle, goals, and pertinent medical history.

4. Objective data: Results of objective testing and the PT's or PTA's observation of the patient. Examples include physical status, such as strength, endurance, skin condition, active range of motion (AROM), or passive range of motion (PROM); neurological status; functional status, such as mobility, transfers, ambulation, activities of daily living, and abilities at work, school, and home; mental status, such as cognition, orientation, communication problems, judgment, and ability to follow directions; status of appropriate reflex responses, such as presence of primitive reflexes and automatic reactions; status of muscles and alignment, including muscle tone and symmetrical alignment; and functional abilities, such as the level of function and any need for assistive devices.

5. Evaluation: The PT's interpretation of the results of the testing and observation.

6. Diagnosis: The physical therapy diagnosis identifying the impairments and functional limitations. The medical diagnosis is provided by the referring physician and should be clarified by the treating PT to ensure the codes are correct. Then the PT will determine the correct treatment codes for the skilled PT services, which may be different from the medical diagnoses codes.

7. Goals: Anticipated goals and expected outcomes related to resolving the diagnosis, written in measurable and functional terms and working toward discharge.

8. Treatment plan or recommendation: Treatment plans related to accomplishing the goals, including specific interventions, their frequency and duration, a statement regarding the prognosis (the patient's rehabilitation potential or expectations of treatment effectiveness), an estimate of the length of time the patient will be receiving physical therapy treatment, and a schedule or plan for evaluating the effectiveness of the treatment. Again, the treating therapist must be aware of the requirements of the third-party payer to meet the goals outlined in the POC and to increase the functional capabilities of that patient.

9. Physical therapist designation: Authentication and appropriate designation of the physical therapist, including signature, title, and professional license number (or those requirements outlined in the state practice act).

Reexamination and Re-evaluation

The continuum of skilled physical therapy care that the patient is receiving is conveyed by the PT in the reexamination and re-evaluation reports and then by the PTA or PT in the daily notes. The content of the PT's reexamination and re-evaluation reports is discussed later in this chapter, and the content of the daily notes is discussed in the remaining chapters.

Interim or progress examinations and evaluations are performed by the PT periodically while the patient is receiving physical therapy, especially when it is required by the third-party payer for reimbursement. The content of the progress examination and evaluation includes the following information:

1. Intervention or service provided: Treatment procedures administered, including a summary of the interventions and other services provided by the PT or PTA since the initial evaluation.
2. Patient status, progress, or regression: Subjective data—patient's subjective information about the effectiveness of the interventions. Objective data—a repeat of the testing and observations made in the initial evaluation.
3. Reexamination and re-evaluation: Results or effectiveness of the treatment plan, including the following:
   a. Interpretation of objective test results and observations and a comparison with data from the initial evaluation
   b. Statement addressing the accomplishment of the goals set in the initial evaluation and any new goals set (for patients under Medicare Part B, the appropriate "G" codes must be addressed here; see Chapter 3)
   c. Information regarding any change in the patient's status
   d. Treatment plan written by the PT indicating whether the initial plan is to be continued or changed
   e. Signature, title, and license number of the physical therapist

Summation of Care

This discharge examination and evaluation is the patient's final evaluation and the final note about the patient in the medical record. This note must be written by the supervising PT. A properly written discharge note follows APTA's guidelines and should include the following information:

1. Brief summary of the treatment that was provided (intervention procedures administered)
2. Relevant information provided by the patient (subjective data)
3. Interpretation of repeated testing and observations and a comparison with data from the latest interim evaluation and the initial evaluation (objective data and results or effectiveness of interventions)
4. Statement regarding the accomplishment of anticipated goals and expected outcomes (results or effectiveness of the treatment plan)
5. Further interventions or care needed following discharge
6. Plans for follow-up or monitoring following discharge
7. Signature, title, and professional license number of the PT[2]

Discharge Notes

Physical therapy professionals disagree about the definitions of *discharge evaluation* and *discharge summary.* Some believe the evaluation and the summary are the same, whereas others consider them different types of documents.

If a discharge summary is considered the same as a discharge evaluation, then the evaluation/summary will have content that interprets the test results and identifies the plans for the patient following discharge. Decisions about the patient's care following discharge may be made based on the information in the discharge evaluation/summary. In this case, only a PT can write a discharge summary.

When a patient's treatment has been discontinued, the PTA may write the discharge summary or note. This note only *summarizes* the care given to the patient and the patient's response to the interventions, and it objectively states the functional status of the patient at the time of discharge. There can be *no interpretation of the data or evaluation of the patient's status,* the

PTA can make no plan for the patient's care following discharge if identified, and no decisions can be made by the PTA based on changes in the POC. If the PTA writes a discharge summary of this nature, there still must be a discharge evaluation written by the PT as the final note in the patient's medical record. In any situation, the *final documentation in the patient's physical therapy chart must be written by the PT.*[2]

PTA Involvement

Although the PTA does not perform evaluations, he or she may assist the PT with the evaluation procedure. The PTA may take notes and help gather the subjective data. The PTA also may take measurements, perform some tests, and record the results. However, the PTA may not interpret the results. Performing the tests and recording the results constitute *data collection.* Interpreting the results involves making a judgment about their value. This is called *evaluating.* Examples of tests and measurements that are part of a PTA's data collection skills include girth measurements, manual testing of muscle groups, goniometry measurements to assess ROM, and assessment of vital signs. While it is not the intent of this textbook to completely review the responsibilities of the PT versus those of the PTA in all areas of practice, readers should review the supervision algorithm provided by the American Physical Therapy Association that delineates the responsibilities of the PT versus the PTA (see Fig. 6–2).

During the course of a patient's treatment, the PTA is often expected to repeat the measurements and tests to record the patient's progress since the initial examination and evaluation. These objective data are more reliable when the same person performs the tests and measurements in a consistent manner throughout the course of the patient's treatment. In addition, assisting the PT with the evaluation offers the PTA and patient an opportunity to become acquainted so the patient will feel comfortable working with the PTA as the treatment plan is carried out.

When writing daily notes, the PTA refers to the problems, goals and outcomes, and treatment plans outlined in the initial and interim evaluation reports. Daily notes should record the effectiveness of the treatment plan by comparing the patient's progress toward accomplishing the goals and outcomes with the status of the patient at the initial evaluation. It is important to note that the PTA must perform such assessment within the PT's POC.

Documentation Responsibilities

The documentation content is found in the examination and evaluation reports and in the daily notes. The PT is responsible for the evaluations, consultations, and decision-making required for the patient's physical therapy health care. Therefore, the PT's documentation responsibilities are to record the following information:

1. Initial evaluation, which includes the goals and outcomes and the treatment plan
2. Interim or progress evaluations performed
3. Changes in the treatment plan
4. Discharge information[2]

The PT may also write daily notes, but the primary documentation responsibility of the PTA is to record the daily or interim notes.

The PTA must be familiar with the content of the PT's examination and evaluation reports. The reports inform the PTA of the patient's medical and physical therapy diagnoses. The PTA follows the treatment plan outlined in the evaluations and directs all treatment sessions toward accomplishing the goals and outcomes listed in the evaluations.

Person-First Language

Documentation should follow standards set forth by APTA's *Guide to Physical Therapist Practice* and other expected methods to protect the patient and use language appropriate for the care given. Any documentation should address information related to a patient in "person-first" language. The meaning of this statement relates to the person and the disabling characteristic for which the individual is receiving medical treatment. The disability should not define the person; instead, emphasis should be placed on the person's identity, not on his or her physical limitations. This is also emphasized in the ICF framework to address the patient's functional deficits and not the diagnosis or disease to determine how best to treat the patient.

PTA Supervision Algorithm
(See Controlling Assumptions)

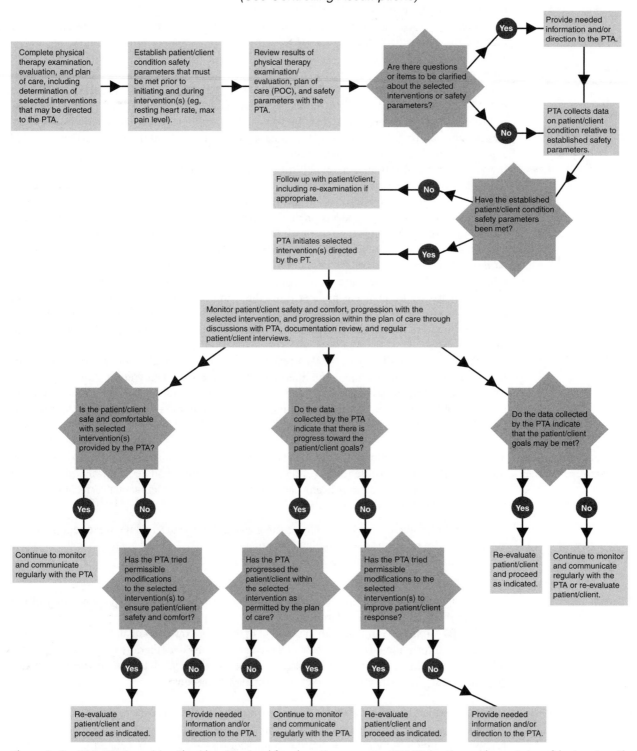

Figure 6—2 APTA PTA Supervision Algorithm. (Reprinted from http://www.apta.org/PTA/PatientCare, with permission of the American Physical Therapy Association. This material is copyrighted, and any further reproduction or distribution requires written permission from APTA. APTA is not responsible for the accuracy of the translation from English.)

Examples of terminology that should *not* be used when documenting patient care include:

- The paralyzed patient
- The hemiplegic patient
- CVAs
- Amputees
- The MS patient
- The TBI student

Instead, use person-first words or expressions similar to those in the following list:

- The male patient with a T12 spinal cord injury
- The person who is disabled
- The woman who has had an Ⓛ CVA
- Mr. Jiminez, who is paralyzed
- Mrs. Sanchez, a 62-year-old woman with spina bifida[1]

Through the proper use of person-first language in documentation, the patient remains a viable member of the team and is not delegated to an inferior position in which he or she is identified solely by a disease or disability.

SUMMARY

The documentation content about a patient's treatment is found in the written evaluation reports and in the daily notes. The PT performs and writes initial, interim, and discharge examination/evaluation reports. The PTA can assist the PT in an evaluation but cannot perform one. The PTA documents the daily notes, which is the focus of this book.

In addition, it is important for the treating therapist to document how progress is accomplished to meet the needs of the patient in restoring function, for proper reimbursement, and in meeting the requirements of the third-party payer. Documentation is the mainstay of the therapist's ability to determine how he or she is best meeting the needs of the patient to restore the patient to the highest functional level possible, to provide appropriate feedback and communication to the health-care team involved in the patient's care, and to provide the necessary communication link between the supervising PT and the PTA. In addition, documentation should use person-first language to focus on the patient and still define the functional limitations brought on by the disease or disorder. By following the proper documentation techniques outlined in APTA's *Guide to Physical Therapist Practice* and the requirements outlined by different third-party payers, the treating therapist can be assured of appropriate reimbursement for his or her skilled services.

REFERENCES

1. American Physical Therapy Association. (2014). *Guide to physical therapist practice* (3rd ed., Chapter 1). Alexandria, VA: Author. Retrieved from http://guidetoptpractice.apta.org
2. American Physical Therapy Association. (2014). Underlying concepts. In *Guide to physical therapist practice* (3rd ed., Chapter 1). Alexandria, VA: Author. Retrieved from http://guidetoptpractice.apta.org/content/current
3. American Physical Therapy Association. (2014). Defensible documentation for patient/client management. In *Guide to physical therapist practice* (3rd ed., Chapter 1). Alexandria, VA: Author. Retrieved from http://www.apta.org/Documentation/DefensibleDocumentation

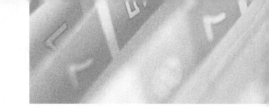

Review Exercises

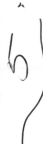

1. According to APTA's *Guide to Physical Therapist Practice,* what **five** elements are included in physical therapy patient management?

2. The medical record should include multiple categories, 11 in all. List **five** of the categories.

3. What is the PTA's **responsibility** regarding the discharge summary?

4. The discharge note should include certain information. List **three** items that should be included in the note.

5. **What** is person-first language?

PRACTICE EXERCISES

Practice Exercise 1 ➤ *Identify the documentation responsibilities of the PT and the PTA. Write "PT" next to the items that are the responsibility of the PT only. Write "PTA" next to items that are documentation tasks for the PTA. Write "PT/PTA" next to items that can be done by either the PT or the PTA, or by both.*

_____ Initial examination and evaluation

_____ Discharge examination and evaluation

_____ Daily notes

_____ Change in treatment plan

_____ Reexamination and re-evaluation

_____ Objective notes

Practice Exercise 2 ➤ *Through the proper use of person-first language in documentation, the patient is not identified solely by his or her disease or disability. In the list below, place a "P" next to statements that use person-first language.*

_____ Mr. Pena's amputated arm needs a dressing change.

_____ The CVA patient in room 201 with a right hemiparesis needs exercises.

_____ Mrs. Sanchez, who has a left transtibial amputation, needs to learn wrapping techniques.

_____ Jasmine, the patient with a T1 SCI, needs to be checked for decubiti.

_____ The MS patient with the bilateral AFOs needs a skin check.

_____ Mr. Rodriguez's Parkinson's symptoms are getting worse.

_____ Shelby, the patient with spina bifida, is learning to crawl on the floor.

_____ The TBI patient in the wheelchair needs to go back to bed.

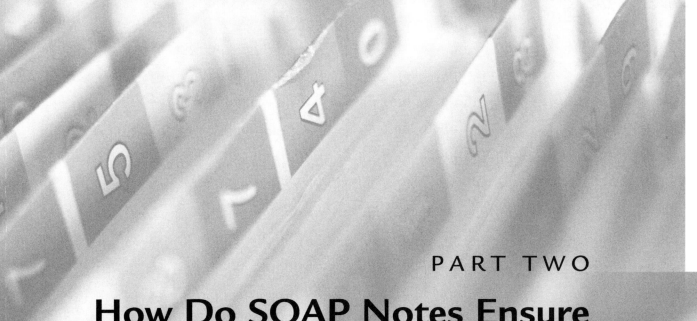

PART TWO

How Do SOAP Notes Ensure Good Patient Care?

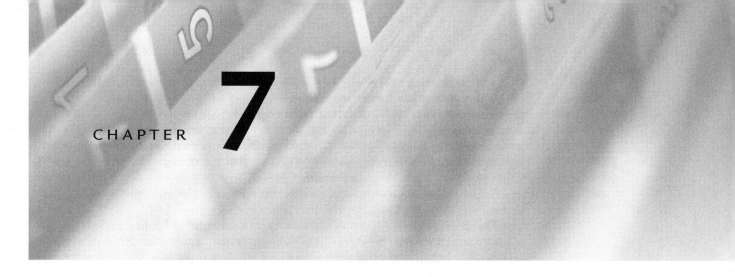

CHAPTER 7

How Does Documentation Relate to Patient Issues?

LEARNING OBJECTIVES

After studying this chapter, the student will be able to:

☐ Compare and contrast functional levels and activity limitations

☐ Differentiate between medical and educational therapy services

☐ Assess specific types of communication related to patient treatment and determine the scope of practice/work responsibilities related to the PT's and PTA's treatments

☐ Discuss general requirements related to patient confidentiality and relate these requirements to HIPAA and FERPA practices

☐ Be able to develop a report for any incident causing injury to a patient during a treatment session or while the patient is under the care of the PTA and identify the time frame for creating such a report

INTRODUCTION

In the chapters in Part Three, we will review what information should be included in each section of the SOAP note to document the progress of the patient. In addition, we will discuss the importance of documenting the patient's progress through the prescribed plan of care (POC) to meet third-party payer requirements for reimbursement. With this knowledge come additional responsibilities to ensure that all facets of patient care are addressed, not just those related to documentation. In this section, we will address those additional responsibilities, which include, but are not limited to, the following:

- Determining whether the care being provided is medically or educationally appropriate
- Addressing and documenting maintenance therapy
- Adhering to the patient confidentiality practices set forth in the Health Insurance Portability and Accountability Act (HIPAA)[1] and Family Educational Rights and Privacy Act (FERPA)[2]
- Documenting telephone communications
- Following appropriate procedures for filing incident reports
- Addressing and documenting patient noncompliance and refusal of care

When addressing such issues, the PT and PTA must determine whether the therapy being provided is appropriate for the setting and the patient's functional abilities, is meeting all prescribed guidelines, and is protecting patient rights as required by law.

In addition to these issues, frequent changes related to health-care and physical therapy services are being proposed continually, making it difficult to keep current with services being provided to patients. For more current information related to changes, the reader can visit the Centers for Medicare & Medicaid Services (CMS) website: (https://www.cms.gov/Regulations-and-Guidance/Regulations-and-Policies/QuarterlyProviderUpdates/index.html?redirect=/QuarterlyProviderUpdates).

The site's Quarterly Provider Update includes all changes to Medicare instructions that affect medical providers, provides a single source for national Medicare provider information, and gives medical providers advance notice on upcoming instructions and regulations.

OUTCOMES AND TREATMENT

There are two primary settings for treating a patient through therapeutic intervention: a medical setting and an educational setting. It is important to be able to determine whether the necessary treatment meets a medical goal or an educational one. The PT and PTA can use functional levels and limitations to help determine some of these goals, depending on the environment in which services are being provided. Each setting has prescribed requirements that must be met to address patient progress.

In a medical setting, the PT or PTA must address the goals that are affected by the medical problem preventing the patient from returning to the highest functional level possible. In a medical setting, the POC is developed based on the initial evaluation, and the PTA follows that POC through the discharge process. The PT monitors the POC, revises it as progress continues, and discharges the patient when goals have been met. Conversely, in an educational setting, the PT develops an individualized education plan (IEP) based on the evaluation, and the PTA follows that IEP until the student has met all of the goals set and no longer needs therapy services, the student reaches the age of 21 (when the school is no longer responsible for providing services to the student), or the student's educational goals are hindered by a medical problem that will be addressed in a medical setting.

One fundamental difference between therapy provided in a medical setting and therapy provided in an educational setting is the time period during which treatment is allowed. Treatment in a medical setting is limited to a prescribed timeline determined by the third-party payer, based on the medical diagnosis. In an educational setting, therapy may continue throughout the time period in which the student attends school, if required guidelines are met. In either setting, patient confidentiality remains important for the time period in which the patient receives treatment. Following discharge, records related to patient care are kept according to the timeline set by the facility. In addition to determining the setting in which therapeutic intervention is provided, the evaluation process must also determine whether such services are necessary and appropriate.

Medical Necessity

Medical necessity determines the type and frequency of physical therapy intervention. The treatment must be "reasonable and necessary" to receive reimbursement. The medical condition that resulted in the referral may not be the sole reason for physical therapy. For example, a patient who has experienced a stroke does not automatically have a medical reason for physical therapy. The fact that the patient now has left-sided paresis and can no longer ambulate independently would be the reason for the referral. It is important to document the actual reasons for the physical therapy referral and the reason skilled physical therapy services will benefit the patient and return him or her to a higher functional level. It is also important to emphasize the reason it is necessary for a PT or PTA to provide skilled therapeutic intervention, instead of the family providing support with minimal physical therapy intervention. For example, a patient has limited range of motion, and skilled physical therapy services have been ordered. However, with an initial training session for teaching range-of-motion exercises to the family, the family is able to provide range-of-motion intervention for the patient. Consequently, skilled physical therapy services are not necessary. Skilled physical therapy services mean just that: A PT or PTA is needed to provide services to restore the patient to the highest functional level possible. If the family can be taught the skills needed to restore the patient to the highest functional level possible, then skilled physical therapy services are not necessary and will not be reimbursed.

Educational Necessity   Physical therapy provided in a school setting can be very different from that provided in a medical setting. The student may qualify for physical therapy in the school system if he or she cannot move about in the school environment, cannot ambulate independently, or has balance and coordination problems.

For example, the PT receives a referral for physical therapy for a 5-year-old child with Down syndrome. The child can ambulate independently and moves throughout the school environment without assistance, but he cannot climb the ladder to go down the slide. The parent is demanding that her child receive physical therapy services for this reason and because he has Down syndrome. Following the PT's evaluation, it is determined that the child can ambulate independently, run with good control (although awkwardly), and ascend and descend stairs with the aid of two handrails and by marking time (going up or down one step at a time instead of using a reciprocal gait pattern). Because the child can ambulate and move about the school environment independently, he does not qualify for physical therapy in the school setting. Down syndrome cannot be the sole reason he receives therapy. Because he has difficulty using some of the playground equipment and demonstrates some coordination problems, the PT might refer him for an adaptive physical education evaluation instead.

From this review of both types of settings, it is important to note that outcomes in either setting are directly related to the following:

- The patient's prior level of function (PLOF)
- The medical and physical therapy diagnoses
- The patient's functional/activity limitations
- The assessment of the referred problem
- The development of a treatment plan
- Input from the patient, family, and medical or educational staff for functional goals

Patient's Limitations   When dealing with referrals for physical therapy, the PT and PTA must be cognizant of the patient's limitations. Such limitations may or may not be directly related to the physical therapy diagnosis and may or may not affect the patient's functional level. The physical therapist decides whether the limitation the patient is experiencing can be improved through the physical therapy POC. If not, the limitation could interfere with or decrease the success of physical therapy. Any limitation must be evaluated to determine whether it will affect efforts to return the patient to the previous level of function or whether it makes physical therapy intervention inappropriate, regardless of the setting.

Maintenance Therapy   One determinant that would cause a discontinuation of physical therapy services relates to the necessity for and reimbursement of those services. For an adult patient who does not show any progress, who has met the goals and objectives of therapy, or who has received the maximum amount of therapy allowed by the paying entity, therapy is considered a maintenance service and is no longer "reasonable and necessary." Therefore, physical therapy is no longer appropriate for the patient, and the patient will be discharged from services. The agency providing therapy services must be cognizant that reimbursement will no longer be provided for patients if services are no longer appropriate. However, even though there may no longer be financial support from a third-party payer, the patient may elect to cover the cost of treatment him- or herself, or services may be provided on a pro bono basis.

Maintenance therapy is not a determinant against physical therapy services for pediatric patients. Through the support of numerous state and federal agencies, pediatric patients may receive physical therapy services from birth through 21 years of age. From birth to 3 years of age, patients may be enrolled in an early intervention program. From 3 to 21 years of age, they may receive services through the public school system, as discussed previously. Even if the patient does not show improvement in function in the school setting, physical therapy services still can be provided if the PT determines they are necessary. The only requirement relates to the student's access to, and ability to move safely in, the school environment. Even with no improvement noted in function, the treating therapist still can document that skilled services are necessary for training for safe transfers with school staff; appropriate positioning for schoolwork, eating, and rest time; and alternative methods for transporting the student within the school environment.

**PATIENT
CONFIDENTIALITY
ISSUES**

All medical records and information regarding the patient's condition and treatment are confidential. Only health-care professionals who provide direct care to the patient have access to the patient's medical and treatment information. Any individual not providing direct care to the patient must be authorized by the patient to receive information about his or her medical care and condition. This is an ethical principle commonly called the *rule of confidentiality.* In the medical setting, a patient's information is guarded by HIPAA; in an educational setting, the student's information is guarded by FERPA.

HIPAA Requirements

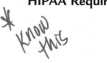

The Health Insurance Portability and Accountability Act of 1996 (HIPAA),[1] which includes the Standards for Privacy of Individually Identifiable Health Information (also known as the Privacy Rule), was mandated by the federal government to protect individuals and all information related to an individual's health care. These standards were revised by the Department of Health and Human Services (HHS) on January 17, 2013. Please refer to the following website for additional information: http://www.hhs.gov/about/news/2013/01/17/new-rule-protects-patient-privacy-secures-health-information.html. These new standards gave patients more control over their medical records and more protection regarding who had access to them.

HIPAA includes provisions regarding electronic transactions and covers all health plans, health-care providers, and individuals or facilities that conduct administrative transactions (e.g., billing). Reasonable safeguards must be initiated to protect the patient, including the following:

- While discussing a patient's condition with family members or other health-care providers, move the conversation to a private conference room or office.
- Avoid using the patient's name or even a description of the patient in hallways and elevators, and post signs to remind employees to protect the patient's confidentiality.
- Isolate and lock filing cabinets or records rooms.
- Provide additional security, such as computer passwords, to secure personal information.

In addition, HIPAA:

- Provides patients with access to their medical records and the right to have errors corrected within 30 days of a written request. Patients may be charged for the costs of copying and postage.
- Calls for patients to be provided with information about how their medical records are kept and how their rights are protected regarding the medical care they receive and the individuals who have legal access to that information.
- Calls for patients to be provided with information about the method of disbursement of their medical information and an acknowledgment when that information is shared with the patient's written permission.
- Protects patients from the marketing of any information related to their medical care without written authorization while allowing patients access to disease-management information.
- Informs patients that state regulations can overrule HIPAA in circumstances such as the reporting of an infectious disease outbreak to public health authorities.
- Gives patients the right to file a complaint with the Office of Civil Rights (OCR) when they feel their rights regarding their medical information have not been honored (complaints can be filed by calling 1-866-627-7748 or accessing www.hhs.gov/ocr/hipaa).

As of October 1, 2015, all facilities that follow HIPAA guidelines must now use ICD-10 coding for all medical and physical therapy diagnoses. Refer to Chapter 3 for a review of ICD-10 coding.

Employers and employees must also follow guidelines related to sharing medical information:

- Written policies and procedures must be in place to protect patient medical information from individuals who might have access to such information.

- Employees must be trained in privacy policies and procedures, and disciplinary procedures must be in place in case those procedures are violated.
- Disclosure policies related to emergency situations, public health needs, judicial proceedings, and certain law enforcement activities must be relayed to employees.
- Employees must be trained to disclose any information that may affect national defense or security.

Under HIPAA, protected health information may be disclosed to a covered entity without the patient's authorization for the following purposes or situations:[1]

- Release of medical records to the patient (unless required for access or accounting of disclosures)
- Treatment, payment, and health-care operations
- Opportunity to agree or object
- Incident to an otherwise permitted use and disclosure
- Public interest and benefit activities
- Limited data set for the purposes of research, public health, or health-care operations (limited data include nondescript patient information—e.g., date of birth, date of death, age, sex, date of service, town, zip code—that do not include an identifying factor related to a specific individual)

Covered entities (e.g., health-care providers, health plans, health-care clearinghouses) should use professional ethics and best judgment in deciding which of the following permissive uses and disclosures to make:[1]

- A covered entity must obtain the patient's written authorization for any use or disclosure of protected health information that is not for treatment, payment, or health-care operations or other uses permitted or required by the Privacy Rule. (HIPAA's Privacy Rule establishes national standards to protect medical records and other personal health information and applies to health plans, health-care clearinghouses, and those health-care providers that conduct certain health-care transactions electronically.) The Privacy Rule requires appropriate safeguards to protect the privacy of personal health information, and it sets limits and conditions on the uses and disclosures that may be made of such information without patient authorization. The Privacy Rule also gives patients rights over their health information, including the rights to examine and obtain a copy of their health records and to request corrections.[3]
- A covered entity may not condition (i.e., stipulate, order, state) treatment, payment, enrollment, or benefits eligibility on an individual granting an authorization, except in limited circumstances.
  - An authorization must be written in specific terms. It may allow use and disclosure of protected health information by the covered entity seeking the authorization or by a third party.
  - Examples of disclosures that would require an individual's authorization include disclosures to a life insurer for coverage purposes, disclosures to an employer of the results of a pre-employment physical or lab test, or disclosures to a pharmaceutical firm for their own marketing purposes.
  - All authorizations must be in plain language and contain specific information regarding the information to be disclosed or used, the person(s) disclosing and receiving the information, expiration of the authorization, right to revoke in writing, and other data.

FERPA Requirements In the educational setting, a student's information is guarded by FERPA. To disclose student records under FERPA guidelines, a school must:[2]

- Have a student's or parent's consent prior to the disclosure of education records.
- Ensure that the consent is signed and dated and states the purpose of the disclosure.

A school may disclose education records without consent when:[2]

- The disclosure is to school officials who have been determined to have legitimate educational interests as set forth in the institution's annual notification of student rights.
- The student is seeking or intending to enroll in another school.
- The disclosure is to state or local educational authorities auditing or enforcing federal- or state-supported education programs or enforcing federal laws that relate to those programs.
- The disclosure is to the parents of a student who is a dependent for income tax purposes.
- The disclosure is in connection with determining eligibility, amounts, and terms for financial aid or enforcing the terms and conditions of financial aid.
- The disclosure is pursuant to a lawfully issued court order or subpoena.
- The information disclosed has been appropriately designated as directory information by the school.

It is important to note that while FERPA guidelines mirror those of HIPAA, they apply to students younger than 21 years of age if those students are enrolled in kindergarten through 12th grade. For that reason, it is important to obtain permission from the student if an individual outside of the school system wants access to such records. Such permission should be in writing, state the specific purpose of the request, and list a date after which the request is null and void. Written policies must be in place at each educational institution that further delineate the requirements for someone to obtain, view, or use student records related to any medical intervention. For students enrolled in a postsecondary educational institution, FERPA guidelines provide the same protections for students older than 18 years of age. The student must provide written permission for the school to share his or her educational files with anyone, including his or her parents.

General Requirements The patient provides authorization for sharing his or her medical or educational information by signing a release of information form for each health-care organization or educational facility, or by naming each person to whom the information can be released. Figure 7–1 is an example of a release of information form.

The PTA may not provide information about the patient or student to anyone without first knowing whether the person is authorized to receive the information. This includes the patient's spouse, parent, any other relative, neighbor, or friend. Once authorization is obtained, then the facility's procedure for releasing information is followed.

The individual's record is kept in a secure location, such as behind the nursing station counter or in a secure office with limited access, to prevent unauthorized individuals from reading it. The PTA respects this rule of confidentiality by returning the record to its proper location or by passing it on to another authorized person. The record must never be left lying unattended on a counter or desk or visible on a computer screen. Also, never leave documents with an individual's confidential information unattended at a copy machine. If you must make photocopies of any part of an individual's record, remain with the documents at all times and make sure to remove all of the documents from the copy machine when you are finished. Any discussion about the individual's condition must occur in private areas and only with the individual, legal guardian, caregivers, and/or those authorized to receive the information.

Any researcher who wants to gather information from the medical or student record must have the individual's permission. The researcher cannot publish or reveal the individual's name or any other descriptions that would identify the patient or student.

The Patient's Rights Although the health-care or educational facility is the legal owner of the individual's records, the patient or student (or legal guardian) has the legal right to know what is in them. The patient or student must follow the facility's procedure to access his or her records. Usually the procedure simply involves having the patient or student sign a request form. The PTA needs to be knowledgeable about the facility's procedure.

Release of Information Form

Patient Name _____   DOB _____
Address: _____   Social Security # _____

I authorize and request XXX Medical Rehabilitation Center to release records maintained while I was a XXX patient, disclosing information as specified below. This form may be utilized for several parties to eliminate duplicate paperwork.

PURPOSE OF REQUEST:

- _X_ Insurance Reimbursement
- _X_ Subsequent Treatment/Intervention on behalf of patient
- ____ Other (Specify) _____

- ____ Worker's Compensation
- ____ Damage or claim eval. by attorney

INFORMATION TO BE RELEASED:

- _X_ Eval Reports
- _X_ Progress Notes
- _X_ Plan of Care

- _X_ Discharge Reports
- _X_ Physician Order(s)
- _X_ Other (Specify) _____

By placing my initials in the appropriate space, I specifically authorize XXX to include in the records released, information relating to or mentioning the following, if any:

____ Psychological conditions   ____ Drug or alcohol abuse

RELEASE:

*1. Release to: Physician
   Name:
   Address:

*2. Release to: Insurance Company
   Name:
   Address:

*3. Release to: Employer
   Name:
   Address:

*4. Release to: QRC or Disability Case Manager
   Name:
   Address:

5. Release to: Attorney Law Firm
   Name:
   Address:

6. Release to: Patient
   Name:
   Address:

7. Release to:
   Name:
   Address:

8. Release to:
   Name:
   Address:

*When a therapist requests courtesy copies, the above parties signified by an asterisk (*) will automatically receive copies of medical records.

REVOCATION

I understand that I may revoke this authorization at any time. If I do not expressly revoke this authorization sooner, it will automatically expire 1 year from the date of this authorization; or under the following conditions:

a.) authorization may extend beyond 1 year if this is a worker's compensation case.

b.) other (specify) _____

COPIES

A photocopy of this authorization _X_ may   may not be accepted by you in place of the original.

SIGNATURE

_____   Date
Signature of patient or person
authorized to sign for the patient

If signed by someone other than the patient, state how authorized _____

REFUSAL

I do not wish to authorize release of information to the following individual party(ies)

Name of party or parties

Signature   *Date*

Figure 7—1   An example of a release of information form.

COMMUNICATION GUIDELINES: TELEPHONE REFERRALS

The PTA may participate in three common types of telephone conversations requiring documentation in accordance with the facility's policies and procedures:

1. Taking verbal referrals for physical therapy treatment from another health-care or education provider
2. Receiving information directly from the patient or from a representative of the patient
3. Receiving inquiries about the patient's medical condition or about the physical therapy treatment from interested people, provided that the patient has signed a release of information form enabling the sharing of such information

Other Types of Referrals for Physical Therapy

Other health-care providers or their staff members may telephone referrals for physical therapy services to the department or school. A nurse, or a receptionist acting under the physician's direction, may make telephone orders for physical therapy services. One PT may call and refer a patient to another PT with expertise in the treatment of a patient's particular condition. Another health-care provider, such as an occupational or speech therapist, may telephone a referral when physical therapy is indicated.

When receiving a referral over the telephone, the PTA should follow the facility's procedure for documenting the call. Carry a pen and notebook in your pocket at all times to allow quick note taking when answering the telephone. Take notes to gather information to document later. Use the facility's form for recording telephone referrals. A copy or a similar form with the information from the call is sent to the referring provider for signature. This signature proves that the conversation and referral did take place. Typically, the documentation requirements for a telephone referral include the following:

- Date of the call
- Name of the person calling in the referral and the person's relationship to the patient or student
- Name of the primary care physician
- Name of the PTA answering the telephone and receiving the verbal referral
- Details of the referral and accompanying information regarding the patient or student
- Comments regarding plans to send written verification of the telephone referral to the referring party
- Comments indicating that the referral will be brought to the attention of the PT

Information From or About the Patient

The PTA may speak with a patient or family member over the phone when the person calls to report a change in the patient's condition or ability to keep a therapy appointment. If the call is about a change in the patient's condition, the PTA should refer the caller to the PT or the patient's physician. If it is an emergency situation, the PT or PTA should advise the caller to transport the patient to the emergency room (if this is the policy of the facility) or to call 911 for an ambulance. Documentation about this call may include the following:

- Date and time of the call
- Name of the person calling and his or her relationship to the patient
- Name of the PTA taking the call
- A summary of the conversation, including the response of the PTA, the referral of the call to the PT, and so on
- Comments regarding the apparent emotional state of the caller (e.g., tone of voice, disposition, orientation)

Request for Information About a Patient

Often individuals other than those providing direct patient care have an interest in the patient's condition and treatment and may call to inquire about the patient's progress. Attorneys, insurance representatives, parents of children younger than 18 years of age, other relatives, friends, and neighbors are examples of people who might call the physical therapy department in the medical or educational facility. For example, a patient who was injured while working may have lawyers, a rehabilitation manager, an insurance representative, and an employer, all of whom may want to know about the patient's medical care. A student who has multiple medical conditions, receives outside medical care, or is involved in litigation may have other individuals seeking information about his or her medical services in the school setting. When the PTA answers the telephone and the caller asks about a patient's condition, the PTA must follow the rules of confidentiality as they relate to each of the different callers.

PROTECTING THE PATIENT

Along with maintaining patient confidentiality, the PT and PTA have a responsibility to protect the patient in other ways. These ways include, but are not limited to, informed consent, proper use of treatments and related appliances, proper use and filing of an incident report, and legal responsibilities related to the treating therapist.

Informed Consent

Informed consent can be defined as "a legal procedure to ensure that a patient or client knows all of the risks and costs involved in a treatment. The elements of informed consent include informing the client of the nature of the treatment, possible alternative treatments, and the potential risks and benefits of the treatment. In order for informed consent to be considered valid, the client must be competent and the consent should be given voluntarily."[4]

Consequently, informed consent means more than giving permission to treat. In addition, all aspects of the treatment plan, including the purposes, procedures, expected results, and any possible risks or side effects of treatment, must be explained to the patient and/or his or her caregiver. If possible, it is usually best to have the patient participate in designing the plan.

The patient or the patient's representative then decides whether to accept the treatment plan or refuse it. This policy and procedure ensure that the patient is not being coerced into any course of action. This consent may be informal and verbal or formal and written. In the case of the student, the school will develop an IEP so that all parties understand:

- The services that will be provided
- Why the services are being provided
- The time limit for provision of such services
- The frequency of treatment

In addition, such services will be re-evaluated on an annual basis.

When the patient gives a verbal consent, the PT documents the consent in the initial evaluation. In all medical facilities, a formal informed consent form or document must be signed before treatment is initiated. When a patient is receiving physical therapy, the PT designs the treatment plan and reviews the plan with the patient. Thus, the appropriate person to obtain the informed consent signature is the PT, not the PTA. Once signed, this form is part of the medical record.

An informed consent document from a medical facility should contain the following:[1]

1. A description of the physical therapy diagnosis and the proposed treatment plan, written in language that the patient or the patient's representative can understand
2. Name and qualifications of the responsible PT and other physical therapy personnel likely to be providing the care
3. Any risks or precautions associated with the treatment procedures that the patient should consider before deciding to agree to or refuse the treatment
4. An explanation of any alternative treatments that would be appropriate, including risks or precautions that need to be considered if the alternative treatment is used
5. The expected benefits of the proposed treatment plan and the expected outcomes if the physical therapy problem is not treated
6. Responsibilities of the patient or representative of the patient in the treatment plan
7. Answers to patient's questions

Other Documentation Issues

Using Appropriate Ink

Use of black ink is a common guideline in medical documentation. Black ink traditionally has been used because it photocopies more clearly than other ink colors. However, photocopy technology has progressed so that other ink colors now copy clearly and print black. Some facilities have legal documents signed in blue ink to distinguish the original from the copy. While colors such as green, mauve, or taupe may copy well, they remain inappropriate for a medical record. The PTA should follow the facility's procedure.

Falsifying Information   In every case, it should be difficult for someone to change or alter the written note. To ensure that no opportunities exist for changing or falsifying the information, follow these guidelines:

1. Do not use erasable pens.
2. Do not erase errors or utilize correction fluid or tape, such as White-Out®.
3. Draw a line through the error, date and initial directly above the error, and add the correct information (e.g., "patient ambulated with ~~crutches~~ ML/3-4-17 standard walker").
4. Do not leave empty lines or spaces at the end of a sentence, a section, or a completed therapy note. Empty spaces provide the opportunity for someone to add or change information, thus falsifying the record. Draw a horizontal line through empty spaces (see Fig. 7–2).

Timeliness   Complete the documentation as soon as possible after treating the patient while the information is fresh in your mind. A daily note written immediately after the patient treatment session is the most accurate note. However, it is more likely that the PTA moves from one patient to the next and treats a full day's schedule of patients before being able to document those sessions. Carry a small notebook or 3 x 5 index cards to take notes while treating patients so that each patient's daily note will be accurate and thorough.

The specific time of a treatment should be indicated using the 24-hour clock, or "military time," which is denoted as a four-digit number without a colon. If a patient has more than one treatment in the same day, then each treatment time is documented separately after the date ("3-4-17, 0900"; "3-4-17, 1530"). This allows another health-care provider, such as the occupational therapist, nurse, or speech pathologist, to document in the daily note section of the chart between the physical therapy morning and afternoon notes, thus illustrating the continuum of care throughout the day (see Fig. 7–3).

An addendum is made when information is added to a note that has already been written and signed. To add more information later, date the new entry and state "addendum to physical therapy note dated 6-21-17." Refer to Figure 7–4 as an example of a progress note that follows legal guidelines for adding information.

Incident Reports   An *incident* is anything that happens to a patient, student, employee, or visitor that is

- Out of the ordinary.
- Inconsistent with the facility's usual routine or treatment procedure.
- An accident or a situation that could cause an accident.

The patient will be seen 2X/wk for six weeks. Will contact PT for supervisory visit after six visits.

_____ Takahiro Therapist, LPTA

Figure 7–2   An example of line used to cross out an empty space.

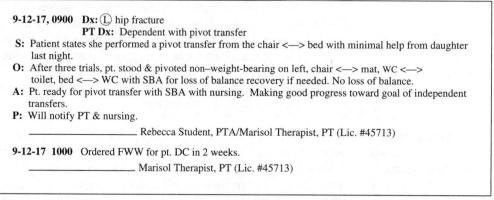

9-12-17, 0900   Dx: Ⓛ hip fracture
　　　　　　　　PT Dx: Dependent with pivot transfer
S: Patient states she performed a pivot transfer from the chair <—> bed with minimal help from daughter last night.
O: After three trials, pt. stood & pivoted non–weight-bearing on left, chair <—> mat, WC <—> toilet, bed <—> WC with SBA for loss of balance recovery if needed. No loss of balance.
A: Pt. ready for pivot transfer with SBA with nursing. Making good progress toward goal of independent transfers.
P: Will notify PT & nursing.
　　　　　　　　_____ Rebecca Student, PTA/Marisol Therapist, PT (Lic. #45713)

9-12-17 1000   Ordered FWW for pt. DC in 2 weeks.
　　　　　　　　_____ Marisol Therapist, PT (Lic. #45713)

Figure 7–3   An example of a patient's progress note showing more than one therapy session in one day.

9-12-17, 0900 Dx: Ⓛ hip fracture
PT Dx: Dependent with pivot transfer
S: Patient states she performed a pivot transfer from the chair <—> bed with minimal help from daughter last night._____
O: After three trials, pt. stood & pivoted non–weight-bearing on left, chair <—> mat, WC <—> toilet, bed <—> WC with SBA for loss of balance recovery if needed. No loss of balance._____
A: Pt. ready for pivot transfer with SBA with nursing. Making good progress toward goal of independent transfers._____
P: Will notify PT & nursing.
_____ Rebecca Student, PTA/Marisol Therapist, PT (Lic. #45713)

9-12-17 1000 (bs): Pt's. vital signs were taken following the PT session. BP was 135/85, temp was 99°, resp. 15/minutes, and pulse 80 BPM. Blood work was completed for pro time and potassium levels per physician order.
_____ Rebecca Student, PTA/Marisol Therapist, PT (Lic. #45713)

Figure 7—4 An example of a progress note with an addendum.

All medical and educational facilities should have a policy and procedure for documenting incidents in an *incident report*. During the first or second day of an internship or a new job, the student or newly employed PTA should read the facility's instructions for completing and filing an incident report and knowing the time period in which it should be filed.

Purpose of an Incident Report

An incident report is used for risk management and legal protection. Following the policy and procedure for reporting incidents protects everyone who uses the facility (i.e., all patients, students, employees, and visitors) from future incidents. The procedure describes a method for providing a prompt response to medical needs, identifying and eliminating problems, and gathering and preserving information that may be crucial in litigation. The report contains information that identifies dangerous situations that either caused or could cause an injury.

Risk managers use this information to change the situation, thereby reducing the risk for injury. The incident report alerts the administration and the facility's lawyer and insurance company to the possibility of liability claims. It "memorializes important facts about an alleged incident [and] create[s] a record for use in further investigation."[5] As with physical therapy practice in general, "If it isn't written, it didn't happen."

Legal Responsibility When an Incident Occurs

Any eyewitness must fill out and sign the incident report. If more than one person witnessed the incident, each eyewitness completes the report. Each person documenting the incident must follow the facility's procedure. The incident report is completed on a form unique to the facility. Most medical facilities use similar forms, which typically ask for the following information:

1. Name and address of the person involved in the incident: If the person involved is a patient, then the form may request the patient's address, date of birth, gender, admission date, and status before the incident. The patient's medical diagnosis and physical therapy diagnosis are recorded along with a brief summary of the care the patient has received. When the person involved is a student, employee, or visitor, his or her home address is provided. For students, the medical diagnosis and physical therapy diagnosis are recorded along with a brief summary of the therapy services the student has received.

2. An objective, factual description of the incident: The PTA completing the incident report does not express an opinion, blame anyone or anything, or make suggestions about how the incident might have been prevented. The incident is to be described as the eyewitness saw it, not as someone else described it. No secondhand information is to be included in the report. The circumstances surrounding the incident, the condition of the affected person after the incident, and the course of action taken are described.

3. Identification of all witnesses to the event: The report includes the addresses of the witnesses, if known, as well as the model number and manufacturer of any equipment involved.

Each facility has a time period within which the report should be submitted. This can range from 24 hours to 3 days following the incident. Because the incident report is not considered part of the medical record, it is placed in a file separate from the patient's medical or student record. The PTA must document the incident in the patient's chart or student record; however, the PTA does not mention that an incident report was completed. The report is a confidential, administrative document for use in case of litigation and for risk-management review and action. Box 7–1 summarizes the "dos and don'ts" of incident reporting.[2] Figure 7–5 is an illustration of a completed incident report. (The names and the situation are fictitious.)

Documenting Patient Refusal of Treatment

As discussed in this section and in Chapter 6, after receiving information about all aspects of the treatment, the patient or a representative of the patient must consent to the treatment plan. The patient does have the right to disagree with the plan and to change his or her mind later and refuse treatment. In an educational setting, the patient's consent is given through the development of the IEP, and any changes to this agreement must be made in writing and with an additional meeting scheduled to discuss such changes.

When a patient refuses treatment in a medical setting, there are several things the PTA can do:

1. Use active listening skills, interview, and talk with the patient to try to determine the reason for refusal. The patient may have a very good reason that it would not be appropriate to receive treatment at that time. For example, a man in a nursing home refuses therapy without explaining why. After the PTA spends some time talking with him, he reveals that his dog passed away the previous evening. This man is grieving his loss and would not be able to concentrate on his therapy activities that day.
2. If there does not seem to be a reason for the refusal, make sure the patient fully understands the purpose of the treatment and the expected outcomes if the problem is not treated.
3. If the patient continues to refuse, recognize the patient's right to refuse, document the refusal in the patient's chart, and notify the PT.

The PTA documents the patient's statement of refusal of treatment and the reason for refusal. The PTA describes his or her response and action taken. A statement about notifying the PT is included. The documentation may read as follows:

8-3-17, 1300:

Pt. refused treatment this p.m. After being encouraged to attend at a later time, pt. stated her sister was visiting from out of state and the only time she would be able to visit with her was this afternoon. She expected her soon and anticipated the visit would last all afternoon. Agreed to cancel treatment this p.m. and scheduled pt. for tomorrow a.m. Will notify PT.

—Simon Roberts, PTA

2-22-17, 0900:

Pt. refused treatment today when PTA arrived in room. Pt. stated she did not want to work with male therapist because of her religious beliefs. Pt. did not disclose this issue to supervising PT during initial evaluation. PTA agreed to cancel treatment session. PTA will communicate with PT regarding a change in therapists to address pt. cultural issue.

—Simon Roberts, PTA

Box 7–1	Summary of Dos and Don'ts of Incidence Reporting

1. DO notify your PT.
2. DO know your facility policy and procedure for reporting an incident.
3. DO write legibly and use professional terminology.
4. DO include the names and addresses of employees or visitors who know something about the incident.
5. DO give the completed report to your supervising PT to route for the necessary signatures.
6. DON'T mention that you've filed an incident report in the patient's chart.
7. DON'T photocopy an incident report.
8. DON'T write anything in the report that implicates or blames anyone for the incident.
9. DON'T use the report to complain about coworkers or other employees or an issue with the facility.
10. DON'T talk about the incident with uninvolved personnel. Remember *confidentiality*.
11. DON'T acknowledge any incident or give any information to the patient or other individuals until you've checked with your PT or a supervisor.

Source: Adapted from Hilton, D. (Ed.) (1988). *Documentation: A clinical pocket manual* (pp. 135–136). Springhouse, PA: Springhouse.

PREDISPOSING CONDITIONS

Diagnosis: Fx Ⓡ hip   hypertension

Mental Status (i.e., Oriented, Alert/Confused, etc.): -alert & oriented

List pertinent medications if applicable: Tylenol   lanoxin   tenex

Follow up measures to Incident:

MD & family notified, vital signs checked every 2 hours for 12 hours

Was a Medical Device Involved?   ☐ Yes   ☒ No   Manufacturer's Name and Address (if Available on Equipment or Packaging):

Type _____   Model No. _____

Serial No. _____   Lot No. _____

Incident Reported By: Kayla McLaughlin   Title: PTA

Date of Report:	Signature & Title of Person Preparing Report:
11/21/17	Kayla McLaughlin/PTA

Reviewed by DON: Virginia McDormel/RN   Reviewed by Administrator: Miguel Rivera
(Signature)   (Signature)

Date: 11/22/17   Charted: ☒ Yes ☐ No   Date: 11/23/17

Reviewed by Medical Director: Dr Silvio Castillo   Date: 11/30/17
(Signature or initials)

DO NOT WRITE BELOW THIS LINE-TO BE COMPLETED BY ADMINISTRATOR/DON

Vulnerable Adult Report Made?   ☐ Yes ☒ No

Incident Reported To (Circle as many of the following as applicable.):

Local Welfare Agency   Local Police Department   County Sheriff's Office   Office of Health Facility Complaints

Other (Explain) _____

Date Report Called in (Within 5 Days): _____   Approximate Time: _____ ☐ a.m. ☐ p.m.

Name of Person Spoken to: _____   Reported By: _____

Date Report Mailed: _____   To Whom: _____

incident.rep

Figure 7—5A An example of the front of a completed incident report.

ABC HEALTH CENTER
INCIDENT REPORT

Resident/Visitor #1 Jemma Ramunto	Resident/Visitor #2 n/a
Address: 7700 Grand Ave. Duluth	Address:
Phone #: 628-2341 DOB 1/17/35	Phone #: DOB
Date: 11/21/17 Time 1430	Location of Incident: P.T. Dept

Description of Incident:

Pt was standing in parallel bars with PTA holding on with transfer belt, Pt performing Ⓡ L/E standing exercise, she became pale and dizzy, could not walk back to chair, was lowered to floor by PTA. Never lost consciousness, felt much better once reclined. With assist of PT was lifted into w/c

Assessment: Describe injury (if any) in detail:

Skin tear on Ⓡ forearm when arm hit bar while lowering small 1.5X 2.0 open area with small amount of blood

Name/Title of All Witnesses:	Safety Measures in Use:
Olivia Smith-Carter/PT Kayla McLaughlin/PTA	Transfer Belt: X Siderails: Restraint: does not use Type:

Intervention: None Required	At Facility X

Describe:

Vital signs checked and charted in nursing chart, skin tear was cleansed & protective covering in place. ROM to U/E & Ⓛ L/E WFL s̄ pain! Ⓡ L/E ROM within hip precaution limits 3 pain

Resident #1

Hospitalized: Yes____ No X	Date n/a Time____ am/pm	Hospital n/a
Physician Name: Preet Batra	Notified by: Dana Olson/RN Date 11/21/17 Time 1300	
Family Name: Robert Ramunto/son	Notified by: Dana Olson/RN Date 11/21/17 Time 1315	

Resident #2 n/a

Hospitalized: Yes____ No____	Date____ Time____	Hospital____
Physician Name:	Notified by:	Date____ Time____
Family Name:	Notified by:	Date____ Time____

Figure 7—5B   An example of the back of a completed incident report. The names and situation are fictitious.

SUMMARY   The PT and PTA are responsible for documenting numerous events and tasks during the course of a day. The PTA must know the facility's procedures for documenting various types of conversations, maintaining patient confidentiality, obtaining informed consent, understanding and writing incident reports, and documenting the patient's refusal of treatment.

REFERENCES
1. Health Insurance Portability and Accountability Act (HIPAA). (n.d.). Retrieved from http://www.hhs.gov/ hipaa/index.html
2. Family Educational Rights and Privacy Act (FERPA). (2011). Retrieved from http://www2.ed.gov/policy/gen/ guid/fpco/ferpa/index.html
3. The Privacy Rule. (n.d.). Retrieved from http://www.hhs.gov/hipaa/for-professionals/privacy/index.html
4. Cherry, K. (2016). What is informed consent? Retrieved from https://www.verywell.com/what-is-informed-consent-2795276
5. Hilton, D. (Ed.). (1988). *Documentation: A clinical pocket manual* (p. 135). Springhouse, PA: Springhouse.

Review Exercises

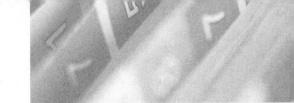

1. **Explain** the **difference** between medical and educational necessity.

2. List **three** requirements you must follow to protect patient confidentiality.

3. Your patient's neighbor brought her to therapy today. She wants to know how her friend is doing and why she is receiving PT. **What,** if anything, can you tell her and **why?**

4. What is **HIPAA?**

5. What is **FERPA?**

6. What are **two differences** between HIPAA and FERPA?

7. You are working with a student in an elementary school. **How** would you know that you have informed consent to treat a student in this setting?

8. An attorney representing your patient in a lawsuit calls you and wants an update on the patient's progress. **What** is your best response?

9. What is an **incident report,** and why is it important in patient care?

10. **Who** is responsible for completing an incident report, and **why** is it not filed in the patient's medical record?

Practice Exercise 1 ➤ *In the following list of statements, identify the statements that the PT might write in a SOAP note with "PT," those that the PTA might write with "PTA," and those that either might write with a "B."*

1. _____ The patient stated his pain had decreased from 8/10 to 6/10 following treatment today.

2. _____ The patient was discharged on 2-7-17 for noncompliance.

3. _____ PROM is WFL in the Ⓡ UE.

4. _____ The patient's wife stated that he did not sleep last night because of ↑ pain in his right knee.

5. _____ The patient was able to walk with CGA for 100 ft using a FWW on linoleum with a non-reciprocal gait pattern.

6. _____ The next supervisory visit with the PT will be on 4-21-17.

7. _____ Will refer patient to OT services for an evaluation.

8. _____ Re-evaluation will be done on the next visit on 3-23-17.

9. _____ Strength in the Ⓛ LE hip flexion is 3/5 with PROM/AROM WNL.

10. _____ Will review progress and POC in next department team meeting.

Practice Exercise 2 ➤ *Identify the statements that indicate **medical necessity** or **educational necessity**, or **both**, by marking them with an "M," "E," or "B."*

1. _____ Pt. will ↑ strength from 3/5 to 4/5 in triceps by 3rd visit for ADL function.

2. _____ Pt. will ambulate independently, within the school building, using a posterior walker and a reciprocal, heel-toe gait pattern, s̄ LOB.

3. _____ Pt. will transfer from wheelchair to desk Ⓘ c̄ SBA.

4. _____ Pt. was shown the HEP and successfully performed a correct return demo of all ex.

5. _____ Pt. stated that she could not lift the 5-lb weight in shld flex and used ↓ weight to 2 lb for ADL function.

6. _____ Pt. will demo a safe and Ⓘ transfer from the chair to a mat in gym area.

7. _____ Pt. will receive PT services 3X/week in the classroom and gym setting.

8. _____ Pt. has ↑AROM in Ⓑ UE shld abd from 100° at IE to 115° today.

Practice Exercise 3 ➤   *From the statements given, identify the statement that will **protect** patient confidentiality under HIPAA guidelines by marking it with a "P." If the statement violates patient confidentiality, mark it with a "V." **Explain** why each statement protects or violates patient confidentiality.*

1. _____ Calling the patient by her first name to notify her you are ready for her treatment.

_____

2. _____ Having all patients sign in at the front desk.

_____

3. _____ Telling the friend what is wrong with her neighbor.

_____

4. _____ Telling the parents what progress their child has made during therapy.

_____

5. _____ Sending patient information to the referring doctor.

_____

6. _____ Receiving a patient referral by telephone.

_____

7. _____ Letting the patient look at his chart.

_____

8. _____ Giving the patient a diagnosis in the waiting room.

_____

9. _____ Allowing the speech-language pathologist to review the therapy notes on your patient.

_____

10. _____ Reporting the patient's noncompliance in a team meeting.

_____

Practice Exercise 4 ➤   *Identify the statements that warrant an incident report by marking them with an "I."*

1. _____ The patient slipped through the gait belt but was caught by the therapist before falling.

2. _____ The patient fainted while sitting on the edge of the bed but did not fall off the bed.

3. _____ The patient fell on the floor while walking in the hallway.

4. _____ The patient received a minor burn from the UV lamp.

5. _____ The patient felt dizzy and was moved to a chair while walking.

6. _____ The patient fell out of bed and was found on the floor.

7. _____ The patient fainted while on the commode and was found leaning against the wall.

8. _____ The patient left the facility, against medical advice (AMA).

9. _____ The patient mentioned that she had stubbed her toe last night.

10. _____ The patient fell down the hospital stairs while using crutches.

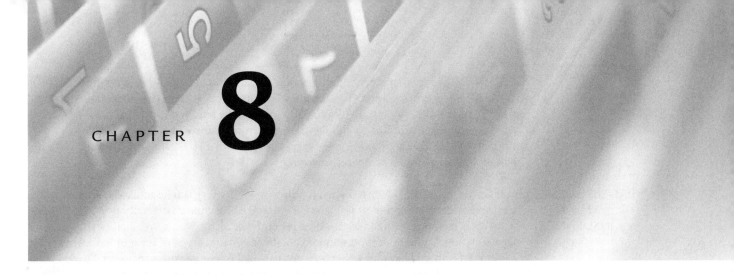

CHAPTER **8**

Your Documentation Related to Legal and Ethical Issues

LEARNING OBJECTIVES

After studying this chapter, the student will be able to:

☐ Organize information to present documentation at state and federal court hearings

☐ Describe professional liability and its importance in the legal setting

☐ Define what a deposition is

☐ Explain the PTA's responsibilities when testifying in a legal setting

☐ Describe ethical standards of practice for the PTA

INTRODUCTION

Part of a therapist's responsibility in documentation is to provide information and to appear, when requested, in a civil, state, or federal court proceeding on behalf of a patient or the medical facility for which he or she works. Any therapist who provides documentation can be subpoenaed (that is, ordered, in writing) to produce documentation or to testify in a court proceeding for the prosecution or the defense. As seen in the example in Chapter 1, PTs and PTAs can be called for either side. It is imperative that patient documentation be comprehensive, reproducible, and able to stand on its own in a court hearing.

Generally, most medical records should be kept for 3 to 6 years. However, some medical facilities keep them longer, even indefinitely. For liability purposes, it is important for the PTA to know how long records should be kept according to state statutes and individual medical facility policies. Generally, HIPAA guidelines require medical facilities to retain their patient records for 7 years.[1] Following a patient's death, the record must be kept for 3 years.[1] Records related to minors should be retained until the minor reaches legal age (depending on the state) or until the statute of limitation for that state is reached. FERPA guidelines require records related to a student's name, address, birth date, academic work completed, level of achievement, and attendance record be kept for 100 years.[2] However, with the increased use of EHRs, some of these policies have changed for those facilities that use them. In addition, the continued ability to ensure HIPAA requirements requires an ongoing effort at all facilities. While the retention requirements remain the same for EHR storage, dependent on the medical facility and state requirements, EHRs have created difficulties for some facilities to maintain privacy. Because of issues related to online access, HIPAA, while not requiring a specific timeline for record storage, does require record protection utilizing the Privacy and Security Rules. The HIPAA Privacy Rule protects the privacy of individually identifiable health information, called protected health information (PHI), as explained in the Privacy Rule. The Security Rule protects a subset of information covered by the Privacy Rule, which is all individually identifiable health information a covered entity creates, receives, maintains or transmits in electronic form. The Security Rule calls this information "electronic protected health information" (e-PHI). The Security Rule does not apply to PHI transmitted orally or in writing.[3]

PROFESSIONAL LIABILITY INSURANCE

Like the PT, the PTA also must maintain professional liability (malpractice) insurance to provide legal protection in case of litigation. This type of insurance is usually provided through the medical facility at which the therapist is employed. However, some facilities (e.g., small outpatient clinics, clinics in rural settings) do not provide this type of insurance, in which case the PT or PTA should have his or her own professional liability insurance policy. Several companies offer such insurance, such as the Healthcare Providers Service Organization (HPSO; http://www.hpso.com) and the Professional Liability for Allied Health Professionals/Lockton Affinity (http://www.ahc.lockton-ins.com/pl). The annual fee for professional liability insurance ranges from approximately $100 to $200, depending on the company, the PTA's number of years in practice, whether the PTA is self-employed, and whether the PTA practices in more than one medical facility.

Professional liability insurance should cover the employed or student therapist on and off the job. This type of coverage protects the treating therapist if litigation occurs and provides legal representation if the medical facility does not do so. Standard coverage includes the following[4]:

- Up to $1,000,000 professional liability coverage for each claim
- Up to $3,000,000 aggregate professional liability coverage
- Occurrence-based coverage
- Defense cost payment
- Deposition representation
- Defendant expense benefit
- License protection
- 24-hour coverage

Depending on the company, additional coverage may include the following:

- Assault coverage
- Personal liability coverage
- Personal injury coverage
- First-aid expenses
- Medical payments
- Damage to the property of others

Based on the 2016 claim report from HPSO, the most common reason for litigation in physical therapy practice is fractures caused during patient treatment. The most common types of claims were against physical therapy practices and physical therapists, with physical therapist assistants named as part of the suit. Allegations for litigation included, but were not limited to, improper management of the surgical patient, improper management of the patient over the course of treatment, and improper performance using therapeutic exercise.

Recommendations for risk control in physical therapy practice include the following:

- Appropriate clinical support and supervision
- Delegation of PT services only to the appropriate level of staff
- Recognition of patients' medical conditions
- Utilization of appropriate safety devices
- Presence in the therapy area
- Close observation of high-risk patients to prevent falls
- Knowledge and understanding of the scope of practice parameters for the state in which you practice
- Knowledge of the levels of supervisory responsibilities of the PT
- Ensuring that clinical practices comply with standards endorsed by physical therapy professional associations[5]

LEGAL ISSUES

Any professional interaction with the public brings challenges that may result in litigation. This is especially true when working with individuals in the medical arena. Because of this increased risk for litigation related to patient treatment, the PTA must be cognizant of proper treatment and documentation if he or she is subpoenaed for a deposition or to testify in a court of law. For this type of situation, appropriate and timely documentation is critical in determining whether or not the treating therapist is liable for the unintended result of the intervention provided. The documentation should describe the patient's consent for treatment, the type of treatment the patient received, and the patient's response to that treatment. Because of the increasing opportunities to be called to testify, the PTA must ensure that documentation for each client is complete in order to be prepared for such a development.

Testifying in Court

A summons to appear in court can be very intimidating, but if the PTA has documented the care given to the patient appropriately and has acted within his or her scope of practice, then there should be nothing to worry about. During the court proceedings, the PTA is called to testify and swears to tell the truth when giving an account of the situation as he or she remembers it. One of the primary mistakes people make when requested to testify in court is to provide too much information. It's best simply to answer the questions that are presented in a clear and concise manner, without elaboration. As therapists, we tend to want to help, and this can be a poor idea in any legal setting. The best rule of thumb is to answer only the question that was asked. For example, if the attorney were to ask a question requiring an answer of only yes or no, then the PTA should give that answer only, without expanding on the response. It is important not to elaborate on any one question and to let the documentation speak for itself. The purpose of the testimony is to provide an accurate account of the treatment received by the patient, defend the care that was provided, and prove that the PTA treated the patient within his or her scope of practice and followed the POC set by the supervising physical therapist and the medical facility in which they practice.

In addition, the PTA must tell the truth, the whole truth, and . . . well, you get the idea. The truth is best supported by accurate, comprehensive, and understandable documentation. Testimony about a particular patient may not occur for months or even years after treatment. It is important to be able to read the documentation because it will be impossible to recall every detail about every patient. The documented notes are projected onto a screen for everyone to see and read. Penmanship and spelling do matter! If the penmanship is illegible, the patient, facility, or the PTA could be in unnecessary jeopardy. With the increased use of EHRs, however, this is becoming less of an issue, and the printed report or screen shots of the report are more legible than those handwritten. Any documentation related to patient care must be provided. For example, any note completed on behalf of the patient and the care that he or she has received can be entered into court as a document of record. The method of documentation does not matter. Whether the notes were handwritten, transcribed from a recorder, or placed on a computer, any and all forms must be produced in response to a subpoena.

Depositions

A deposition, also known as an examination before trial (EBT), is the act or fact of taking sworn (under oath) testimony from a witness outside of court. The deposition is written down by a court reporter for later use in court. It is a part of the pretrial discovery process whereby litigants obtain information from each other in preparation for trial.[4] Some jurisdictions recognize an affidavit—"any written document in which the signer swears under oath before a notary public or someone authorized to take oaths (like a county clerk) that the statements in the document are true"[5]—as a form of a deposition.

Depositions are taken for the purpose of discovering the facts upon which a party's claim is based and can be used to discover a witness's testimony prior to trial, to discredit a witness if the witness changes his or her testimony prior to litigation, or to obtain financial information. The deposition can also be used to preserve the testimony of a witness who will be unable to appear at trial. In addition, some depositions may be taken by using a digital video deposition system in which the individual may be deposed from a remote location, a more cost-effective solution to the problem of having to travel and take time away from work. This type of deposition can be scheduled for any time or date, can be reviewed for changes, and becomes part of the permanent record.

At a deposition, the lawyers for both the prosecution and the defense are present, and both lawyers can question the person testifying. The PTA is sworn in during the proceeding to ensure the accuracy of his or her responses. The main differences between a court hearing and a deposition are the environment in which the deposition is held and the fact that the PTA is able to review the information and make changes before it is entered into the record. Most depositions are held in a lawyer's office, public building, conference room, and so on. The proceedings are taped and/or documented by a court reporter. Again, because this is a legal proceeding, it is important for the PTA to answer only the questions that are asked and not elaborate by providing more detail than necessary. Answers should remain concise and to the point, and the PTA should expect his or her documentation to support the care given.

Statements   Sometimes a general statement will be requested from the PTA. A court setting or deposition usually isn't required for this, nor is it supplied under oath. The general statement may be part of an information-gathering process to determine whether a court hearing is necessary or whether an arbitration hearing might be possible.

In an arbitration hearing, the participants testify under oath and all parties agree to abide by the results of the arbitration decision. Because this is not a court hearing, substantial court costs are not incurred and issues are settled more quickly. Again, regardless of the circumstances, the PTA must answer only the questions asked and not elaborate any further.

ETHICAL ISSUES   When giving any statement related to the care of a patient, you must determine whether the patient's rights and confidentiality are being protected and confirm that HIPAA and FERPA guidelines are being met. Under these guidelines, any medical information related to the patient's care or the student's information can be used in a deposition or court hearing. In addition, any medical or educational information is accessible to the patient or student with a written request. Patients have the right to have copies of their medical records, can request changes in those records, and can decide with whom those records can be shared. A student may request copies of his or her educational records but may have to meet additional guidelines set by the educational institution in order to be given the records. With the evolution of HIPAA in 1996 and FERPA in 1974, patient confidentiality requirements make adherence to these guidelines paramount. (For additional information on HIPAA requirements, visit https://www.cms.gov/Regulations-and-Guidance/Regulations-and-Policies/QuarterlyProviderUpdates/index.html?redirect=/QuarterlyProviderUpdates.)

In addition, the PTA is bound by professional ethics and conduct, as outlined in ATPA's *Guide to Physical Therapist Practice*.[7, 8] APTA's code of ethics for PTAs is listed in Box 8–1. Additional documentation regarding ethical conduct and professionalism for the physical therapist assistant can be found on the APTA website.[9,10] It is the duty of all PTAs to be conversant with these documents provided by APTA and to follow them in their practice settings to provide appropriate care for the patients they treat. By following these guidelines for ethical conduct, the PTA provides appropriate and ethical care for patients in following the POC outlined by the supervising PT. Through proper documentation, this appropriate and ethical care is outlined for the patient, the third-party payer, and other government entities that provide accreditation for such medical facilities. It is imperative that the PTA communicates on a regular basis with the supervising PT to ensure that the POC remains appropriate and that the PTA continues to work within the scope of practice as outlined in the state practice act. It is the responsibility of the PTA to ensure that he or she has reviewed those regulations for every state in which he or she has a license to practice. By graduating from an accredited physical therapist assistant school, the PTA further receives an introduction to and follow-through of such ethical conduct.

These ethical standards apply nationwide and should be followed no matter the type of medical or educational facility at which the PTA works, the number of hours a PTA works, or who the supervising PT might be. As for the PT, these standards of ethical conduct are in place to protect the patient, ensure that appropriate care is provided, and maintain treatment under a POC developed and supervised by a licensed PT.

| Box 8-1 | Standards of Ethical Conduct for the Physical Therapist Assistant |

HOD S06-09-20-18 [Amended HOD S06-00-13-24; HOD 06-91-06-07; Initial HOD 06-82-04-08] [Standard]

Preamble

The Standards of Ethical Conduct for the Physical Therapist Assistant (Standards of Ethical Conduct) delineate the ethical obligations of all physical therapist assistants as determined by the House of Delegates of the American Physical Therapy Association (APTA). The Standards of Ethical Conduct provide a foundation for conduct to which all physical therapist assistants shall adhere. Fundamental to the Standards of Ethical Conduct is the special obligation of physical therapist assistants to enable patients/clients to achieve greater independence, health and wellness, and enhanced quality of life.

No document that delineates ethical standards can address every situation. Physical therapist assistants are encouraged to seek additional advice or consultation in instances where the guidance of the Standards of Ethical Conduct may not be definitive.

Standards

Standard #1:

Physical therapist assistants shall respect the inherent dignity, and rights, of all individuals.

1A. Physical therapist assistants shall act in a respectful manner toward each person regardless of age, gender, race, nationality, religion, ethnicity, social or economic status, sexual orientation, health condition, or disability.

1B. Physical therapist assistants shall recognize their personal biases and shall not discriminate against others in the provision of physical therapy services.

Standard #2:

Physical therapist assistants shall be trustworthy and compassionate in addressing the rights and needs of patients/clients.

2A. Physical therapist assistants shall act in the best interests of patients/clients over the interests of the physical therapist assistant.

2B. Physical therapist assistants shall provide physical therapy interventions with compassionate and caring behaviors that incorporate the individual and cultural differences of patients/clients.

2C. Physical therapist assistants shall provide patients/clients with information regarding the interventions they provide.

2D. Physical therapist assistants shall protect confidential patient/client information and, in collaboration with the physical therapist, may disclose confidential information to appropriate authorities only when allowed or as required by law.

Standard #3:

Physical therapist assistants shall make sound decisions in collaboration with the physical therapist and within the boundaries established by laws and regulations.

3A. Physical therapist assistants shall make objective decisions in the patient's/client's best interest in all practice settings.

3B. Physical therapist assistants shall be guided by information about best practice regarding physical therapy interventions.

3C. Physical therapist assistants shall make decisions based upon their level of competence and consistent with patient/client values.

3D. Physical therapist assistants shall not engage in conflicts of interest that interfere with making sound decisions.

3E. Physical therapist assistants shall provide physical therapy services under the direction and supervision of a physical therapist and shall communicate with the physical therapist when patient/client status requires modifications to the established plan of care.

Continued

Box 8–1	Standards of Ethical Conduct for the Physical Therapist Assistant—cont'd

Standard #4:

Physical therapist assistants shall demonstrate integrity in their relationships with patients/clients, families, colleagues, students, other health care providers, employers, payers, and the public.

4A. Physical therapist assistants shall provide truthful, accurate, and relevant information and shall not make misleading representations.

4B. Physical therapist assistants shall not exploit persons over whom they have supervisory, evaluative or other authority (eg, patients/clients, students, supervisees, research participants, or employees).

4C. Physical therapist assistants shall discourage misconduct by health care professionals and report illegal or unethical acts to the relevant authority, when appropriate.

4D. Physical therapist assistants shall report suspected cases of abuse involving children or vulnerable adults to the supervising physical therapist and the appropriate authority, subject to law.

4E. Physical therapist assistants shall not engage in any sexual relationship with any of their patients/clients, supervisees, or students.

4F. Physical therapist assistants shall not harass anyone verbally, physically, emotionally, or sexually.

Standard #5:

Physical therapist assistants shall fulfill their legal and ethical obligations.

5A. Physical therapist assistants shall comply with applicable local, state, and federal laws and regulations.

5B. Physical therapist assistants shall support the supervisory role of the physical therapist to ensure quality care and promote patient/client safety.

5C. Physical therapist assistants involved in research shall abide by accepted standards governing protection of research participants.

5D. Physical therapist assistants shall encourage colleagues with physical, psychological, or substance-related impairments that may adversely impact their professional responsibilities to seek assistance or counsel.

5E. Physical therapist assistants who have knowledge that a colleague is unable to perform their professional responsibilities with reasonable skill and safety shall report this information to the appropriate authority.

Standard #6:

Physical therapist assistants shall enhance their competence through the lifelong acquisition and refinement of knowledge, skills, and abilities.

6A. Physical therapist assistants shall achieve and maintain clinical competence.

6B. Physical therapist assistants shall engage in lifelong learning consistent with changes in their roles and responsibilities and advances in the practice of physical therapy.

6C. Physical therapist assistants shall support practice environments that support career development and lifelong learning.

Standard #7:

Physical therapist assistants shall support organizational behaviors and business practices that benefit patients/clients and society.

7A. Physical therapist assistants shall promote work environments that support ethical and accountable decision-making.

7B. Physical therapist assistants shall not accept gifts or other considerations that influence or give an appearance of influencing their decisions.

7C. Physical therapist assistants shall fully disclose any financial interest they have in products or services that they recommend to patients/clients.

7D. Physical therapist assistants shall ensure that documentation for their interventions accurately reflects the nature and extent of the services provided.

7E. Physical therapist assistants shall refrain from employment arrangements, or other arrangements, that prevent physical therapist assistants from fulfilling ethical obligations to patients/clients

> **Box 8–1** **Standards of Ethical Conduct for the Physical Therapist Assistant—cont'd**
>
> *Standard #8:*
>
> Physical therapist assistants shall participate in efforts to meet the health needs of people locally, nationally, or globally.
>
> 8A. Physical therapist assistants shall support organizations that meet the health needs of people who are economically disadvantaged, uninsured, and underinsured.
>
> 8B. Physical therapist assistants shall advocate for people with impairments, activity limitations, participation restrictions, and disabilities in order to promote their participation in community and society.
>
> 8C. Physical therapist assistants shall be responsible stewards of health care resources by collaborating with physical therapists in order to avoid overutilization or under-utilization of physical therapy services.
>
> 8D. Physical therapist assistants shall educate members of the public about the benefits of physical therapy.
>
> *Source:* Retrieved from http://www.apta.org/uploadedFiles/APTAorg/About_Us/Policies/HOD/Ethics/Standards.pdf. Used with permission from APTA.

SUMMARY

It is necessary and important for the PTA to maintain appropriate and comprehensive documentation for any patient included in his or her caseload. Proper documentation, regardless of the format, protects the patient, the treating PTA, the supervising PT, and the medical facility itself. The PTA must be held accountable for appropriate documentation that addresses the scope of practice in the state where he or she is licensed.

It is the responsibility of the PTA to provide treatment under the supervision of a licensed PT and to be able to defend the care given to any patient by following the POC outlined by the supervising PT. The PTA must know and understand the standards of ethical conduct presented by APTA to ensure appropriate and ethical patient care is provided. Through appropriate documentation and by following ethical standards of practice, the PTA can ensure that the care given to the patient will be appropriate and ethical even if the PTA receives conflicting information from the supervising PT. If the PTA provides treatment within his or her scope of practice, as dictated by the practice act of the state where he or she serves, the PTA can ensure that the patient is protected and the care given is accurate. As always, it is the PTA's responsibility to ensure the care he or she gives is appropriate for the patient's condition and within the PTA's scope of practice.

REFERENCES

1. Kasprak, J. (n.d.). *Patient access to medical records.* Retrieved from http://www.cga.ct.gov/2006/rpt/2006-r-0599.htm
2. *Student record storage.* (2005). Retrieved from http://www.psea.org/uploadedFiles/Publications/Professional_Publications/Advisories/StudentRecords07.pdf
3. Health Information Privacy. (2003, February 20). *Summary of the HIPAA Security Rule.* Retrieved from http://www.hhs.gov/hipaa/for-professionals/security/laws-regulations/index.html
4. Healthcare Providers Service Organization. (2012). *Professional liability insurance—Individual coverage through HPSO.* Retrieved from http://www.hpso.com/professional-liability-insurance/coverage-description.jsp
5. Healthcare Providers Service Organization. (2016). *PT professional liability exposures: 2016 claim report webinar.*
6. Deposition. (2016). In *Nolo's plain-English law dictionary.* Retrieved from http://www.nolo.com/dictionary/deposition-term.html
7. American Physical Therapy Association. (2003). *Guide to physical therapist practice* (2nd ed.). Alexandria, VA: APTA.
8. American Physical Therapy Association. *Standards of ethical conduct for the physical therapist assistant.* Retrieved from http://www.apta.org/uploadedFiles/APTAorg/About_Us/Policies/HOD/Ethics/Standards.pdf
9. American Physical Therapy Association. (2011). *Professionalism.* Retrieved from http://www.apta.org/Professionalism
10. American Physical Therapy Association. (2010). *APTA guide for the conduct of the physical therapist assistant.* Retrieved from http://www.apta.org/uploadedFiles/APTAorg/Practice_and_Patient_Care/Ethics/GuideforConductofthePTA.pdf

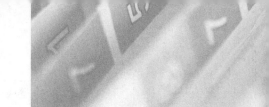

Review Exercises

1. Describe the **importance** of keeping legible and comprehensive notes of patient care.

2. **Why** would a PTA need to testify in a court of law?

3. What are two **differences** between giving a deposition and testifying in a court of law?

4. In the facility in which you work, how **long** should medical records be kept?

1. You have followed the POC outlined by your supervising PT to perform joint mobilization to a patient's right shoulder. You have performed Grade 4 joint mobilizations on the patient's shoulder, causing a tear in the rotator cuff. Even though this treatment intervention is outside your scope of practice, you followed the POC outlined by the PT. Could this be a reason for a patient to bring litigation against you, as the treating PTA? Why or why not?

2. In question 1, which standard of ethical conduct did you violate?

3. Following the treatment session, your patient has requested a copy of her medical records from your facility. Are you allowed to release a copy to the patient? Why or why not?

4. You are working with a patient and stretching the heel cords, following the POC outlined by the supervising PT. Suddenly, you feel the heel cord release and the patient cries out in pain. The back of the ankle suddenly starts to swell. You immediately put ice on the ankle, call the supervising PT to notify him of the injury, and recommend an x-ray of the ankle (per the MD's order) to determine the extent of the injury. You also complete an incident report to document what happened and the treatment given to the patient following the injury. The patient heals well with no further problems, the doctor reviews the x-rays and finds no bone injury, and the patient does not appear to have any further complaints. Two years later, the patient decides to sue your facility because of this injury, claiming he does not have full range of motion in the injured ankle. As the treating PTA, do you think your documentation is valid and will provide appropriate information to outline your treatment intervention and to prove that you were within your scope of practice for this patient's treatment? Why or why not?

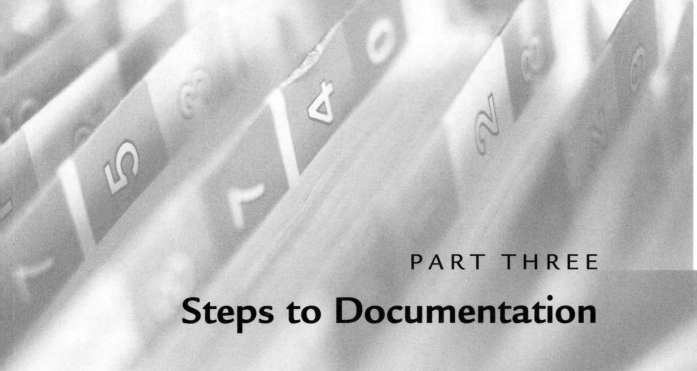

PART THREE
Steps to Documentation

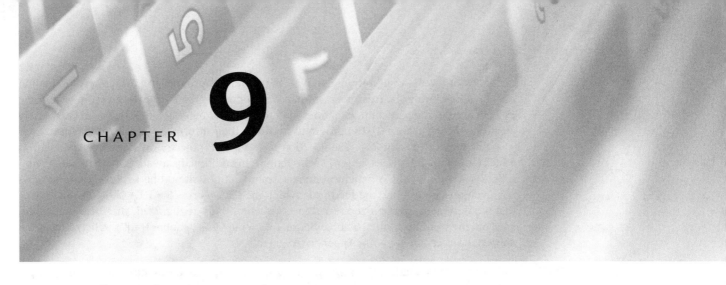

9

Introduction to the SOAP Note

LEARNING OBJECTIVES

After studying this chapter, the student will be able to:
- ☐ Understand each section of the SOAP note
- ☐ Differentiate between the sections of the SOAP note
- ☐ Identify common errors that occur in SOAP note documentation
- ☐ Utilize a SOAP note rubric to help develop a complete note
- ☐ Discuss criticisms related to the use of the SOAP note format

INTRODUCTION

Chapters 5 and 6 provided the basis of the SOAP note documentation process by outlining the differences between the medical diagnosis and the physical therapy diagnosis and by providing a review of the different types of medical records used in documentation, the different formats used to complete documentation, and the responsibilities required for appropriate documentation. This chapter reviews the importance of each part of the SOAP note and the information that should be included within each section.

With most documentation, information gathered about a patient may include both subjective and objective data. Most of this information is gathered at the time of admission or when the patient is first seen by each medical provider. However, information is being gathered continuously throughout the span of the patient's care. Data gathered when the patient is admitted is located in the reports on the initial evaluations performed by the various medical practitioners. For example, Table 5–1 in Chapter 5 reviews the type of information recorded when the patient is admitted to the emergency room, when the patient is taken to radiology, when the patient is admitted to the orthopedic unit, and when laboratory tests are performed. More information is gathered when the patient is first seen by physical therapy, occupational therapy, and social services. Examples of the data gathered in each discipline are highlighted in Table 5–1 in Chapter 5.

For further delineation of patient information, the PT and PTA can report information in a SOAP note format. This type of format includes sections for Subjective data, Objective data, Assessment, and Plans. It is important for the PTA student and newly employed therapist to be able to organize his or her thoughts into a succinct account of the treatment session with the patient after the PT has completed the evaluation and developed the plan of care (POC). The SOAP note provides an excellent medium for learning how to put information related to the patient in an outline format. In this manner, the PTA student is able to develop the necessary skills to communicate how the patient is progressing, assess problems that may develop during the treatment session, develop time frames for progression within the POC, make discharge recommendations, and recommend other health-care treatments. Many electronic health record (EHR) programs organize their information in a similar format.

A general explanation of each section of the SOAP note follows. (See Chapters 10 to 13 for more in-depth discussions of each section.) In addition, be aware that when completing a SOAP note following a patient treatment, abbreviations should be kept to a minimum. If abbreviations are used by the facility in which the PTA works, the PTA should use the ones that are commonly recognized. For those not commonly recognized, the therapist should spell out the word first with the abbreviation following (e.g., "patient [pt.]"). A list of common abbreviations can be found in Appendix A.

SUBJECTIVE DATA

Subjective data include any information the health-care provider gathers about the patient. Subjective data include:

1. Information about the patient's medical history
2. Symptoms or complaints that caused the patient to seek medical attention at this point in time
3. Factors that produced the symptoms
4. The patient's functional and lifestyle needs prior to and following the disease or disorder
5. The patient's goals or expectations regarding medical care

Typically, data relevant to the patient's condition and reason for admission are obtained by interviewing the patient, his or her caregivers or other family members, and/or a significant other. Collecting Subjective data is an ongoing process while medical care is being provided. The information reflects the patient's response to treatment and effectiveness of treatment.

The PT documents Subjective data in the physical therapy examination and evaluation reports. The PTA documents Subjective data in the daily or weekly progress notes. The Subjective section is found at the beginning of the note. Subjective data are critically important in physical therapy examination and evaluation reports. As part of the continuum of care in progress notes, Subjective data provide evidence of treatment effectiveness or progress toward the functional goals as reported by the patient to the treating therapist.

OBJECTIVE DATA

Objective data include information that is *reproducible and readily demonstrable*. Objective data are gathered by carefully examining the patient through the use of data-collecting methods such as measurements, tests, and observations. These methods can be reproduced by any medical professional with the same training as the one who first performed the evaluation.

Objective data include signs of the patient's condition. Reviewing the signs by repeating the measurements, tests, and observations is also an ongoing process for determining treatment effectiveness and patient progress. The PT performs the physical therapy examination and evaluation and uses objective methods to gather data. These data are used to determine the effectiveness of the intervention as it relates to the physical therapy diagnosis. The PTA repeats any measurements, tests, and observations, within the scope of his or her practice, to determine the patient's progress toward accomplishing the treatment goals as outlined in the POC.

ASSESSMENT

The Assessment section is a summary of the Subjective and Objective information. In this section, the PT interprets the information in the Subjective and Objective sections of the SOAP note, makes a clinical judgment, and sets functional outcomes and goals. The PTA summarizes the information described in the two preceding sections and reports the progress that the patient is making toward accomplishing the goals. The PTA uses this section to summarize which of the patient's outcomes have been met and which may need revision by the supervising PT. This section also provides the PTA with a method to address how much progress is occurring compared with the evaluation completed by the PT or compared with previous treatment sessions. This is one of the most important sections that third-party payers read, and it's where they expect to find progress discussed. If the information in this section is not accurate, the treatment session may not be reimbursable.

PLAN   The Plan describes what will happen next. The PTA describes what he or she needs to do before or during the next treatment session or what the patient or caregivers need to do. This section also states when the PT supervisory visit (SV) will occur. It is important that the PTA state the date or time period when the SV will occur and that specific state rules and regulations are followed.

DOCUMENTATION ERRORS   Even though many facilities are transitioning to EHR programs, some clinics still complete handwritten SOAP notes. In those cases, the PTA may make a mistake in the information provided or a spelling error. It is important to know how to make a correction within the document that is legal and appropriate for any facility. If the PTA is writing the note and makes a mistake, the PTA should draw one line through the incorrect information, initial the mistake, and provide the date of the correction (e.g., "with pt. supine: Ⓡ leg bent, Ⓛ completed straight leg raised (SLR), Ⓘ to ~~65°~~ 75°"). Then the PTA may provide the correction if it is not a lengthy one and continue with the written documentation. However, if the PTA needs to make a correction once the note has been written already, or if the note was submitted electronically, the PTA must provide a written or computer-generated addendum. Then a copy of this addendum must be filed in the patient's chart for additional clarification. For mistakes made in an EHR, the PTA must complete an addendum for any changes that must be made. Most EHR programs have an addendum that is easily accessed and added to the current note that needs amending.

EXAMPLES OF SOAP NOTE ORGANIZATION   Thinking about the letters that spell out *SOAP* helps you organize information so that it can be documented in a logical sequence. This organization also makes it easy to find information, as evidenced by the following examples.

Example One   Suppose your 10-year-old daughter has been diagnosed with strep throat and an ear infection. You obtained medication and have started her on the treatment. It is the next morning.

> **11-8-17:**   *Dx/Pr: Strep throat and ear infection.*
>
> ---
>
> **S:**   Pt. reports pain in Ⓡ ear of 6/10 on the verbal rating score (VRS) and being upright makes the pain worse; she feels too tired to go to school today and instead stayed home and slept.
>
> **O:**   Temperature 100.8°F, down 2° from last night, skin color pale. Pt. sat at breakfast table 20 min before needing to lie down and was not able to eat solid food. Pt. took medication, 2 tablets, 8:00 a.m. per instructions on prescription.
>
> **A:**   Pt.'s fever decreasing but temperature not at goal of 98.6°F. Pt. is not able to stay up all day for school and is not able to consume a normal diet.
>
> **P:**   Will call attendance office to excuse pt. from school; will continue medication per dr.'s orders.
>
> —Super Parent, PTA

Example Two   You are a PTA teaching a patient to walk with crutches. This patient had a skiing accident that resulted in multiple fractures of bones in the ankle joint. The ankle has been surgically set and placed in a cast, and the patient is not permitted to bear weight on the foot.

> **11-16-17:**   *Dx: Fx Ⓛ ankle, surgically set and casted c̄ ankle in neutral.*
>
> ---
>
> **Pr:**   NWB on Ⓛ leg, requiring amb c̄ underarm crutches.
>
> **S:**   Pt. states he plans to go home tomorrow and needs to climb a flight of stairs (7 steps) in his house and to manage ramps and curbs to return to work. Stairs have a rail on side.
>
> **O:**   After 3X c̄ SBA for safety and sense of security and c̄ vc, patient Ⓘ ascended 12 steps WB on LE and descended with WB on Ⓡ LE using the railing and axillary crutches, NWB on Ⓛ: and Ⓘ ambulated up and down a 6 ft. ramp using a

swing-to gait pattern and stepped up and down from curbs of various heights (1", 2", 4", and 5") with vc to maintain NWB status on Ⓛ LE. Pt. Ⓘ transferred in and out of his car, accurately p̄ instructions.

A: Pt. accomplished outcome of being able to Ⓘ manage stairs, ramps, and curbs for functioning within his house and for amb in the community for return to work. Will recommend DC to PT because all goals have been met. Reviewed HEP with pt. (pt. able to perform correct return demo of all ex.) PT to re-evaluate pt. progress within POC tomorrow. Recommend follow-up appointment with orthopedic physician.

P: Will communicate with supervising PT that pt. has met all goals and supervising PT will complete re-evaluation tomorrow.

—Aaron Assistant, PTA, Lic # 6879

SOAP NOTE RUBRIC

For the specific guidelines on what should be included within each section of the SOAP note, refer to Appendix C, which presents a SOAP note rubric. This rubric provides the PTA with a summary of what needs to be included in each section of the SOAP note and provides examples for additional clarification.

One definition of *rubric* in *Merriam-Webster's Online Dictionary* is "a guide listing specific criteria for grading or scoring academic papers, projects, or tests."[1] Rubrics are typically used to present material in an organized manner with Likert scale scoring to enable the reader to determine when the full measure of the criteria presented has been met. By using the SOAP note rubric, you can review what parameters should be included in each section of the SOAP note. The rubric also provides instructors with a grading scale to assess students' development of each section of the SOAP note. The rubric is provided to help students learn the process and parameters of each section and to provide feedback appropriate for each of those sections.

For example, if you review the Subjective section of the SOAP note rubric, you will see that each section is divided into six score sections. For each section, the student is awarded points depending on the clarity of information provided in that section. If the note meets the requirements for the Subjective section of the SOAP note, as outlined in Chapter 10, then the student is awarded full credit, or 25 points. Lack of information in this section means a lower score.

Student PTAs may use this rubric (see Appendix C) when reviewing the next six chapters and when developing their own SOAP notes for patient care.

CRITICISMS OF SOAP NOTES

As discussed in previous chapters, there are multiple methods of documenting patient care. Because of how easy the SOAP note format makes organizing material and finding pertinent information related to the patient's POC, it remains the primary method used for documentation today. However, critics of the SOAP format state that the information focuses on the patient's impairments, implying that improvement in these will improve the patient's functional abilities. When Dr. Lawrence Weed introduced the problem-oriented medical record (POMR) and the SOAP note documentation content in the 1960s, he did focus on impairments (see Chapters 1 and 5). Although a SOAP note can be written about functional outcomes, a variety of other formats creates a clearer focus on functional outcomes. Each facility must decide which documentation method works best for their practice setting, whether they use written or EHR documentation, and which provides the best information for the patients they treat. Again, because of its organization and the ease in which it allows information to be documented, the SOAP note format remains the documentation method of choice.

SUMMARY

Through the use of documentation, the treating therapist can provide an accurate account of the patient's treatment sessions. By organizing the note into sections, the treating therapist will be reminded of information that should be included within that treatment note, regardless of the type of documentation used. The SOAP note format lends itself to such an organizational model and provides a treating therapist with the means to document how and why the patient was receiving skilled physical therapy services.

REFERENCE

1. Rubric. (2011). In *Merriam-Webster's online dictionary.* Retrieved from http://www.merriam-webster.com/dictionary/rubric

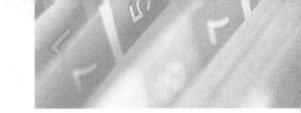

Review Exercises

1. What are the **four** sections of a SOAP note and give a brief **description** of each.

2. **How** can an electronic health record (EHR) mistake be amended?

3. **What** is a criticism to SOAP note formats?

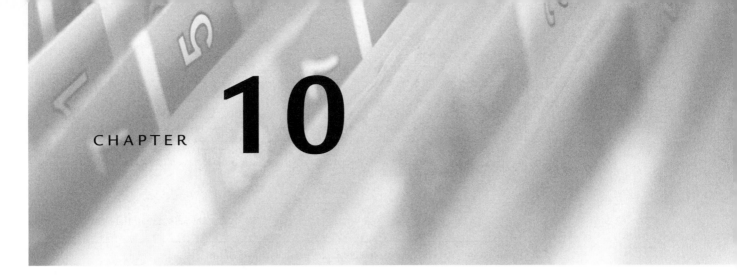

CHAPTER 10

What Are Subjective Data and Why Are They Important?

LEARNING OBJECTIVES

After studying this chapter, the student will be able to:

☐ Select relevant subjective data to document the patient's physical therapy diagnosis and treatment

☐ Identify common characteristics of good listening skills

☐ Organize subjective data for easy reading and understanding

☐ Demonstrate adherence to the recommended guidelines for documenting subjective data

☐ Use appropriate methods to properly document information about the patient's pain

INTRODUCTION

Merriam-Webster's Online Dictionary defines the word *subjective* as "peculiar to a particular individual; modified or affected by personal views, experience, or background; arising out of or identified by means of one's perception of one's own states and processes."[1] Subjective data within a SOAP note, identified by the letter "S," are the information that the patient, his or her caregiver, a family member, or his or her significant other tells the therapist. It is the first introduction to the patient, his or her disease or dysfunction, and the resulting functional limitation that the patient experiences in his or her daily life.

The patient is interviewed and questioned each time he or she is seen for a treatment session. The resulting information is gathered in the Subjective section, along with symptoms of the patient's disease or dysfunction and other information.

SUBJECTIVE DATA

When discussing subjective data and related information, it's important to remember that it must be relevant. Unfortunately, a common mistake in daily notes is the inclusion of information that does not relate to the patient's problem or diagnosis or to the treatment session (Fig. 10–1). Confining the subjective information to only that which is relevant is not an easy task. The PTA and the patient frequently have conversations about a variety of topics. Important information about the patient's problem or diagnosis often slips out during a seemingly unrelated conversation. The PTA must be an alert listener to sort out the relevant information.

11-17-17 Dx: Ⓛ CVA.
PT Dx: Weakness in ⓇUE & LE with unsafe ambulation and dependent in ADLs.
Pt. states not doing exercises at home; has not been going out to church or club meetings because she is afraid of falling. Pt. states she has always been active and wishes she could go to her bridge club meetings. She loves to play bridge and misses her bridge club friends the most. They have been friends since they were girls together in grade school. They just celebrated their 65th year of friendship!

Aaron Therapist, SPTA/ Hai Nguyen, PTA

Figure 10–1   Subjective data section of a daily note containing superfluous information.

Effective listening is a skill that is consciously developed with practice. A new PTA should not expect to have mastered this skill until he or she has been practicing in a clinical setting for more than a few months. To sort out relevant information, the PTA must spend much of the workday listening in a variety of ways. Listening techniques include:

1. Analytic listening for specific kinds of information (e.g., pain, lifestyle, fears)
2. Directed listening to a patient's answers to specific questions (e.g., What positions increase frequency or intensity of pain? What does the patient need to be able to do for his or her day-to-day life?)
3. Attentive listening for general information to get the total picture of the patient's situation (e.g., physical barriers at the patient's home or place of employment)
4. Exploratory listening because of one's own interest in the subject, to provide facts related the listening process
5. Appreciative listening for aesthetic pleasure (e.g., listening to music on headphones while walking during a lunch break)
6. Courteous listening that demonstrates respect for the patient
7. Passive listening through overhearing (e.g., a conversation in the next treatment booth)

Analytic, directed, and attentive listening provide information that may be relevant as subjective data in the daily note (Fig. 10–2). More relevant information may be revealed when exploratory listening is used.

4-19-17 PT Dx: Subdeltoid bursitis with decreased deltoid strength and decreased shoulder ROM interfering with ability to perform work tasks.
S: Pt. reports itching "right where the PT gave my first ultrasound treatment yesterday." Mentioned she is allergic to some perfumes.
O: No skin rash or redness observable in treatment area today. Direct contact US/1 MHz/1.5 w/cm² (moderate heat)/5 min/Ⓡ subdeltoid bursa/sitting/shoulder extended/arm resting on pillow to decrease inflammation. Used ultrasound lotion instead of gel. Gel contains perfume. Pt. correctly performed home exercise program of isometrics for the deltoid, holding for 8 counts (see copy in chart).

Shoulder

AROM:	before tx	after tx
flexion	0–55°	0–60°
abduction	0–68°	0–73°

A: Treatment tissue less sensitive to US (1 w/cm² yesterday). US effective in reducing inflammation. Pt. beginning to progress toward goal of decreased inflammation, improved shoulder mobility to perform work tasks.
P: Will monitor pt.'s response to the US lotion tomorrow and alert PT of the reaction to the gel. Pt. is scheduled for four more treatments.—Samrath Beni, PTA

Figure 10–2   Adding new and relevant subjective information to the medical record through the daily note.

ORGANIZING SUBJECTIVE DATA

The Subjective content in the initial evaluation report may be more complex and detailed than the Subjective data in the daily note. The PT may organize this content into subcategories, such as complaints (c/o), history (Hx), environment, patient's goals or functional outcomes, behavior, and pain level. This helps the PT confine the data to relevant categories only. Organizing the content makes it easy to read and locate information. The example note in Figure 10–3 presents subjective data randomly, making it difficult to get a clear picture of the patient's status. In Figure 10–4, the note is rewritten with the information grouped according to topic.

The PTA needs to document subjective data only if there is an update on previous information or if there is relevant new information. Usually the content is brief. If it falls in more than one topic category, it should be distributed according to topic. However, identifying the topic categories may not be necessary. Daily notes may not contain subjective data when the provided data are not relevant or when the patient is unable to communicate (e.g., the patient is in a coma) and there is no one else present during the treatment to offer subjective data. For additional clarification regarding information that should be included in the Subjective section of the SOAP note, review the SOAP note rubric included in Appendix C.

WRITING SUBJECTIVE DATA
Verbs

When documenting subjective data, use verbs to indicate that the information was provided by the patient. Commonly used verbs include *states, reports, complains of, expresses, describes,* and *denies.* It is not necessary to repeat the word *patient* (or *pt.*) within this section. As in the examples in Figure 10–5, after the term *patient* is used once, it is assumed that all the information in the section was reported by the patient.

Patient Quotations

Occasionally, using direct patient quotations is better than paraphrasing the patient's comments. Quoting makes the intent of the comment or its relevance to the treatment clearer. Here are situations when it is appropriate to quote the patient:

1. To illustrate confusion or loss of memory: *Patient (pt.) often states, "My mother is coming to take me away from here. I want my mother." Pt. is 90 years old.*

Pt. c/o pain in Ⓡ shoulder when Ⓡ arm is hanging down. Lives alone. Pt.'s goal is to play on the college volleyball team this winter. Denies having previous injury or trauma to shoulder. C/o pain when attempting to put on sweater and T-shirts. States he is limited to only a few clothing items he can get into without help. States his shoulder started to ache for no apparent reason. Has been practicing volleyball 6 hr/day for the last 3 weeks.

Figure 10–3 Documentation that randomly presents subjective data, making it difficult to get a clear picture of patient's status.

1. Patient rates pain a 6 on an ascending scale of 1–10 when climbing stairs.
2. Patient gives her pain a 4 on a pain scale of 1–7 where 1 is no pain and 7 is excruciating pain.
3. Patient reports his pain is 3/10 after massage compared to 6/10 before massage.
4. 1_____ x _____1
   1 2 3 4 5 6 7 8 9 10

Figure 10–4 The information in Figure 10-3 rewritten with the information grouped according to topics.

1) Patient states she's allergic to perfume; itched at treatment site following yesterday's treatment.
2) Patient states he is anxious to go fishing; has six steps down to the dock at his cabin.
3) Patient reports he awoke only three times last night; denies having leg tingling and back soreness.

Figure 10–5 Three examples of documentation using the word *patient* once.

2. To illustrate denial: *Pt. insists, "I don't need any help at home. I'll be fine once I get home." Pt. is dependent for transfers and ambulation and lives alone.*
3. To illustrate attitude toward therapy: *Pt. states, "I don't want to play children's games. If I could just go home, I would be fine."*
4. To illustrate use of abusive language: *Pt. yelled to therapist, "Keep your hands off my arm! I'm going to hit you!"*

Information Provided by Someone Other Than the Patient

The patient's caregiver, other family members, or a significant other often provides relevant information. This is especially true for infants and young children and for patients with dementia, speech dysfunction, and altered neurological function (e.g., coma, memory loss).

When someone other than the patient provides the information, begin by stating who provided the information. Be sure to state the reason the patient could not communicate (for example, "All of the following information is provided by pt.'s mother. Pt. is in a coma."). When information is provided by both the patient and another person, specifically note when it is patient-supplied and when it is supplied by the other person (for example, "Mrs. Jones states she did not have to help her husband button his sweater today. Mr. Jones states that today is the first time he has not had to ask for help since his arthritis flared up.").

Pain

When discussing the patient's pain level related to his or her disease or disability, it is important for the patient to rate that pain level and provide the location of the pain. The PTA can assess the patient's pain level through various methods, which will be discussed in the next section. Because these different types of methods are used to rate the patient's pain, the rating may seem more like an Objective statement or as though it is the judgment or opinion of the therapist (i.e., objective data; see Fig. 10–6). However, the documentation of pain is unique because the patient is providing the level of pain he or she is experiencing, the location of the pain, and what exacerbates the pain level as it relates to his or her disease or disability. For that reason, the pain level is an element of Subjective data and is documented in the "S" (Subjective) section of the SOAP-organized daily note.

However, if, in the course of treatment, the pain level changes, then it can be documented in the Objective data section. In this case, the treatment process has affected the pain level, and it would be reported following the treatment session. The pain report in the Subjective section is given prior to treatment. Any changes in pain can be addressed following treatment in the Objective section by reporting the type of intervention that either increased or decreased the pain level. This change in pain also may be addressed in the Assessment section, as will be shown in Chapter 12.

A patient's pain experience and perception of its intensity vary widely among individuals. Consider the example of dental experiences; some dental patients never need local anesthesia to have a cavity filled, whereas others need anesthesia, music played via headphones, and other distractions to make it through the procedure comfortably.

Pain is difficult to describe in words. Not only can patients experiencing similar levels of pain use different words to describe that pain but also different therapists may attribute different meaning to patients' descriptions.

Each facility has its own procedure for documenting pain. Typically, this information is documented in a pain profile. Several types of pain profiles are commonly used, including the verbal rating scale (VRS), checklists, and body drawings.

1. Patient rates pain a 6 on an ascending scale of 1–10 when climbing stairs.
2. Patient gives her pain a 4 on a pain scale of 1–7 where 1 is no pain and 7 is excruciating pain.
3. Patient reports his pain is 3/10 after massage compared to 6/10 before massage.
4.
```
|_____x_____|
 1  2  3  4  5  6  7  8  9  10
```

Figure 10–6 Examples of how the documentation of pain looks like objective data.

Pain Scales   Facilities often use a pain profile based on a numbered scale, usually from 0 to 10 or 1 to 7, with 0 or 1 denoting no pain and 7 or 10 denoting the worst pain imaginable. The patient rates the pain as a number on the scale (see Fig. 10–6). The scale should be described in the note (e.g., "0 = no pain, 10 = worst pain imaginable"; "1 is no pain, 7 is excruciating"). The pain rating may be documented as "5/10" or "3/7" if the definition of the scale has been described earlier in the record or chart or if the scale is one commonly used by that specific facility. When a patient rates pain, it is also important that he or she identify where the pain is located and what activity or exercise decreases or increases the pain level. It is also important for the PTA to note how the previous session affected the patient's pain level.

Checklists   Using a checklist with various words describing pain is another helpful method to document a patient's pain level. The patient simply checks the words that describe his or her pain. This checklist is included in the medical chart, and a note should be included in the Subjective data section of the daily note to instruct the reader to refer to the checklist. Figure 10–7 is an example of a checklist pain profile.

Body Drawings   The patient can also describe his or her pain by marking the location of the pain on an outline of a body drawing (Fig. 10–8). Patients can use symbols or colors to indicate the type and intensity of the pain at each location. Then this form is included in the medical chart for pain documentation and, again, should be noted in the Subjective section.

Regardless of the pain profile or technique used for documenting the pain, consistency in each note is essential. Inconsistent documentation hinders the determination of treatment effectiveness. Information on a pain scale cannot be compared with information on a body drawing. Comparing the initial profile with the pain reports throughout the treatment sessions can identify changes in the pain profile and document progress throughout the skilled therapy sessions.

Consistent documentation of pain provides a clear picture or measurement of treatment effectiveness and helps ensure reimbursement by third-party payers. It is important to understand

There are many words that describe pain. Some of these are grouped below. Check (✔) any words that describe the pain you have these days.

1.	5.	9.	13.	17.
☐ Flickering	☐ Pinching	☐ Dull	☐ Fearful	☐ Spreading
☐ Quivering	☐ Pressing	☐ Sore	☐ Frightful	☐ Radiating
☐ Pulsing	☐ Gnawing	☐ Hurting	☐ Terrifying	☐ Penetrating
☐ Throbbing	☐ Cramping	☐ Aching		☐ Piercing
☐ Beating	☐ Crushing	☐ Heavy		
☐ Pounding				

2.	6.	10.	14.	18.
☐ Jumping	☐ Tugging	☐ Tender	☐ Punishing	☐ Tight
☐ Flashing	☐ Pulling	☐ Taut	☐ Grueling	☐ Numb
☐ Shooting	☐ Wrenching	☐ Rasping	☐ Cruel	☐ Drawing
		☐ Splitting	☐ Vicious	☐ Squeezing
			☐ Killing	☐ Tearing

3.	7.	11.	15.	19.
☐ Pricking	☐ Hot	☐ Tiring	☐ Wretched	☐ Cool
☐ Boring	☐ Burning	☐ Exhausting	☐ Blinding	☐ Cold
☐ Drilling	☐ Scalding			☐ Freezing
☐ Stabbing	☐ Searing			

4.	8.	12.	16.	20.
☐ Sharp	☐ Tingling	☐ Sickening	☐ Annoying	☐ Nagging
☐ Cutting	☐ Itchy	☐ Suffocating	☐ Troublesome	☐ Nauseating
☐ Lacerating	☐ Smarting		☐ Miserable	☐ Agonizing
	☐ Stinging		☐ Intense	☐ Dreadful
			☐ Unbearable	☐ Torturing

Figure 10—7   An example of a checklist pain profile. (Adapted from the McGill Pain Questionnaire.)

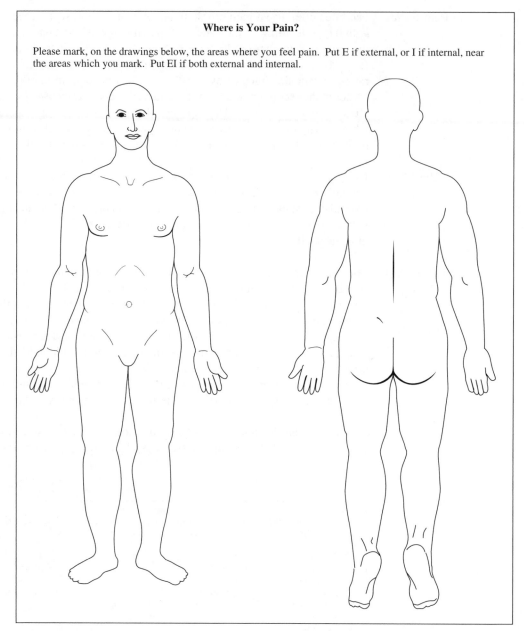

Where is Your Pain?

Please mark, on the drawings below, the areas where you feel pain. Put E if external, or I if internal, near the areas which you mark. Put EI if both external and internal.

Figure 10—8 An example of a body-drawing pain profile.

that although the pain profile provides an *objective* method for documenting pain, pain is documented in the *Subjective* section of the daily note. Students often make the mistakes of documenting pain in the Objective section by not providing an accurate rating in the Subjective data section, not identifying where the pain is located, and not providing a comparison rating or location for the pain level (e.g., stating "5" instead of "5/10 in the right knee").

Examples of Appropriate and Inappropriate Subjective Statements

When writing a Subjective statement, remember the information included in this section and outlined in this chapter. As discussed previously in this chapter, the information needs to be relevant to the patient's care. The following sections contain examples of appropriate and inappropriate statements.

Appropriate
Subjective Statements

- Mr. Jones reported his pain at 6/10 in his right shoulder when he arrived today.
- The patient's wife stated, "My husband was able to walk to the mailbox yesterday for the first time since therapy started."
- The patient stated, "I can reach in the kitchen cupboard to get a coffee cup now and my shoulder does not hurt at all."
- The patient reported that his pain increased to 8/10 following the last treatment session, with the new exercise using the 5-lb weight.

Inappropriate
Subjective Statements

- The patient went to the bar last night and reported he had too much to drink.
- The patient's wife stated, "I am taking my husband with me to the beauty parlor when we leave therapy."
- The patient stated, "I need to pick up some more clothes at the mall when I am through today."
- Mr. Jones said, "My dog was happy for me to come home yesterday."

SUMMARY Information told to a PT or PTA by the patient, significant other, or other caregiver is documented as Subjective data in the daily note. The information must be relevant to the patient's physical therapy diagnosis or treatment. PTs and PTAs use a variety of listening skills to identify relevant information. This information can be paraphrased or quoted verbatim in the daily note. Including information from a patient that has already been documented in previous notes is not necessary. Although appearing more like objective data, comments regarding pain and structured pain profiles are documented within the Subjective data section.

REFERENCE

1. Subjective. (2011). In *Merriam-Webster's online dictionary*. Retrieved from http://www.merriam-webster.com/dictionary/subjective

Review Exercises

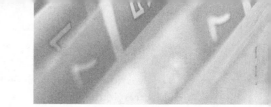

1. What **three types** of listening provide more information than other types of listening for the Subjective section?

2. List **two** of your own examples of subjective statements that are appropriate and **two** of your own examples of subjective statements that are inappropriate for documentation.

3. The following statement was reported to the treating therapist, at the beginning of the treatment sessions. Is it an **appropriate** statement? **Why** or **why not?**
   "The patient reported that she spent 2 hours sitting at the beauty shop yesterday and was too tired to perform her exercises last night, due to increased pain in her low back from 2/10 to 8/10, once she returned home."

4. **Describe** the information documented in the Subjective section of a SOAP note.

5. **Why** is subjective information important in patient documentation?

PRACTICE EXERCISES

Practice Exercise 1 ➤ *While you have studied only subjective data, try to complete the following note with the information you have been given thus far. Think of two events that occurred recently in your life (e.g., a car problem and how you solved it, lost keys and how they were found) and write about them in SOAP format. Organize the information so what is told to you (the subjective data) is in the "S" section, measurable happenings and things you observed (objective data) are in the "O" section, the meaning of your conclusions regarding treatment (assessment data) is in the "A" section, and what you plan to do next is in the "P" section. Write one note in outline form with SOAP headings (Subjective, Objective, Assessment, Plan). Write another note in paragraph form with the information sequenced in SOAP organization but without headings.*

Problem: Lost car keys

Practice Exercise 2 ➤ *You have treated your patient and have taken notes about the treatment session. Identify the "S" sections of the SOAP note.*

1. ____A____ Outcome Ⓘ sit to stand met.

2. ____O____ Observed patient sitting in middle of couch upon arrival for treatment session.

3. ____S____ Patient expresses frustration that she can't get up from the couch without help, especially in evening.

4. _____ Dx: Multiple Sclerosis.

5. ____O____ Gross manual muscle testing (MMT) 3/5 all lower extremity muscle groups, 2/5 at initial evaluation (IE).

6. ____A____ PT Dx: Lower extremity weakness limiting ability to sit ↔ stand and ambulate safely.

7. ____S____ Patient reported his pain in his Ⓛ knee was still an 8/10 after doing his exercises.

8. ____O____ Instructed patient not to sit on couch in evening when fatigued and weak.

9. ____S____ Pt. states pain was 3/10 in the neck following the previous session.

10. ____P____ Will visit patient 2 more times and schedule PT's discharge.

Practice Exercise 3 ➤ *From the information provided, rewrite the subjective section of this note.*

12-26-16: Pt. has met his short-term outcome of Ⓘ crutch walking on level and uneven ground for 30 ft. Says he needs to be able to climb three flights of stairs to get into his apartment. Will work on stair-climbing next session. Used handrail on Ⓛ going up stairs. Pt. ambulated, non–weight-bearing Ⓡ, with axillary crutches, Ⓘ on grass and uneven sidewalk, 300 ft, Ⓡ ankle & foot edema. Circumference equals Ⓛ foot & ankle measurements (see initial evaluation). All Ⓡ ankle AROM WNL, Ⓡ knee flexion PROM 10°–110° (15°–100° last session). Pt. correctly demonstrated Ⓡ knee AROM & gentle stretching exercises (see copy in chart). Ⓡ lower extremity mobility progressing. Will inform PT that pt. will be ready for discharge evaluation next session. Limited lower extremity mobility and non-weight-bearing because of fractured femur, pinned 12-22-16. Pt. states he needs to ambulate Ⓘ to mailbox every day.

— Byana, PTA/Marisol, PT (Lic. #141230)

Practice Exercise 4 ➤ *Identify subjective information in the following list of statements by placing an "S" in the space provided.*

1. _____ Takahiro Tan, PTA (Lic. #010173)

2. ___*S*___ Patient complained of (c/o) itching around wound.

3. _____ 6/10/17

4. _____ Wound healing diameter is 2 cm smaller than at initial evaluation.

5. _____ During gait training, pt. Ⓘ ambulated with axillary crutches, toe-touch gait pattern on Ⓛ lower extremity, on grass, curbs, sidewalk, carpeting, in/out car, stairs.

6. _____ Good posture, good step-through gait.

7. _____ Whirlpool/105°F/sitting Ⓛ heel/to remove dressings/10 min

8. _____ Outcome for independent ambulation in home and community met.

9. _____ Will report to PT re: discharging gait training goal.

10. ___*S*___ Pt. reports he can use his two outside steps at his house Ⓘ.

11. _____ Diameter of wound 4 cm (6 cm at initial evaluation).

12. ___*S*___ Patient reported there was about a teaspoon of drainage that was clear and had no odor when he changed his dressing this am.

13. _____ Wound pink.

14. _____ Goal for healed wound 50% met.

15. ___*S*___ Patient says she feels comfortable and safe on the crutches.

16. _____ Sterile dressings applied per previous treatment procedures.

Practice Exercise 5 ➤ *You have been treating your patient, who had a Ⓡ CVA with Ⓛ hemiplegia, following the treatment plan on the cardex.*

Your patient has progressed, and the cardex needs to be updated, especially because you will be on vacation next week and another PTA will be seeing your patient. The patient reports that her pain level has decreased from a 9/10 during the last session to a 6/10 today, prior to treatment. The changes include the following: 5 repetitions Ⓛ active assistive scapular protraction in supine with active assistive elbow extension facilitated by tapping Ⓡ triceps muscle belly, Ⓡ upper extremity (UE) progressive resistive exercises (PREs), 2 lb, 10x/3 lb, 10×/4 lb as many reps as she can perform (stop at 10), 5-lb cuff wts., for all Ⓡ LE exercises, ambulate in // bars 2× (with max A of 2) to facilitate wt. shift and to control knee, using temporary ankle-foot orthosis (AFO) on ankle, sitting balance now min assist of 1, now Ⓘ with wheelchair (w/c) mobility as brings self to therapy. Standing table discontinued. Other upper extremity exercises the same.

1. Document these new changes by identifying *only* the *subjective* information:

DX: Ⓡ CVA, Ⓛ hemiparesis _____   INITIAL DATE: July 24, 2017

Pain has decreased since last visit from 9/10 to 6/10 for this visit

PRECAUTIONS: ___None___   UPDATE: July 26, 2017

Exercise	set	rep	equipment	assist	Goals
AAROM Ⓛ Scap/supine c̄ Elbow Extension	1	5	w/c	min/1 & AA of elbow	Ⓘ with w/c mobility to and from therapy session from room on rehab unit (approximately 500 feet), D/C standing table
Ⓡ UE PREs	1	10	2, 3, & 4lb wt.	min/1	Same goal/perform with tapping on triceps mm belly
Ⓡ LE	1	5	5 lb wt.	min/1	Same goal
					TDD:
					TDP:
No change in Ⓛ UE ex.					

Patient Name	Age	Sex	MD	PT	RM#	Units
Jennifer Ramunto	54	F	Dr. Raines	Isaiah Morris	502	Rehab Unit

Transfers	Method	Assist	Other
			Ⓘ sit c̄ min Ⓐ

Pregait/Gait

Amb. in // bars 2x with max assist of 2 to facilitate wt shift to Ⓛ and knee control with AFO on Ⓛ ankle.

Practice Exercise 6 ➤   *Place a check mark next to the sentences that would go in the Subjective section of documentation of patient care.*

1. _____ The patient stated that she likes the PTA's new shoes.

2. ___S___ The patient's husband confirmed that the patient took her pain medication a half hour before her physical therapy appointment.

3. _____ The PT stated that the patient will continue working on the current home exercise program (HEP) until the patient can ambulate independently.

4. _____ The patient demonstrated normal ROM in the Ⓡ elbow.

5. ___S___ The patient stated that she has a job interview tomorrow and will not be able to attend her therapy appointment.

6. _____ The patient was able to ambulate independently on uneven surfaces up to 30 ft with axillary crutches.

7. ___S___ The patient's wife said that they are going shopping at the new bookstore after he is done with his therapy.

8. _____ The patient will be seen 1x/wk for PT at the outpatient clinic.

9. _____ The patient became fatigued after walking 20 ft on even surfaces with the FWW.

10. ___*S*___ The patient said that she is motivated to do well in her physical therapy so she can return to her hobby of roller derby.

Practice Exercise 7 ➤ *Make corrections to the "S" section of the following SOAP note. Some sentences may need to be omitted.*

S: He was seen today for a PT session in his home as per the PT's POC. He said that he woke up frequently last night with pain in his lower back of 7/10. The patient was able to sit in a chair for 15 min while doing his exercises. He rated his pain at a 7/10 while performing his exercises. His daughter said that the patient completed all of his exercises 2x, yesterday afternoon.

_____

_____

_____

_____

_____

_____

Practice Exercise 8 ➤ *Write "Pr" next to statements that describe the physical therapy problem or diagnosis and "S" next to statements that fit the Subjective data category.*

1. ___*S*___ Pt. states she has a clear understanding of her disease and her prognosis.

2. ___*S*___ Pt. expresses surprise that the ice massage relaxed her muscle spasm.

3. _____ Muscle spasms Ⓛ lumbar paraspinals with sitting tolerance limited to 10 min.

4. ___*S*___ Pt. describes tingling pain down back of Ⓡ leg to heel.

5. _____ Dependent in ADLs because of flaccid paralysis in Ⓡ upper and lower extremities.

6. ___*S*___ Sue states her Ⓛ ear hurts.

7. _____ Unable to reach behind back because of limited ROM in Ⓡ shoulder internal rotation.

8. ___*S*___ Reports he must be able to return to work as a welder.

9. ___*S*___ Patient states the doctor told her she had a laceration in her Ⓡ VMO.

10. _____ Paraplegic 2° SCI at T12 and dependent in w/c transfers.

11. ___*S*___ States Hx of RA since 1980.

12. ___*S*___ Pt. denies pain with cough.

13. __S__ States injury occurred December 31, 1999.

14. _____ Pt. c/o having to sit for 2 hours in the classroom lectures. *Is this pertinent → to their condition?*

15. _____ Weakness of grip strength and inability to turn doorknobs because of carpal tunnel syndrome.

16. __S__ Describes his pain as "burning."

17. _____ Unable to sit because of decubitus ulcer over sacrum.

18. _____ Unable to feed self because of limited elbow flexion.

19. __S__ Pt. rates her pain a 4 on an ascending scale of 1 to 10.

20. __S__ States able to sit through a 2-hour movie last night.

Practice Exercise 9 ➤

1. For each of the statements in Practice Exercise 8 to which you answered "Pr," <u>underline</u> the impairment and (circle) the functional limitation.

2. For each of the statements in Practice Exercise 8 to which you answered "S," <u>underline</u> the verb in the statement that specified it was subjective.

3. List the medical diagnoses you can find in the statements.

_____

_____

_____

_____

_____

_____

_____

_____

_____

Practice Exercise 10 ➤   *Place "Yes" next to relevant subjective statements and "No" next to those that do not seem relevant.*

_____N_____ 1. Client stated her dog was hit by a car last night and she buried him under her flower bed.

_____Y_____ 2. Client reported he progressed his exercises to 50 push-ups yesterday.

_____N_____ 3. Patient's daughter stated she traveled from Iowa, where it has been raining for 2 weeks.

_____N_____ 4. Patient states he does not like the hospital food and is hungry for some ice cream.

_____Y_____ 5. Patient rates her pain a 4/10 on an ascending scale of 0–10.

_____Y_____ 6. Patient states she is now able to reach the second shelf of her kitchen cupboard to get a glass.

_____Y_____ 7. Patient reports he had this same tingling discomfort in his right foot 3 years ago.

_____Y_____ 8. Client reports experiencing an aching in his "elbow bone" after the ultrasound treatment yesterday.

_____N_____ 9. Patient says she has 10 grandchildren and 4 great grandchildren.

_____N_____ 10. Client states she forgot to tell the PT that she loves to bowl.

_____N_____ 11. Client reports that *NCIS* is his favorite TV program.

_____ 12. Client reports he sat in his fishing boat 3 hours and caught a 7-pound northern pike this weekend.

_____Y_____ 13. Client states he played golf yesterday for the first time since his back injury.

_____N_____ 14. Client states he shot a 56 in golf. (if Par 72, then Y) ☺

_____Y_____ 15. Client states she cannot turn her head to look over her shoulder to back the car out of the garage.

_____N_____ 16. Patient's mother wants to know when her son will come out of the coma.

_____N_____ 17. Client reports he wishes he had not been drinking beer the night of his accident.

_____Y_____ 18. Patient describes his flight of stairs with ten steps, a landing, then five more steps, and the railing on the right, when going up the steps.

_____N_____ 19. Client wishes it would rain, as her prize roses are dying.

_____Y_____ 20. Patient states, "I'm going to Macy's to shop and have lunch today." fxn (Patient is 89 years old and is a resident in a long-term-care facility in a small town in Ohio. She has been placed on some new medication.)

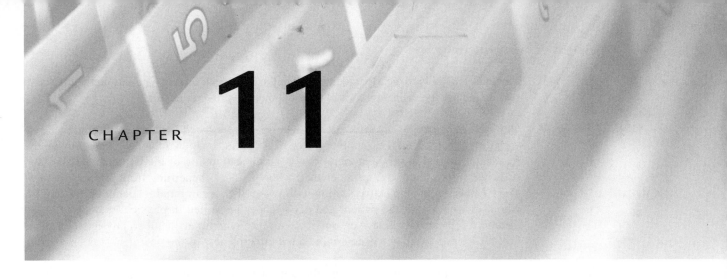

CHAPTER **11**

What Are Objective Data and Why Are They Important?

LEARNING OBJECTIVES
INTRODUCTION
OBJECTIVE DATA
ORGANIZING OBJECTIVE DATA
WRITING OBJECTIVE DATA

SUMMARY
REFERENCES
REVIEW EXERCISES
PRACTICE EXERCISES

LEARNING OBJECTIVES

After studying this chapter, the student will be able to:

☐ Identify objective data and differentiate it from subjective data
☐ Organize objective data for easy reading and understanding
☐ Demonstrate adherence to recommended guidelines for documenting objective data
☐ Document the patient's activities to provide the reader with a picture of the patient's functional capabilities
☐ Document interventions so they are reproducible by another PTA or a PT
☐ Document objective data consistent with the data in the PT's initial evaluation
☐ Identify common mistakes students make when documenting objective data
☐ Explain the differences between subjective and objective information

INTRODUCTION

Merriam-Webster's Online Dictionary defines the word *objective* as "expressing or dealing with facts or conditions as perceived without distortion by personal feelings, prejudices, or interpretations."[1] In the SOAP note format, Objective data are identified by the letter "O" and include only information that can be reproduced or confirmed by another professional with the same training as the person who gathered the initial information. For example, if the initial evaluation measures the range of motion (ROM) in shoulder (SHLD) abduction (ABD) to 170° using a goniometer, another therapist should be able to duplicate that measurement, provided the two individuals have similar training. For this section of the SOAP note, any measurement taken, equipment used, position in which the patient is placed during treatment, and so forth should be reproducible to provide continuity in patient care that is warranted for appropriate reimbursement. This information is gathered by measurable and reproducible tests and observations. It must be described in terms of functional movement or actions. These are the signs of the patient's disease or dysfunction and are recorded in the Objective section of a SOAP note, immediately after the Subjective section.

Whoever reads the Objective data in the PTA's daily note should be able to form a mental picture of the patient, the interventions performed, the patient's response to the interventions, and the patient's functioning before and after the interventions. The PTA should write the Objective data so the words paint a picture of the patient and the treatment session. The reader should also be able to clearly understand that the interventions provided during the treatment session require the skills of a trained physical therapy provider (PT or PTA).

OBJECTIVE DATA

Objective data include any information that can be reproduced or observed by someone else with the same training (i.e., another PT or PTA). When written, Objective data provide the reader not trained in physical therapy with an understanding of the treatment session and sufficient information to determine whether the patient is benefiting from physical therapy. The PTA writes the Objective section with two audiences in mind: (1) another PT or PTA who also works with the patient and (2) a reader untrained in physical therapy (e.g., an insurance representative, lawyer, quality assurance committee member, physician, or other health-care provider) who is determining the effectiveness of the treatment session.

ORGANIZING OBJECTIVE DATA

Six general topics are appropriate for the Objective section of the progress note:

1. The results of measurements and tests
2. A description of the patient's function
3. A description of the interventions provided
4. The PTA's objective observations of the patient
5. A record of the number of treatment sessions provided
6. Any patient education that was included in the treatment session for that day

The information in the Objective section of the progress note is organized to flow from one topic to the next, thus making the information easy to read. Similar information should be grouped together. For example, intervention descriptions, results of measurements and tests, and descriptions of the patient's functioning should be organized into three distinct groups, like this: "Patient (pt.) supine; knees bent, feet flat on mat, pt. completed bridging exercises (ex.), independently Ⓘ, 10x/3 sets for increased core stability."

It is helpful for the treating therapist to "paint a picture" of the treatment session so it is possible to duplicate the session if another therapist needs to treat the patient at a later date. For additional clarification regarding information that should be included in the Objective section of the SOAP note, review the SOAP note rubric included in Appendix C.

WRITING OBJECTIVE DATA

The objective data from the initial evaluation consist of information relevant to the patient's chief complaint and the reason the patient is seeking physical therapy care. These data form the basis for designing the treatment outcomes, goals, and the plan of care (POC). The objective data must consist of measurable, reproducible information so the efficacy of physical therapy treatment procedures can be determined through research of the progress note—for example: "Pt. seated, active range of motion (AROM) in left Ⓛ shoulder flexion (flex) was measured to 90° secondary (2°) to pain (7/10) with 2x/1 set." When appropriate, the PTA should relate the objective data in the progress note to the same information in the initial evaluation report or in previous notes for comparison (e.g., "Pt. seated, AROM in Ⓛ shld flex was measured to 90° 2° to pain (7/10) with 2x/1 set as compared with Ⓛ shld flex to 80° due to pain 10/10 at initial evaluation"). Some objective data can be charted or graphed to provide a quick picture of progress.

Results of Measurements and Tests

All of the activities or areas specifically mentioned in the section on outcomes and goals in the evaluation report should be reassessed and recorded in the progress notes and in the interim and discharge evaluation reports. The PTA determines the patient's progress by readministered the measurements and tests from the initial evaluation that the PTA is trained to perform. These results are then compared with the results either in the initial evaluation report or in previous progress notes, if the patient has been receiving physical therapy for a long period of time. For the comparison to be valid, the retest or measurement must follow the same procedures and techniques that were used when the initial evaluation was performed. The documentation of the results must be consistent. For example, if the measurements were in centimeters in the initial evaluation, they should continue to be documented in centimeters in subsequent reassessments by the PTA.

ROM
MMT
girth
vitals
Standardized tests

The documentation of results may be in the form of either a comment referring the reader to previous results (e.g., "See distance walked in note dated 8-2-17") or an actual written comparison with the results of the previous measurements or tests. Consider the following scenario:

> PTA Takahiro is treating Mr. Vasquez with compression pump therapy to decrease edema in the Ⓛ ankle. Measurements of the circumference of Mr. Vasquez's Ⓛ ankle were taken in the initial evaluation (on 8-10-17) to determine the extent of the edema. Today, after five treatments, PTA Takahiro re-measures the circumference of the ankle and compares his results with the initial evaluation measurements to prove that the edema has decreased and the compression pump intervention is effective. Takahiro could record the measurements in a table format in the Objective section for easy comparison. Figure 11–1 illustrates measurements presented in table form.

> In this example, the reader can easily compare results and see that the edema has decreased and the patient is benefiting from the compression pump intervention. Another PTA could follow the directions and duplicate the measurement procedure. Other measurements and tests performed by PTAs, with guidelines for documenting the results, are described in Box 11–1.

Description of the Patient's Function

The PTA documents improvement by describing the patient's function. For example: "At the initial evaluation, Mr. Wilson could not fit his Ⓛ foot into his running shoe because of the edema in the Ⓛ foot and ankle. Today, he was able to get his Ⓛ foot into the shoe, with the help of a shoehorn." The next day, another PTA could duplicate the assessment by watching Mr. Wilson use a shoehorn to put on his left running shoe. This is a good way to document intervention effectiveness because it "paints a picture" of the patient and describes clearly how the physical therapy interventions are improving the patient's ability to function in his environment. The functional activities must be those specifically mentioned in the goals or functional outcomes in the initial evaluation.

When a comparison of the data shows that the patient's functional status has not changed, be sure all methods for measuring change have been used. For example, a patient may continue to need the assistance of one person for ambulation, but the time it takes the patient to walk from the bed to the bathroom may have decreased. Include the following information when describing the patient's function:

- The patient's functional skill (e.g., ambulation, transferring, stair climbing, lifting, sweeping, sitting, standing, moving from sit to stand or stand to sit)
- Quality of the movement when performing the function (e.g., even weight-bearing, smooth movement, reciprocal gait pattern, correct body mechanics, speed)
- Level of assistance needed (e.g., independent; verbal cues; tactile guidance; supervision; standby assist or contact guard assist; minimal, moderate, or maximal assist; dependent)
- Purpose of the assistance (e.g., verbal cueing for gait pattern, for recovery of loss of balance, for added strength, to monitor weight-bearing, to guide walker)
- Equipment needed (e.g., ambulation aids, orthotics, supports, railings, wheelchair, assistive devices)
- Patient position (e.g., supine, prone, sitting, standing)

	8-10-17	8-15-17
Center Ⓛ lat. malleolus		
1" inferior to center Ⓛ lat. malleolus	6"	4"
1" superior to center Ⓛ lat. malleolus	5.5"	3"
All measurements taken along the superior edge of the marks.	6"	4"

Figure 11–1 Documentation of measurements in a table form.

Box 11–1   Other Measurements and Tests Performed by PTAs With Guidelines for Documenting the Results

Guidelines

All measurements and tests must be performed and documented in the same manner that they were performed and documented in the PT's initial evaluation. The documentation should include, when applicable:

1. Exactly what is being measured or tested, and on which side
2. If a motion is being tested, whether it is active or passive
3. The position of the patient
4. The starting and ending points, the boundaries, and the measurement points above and below the starting point
5. The same scale of measurement (e.g., inches, centimeters, degrees) that was used in the initial evaluation

Measurements

· Tape measurements
· Girth or circumference
· Leg length
· Wound size
· Step and stride length
· Neck and trunk range of motion
· Goniometry of all joints

Tests

· Manual muscle test of muscle groups
· Gross sensory testing

Vital Signs

· Heart rate
· Respiratory rate
· Blood pressure

Standardized Functional Tests*

· Functional Independence Measure (FIM)
· Barthel Index
· Tinetti Assessment Tool
· Peabody Developmental Motor Scales—2nd Edition (PDMS-2)

---

*These are some examples of the many tests available.

■ Distances, heights, lengths, times, weights, and types of surfaces (e.g., 300 feet, 10 meters; 6 minutes; top shelf of standard-height kitchen cabinet; floor to table, a distance of 36 in.; 20 pounds; linoleum, carpet, grass, and uneven surfaces)
■ Environmental conditions (e.g., level surface, carpeting, dim light, outside, ramps, low seat, cold)
■ Cognitive status and any complicating factors (e.g., patient understanding, ability to follow directions, fainting easily, blood pressure or oxygen saturation levels need monitoring, at risk for falls)

Standardized Functional Assessments   Many tools with set protocols and procedures, clear instructions, and methods for rating or scoring a patient's level of function are available. Some examples include the Tinetti Assessment Tool,[2] the Peabody Developmental Motor Scales—2nd Edition (PDMS-2),[3] the Barthel Index,[4] and the Functional Independence Measure (FIM).[5] If a standardized assessment tool is used in the initial evaluation, the PTA, when trained in the use of the tool, can reassess the patient's functional abilities and refer whoever reads the daily note to the copy of the completed assessment form in the chart. The assessment tool describes the function of, and changes in, the rating score as evidence of improvement in functional abilities and progress toward the functional outcome identified in the initial evaluation and the POC. Such tools are very helpful when utilized to determine functional outcomes with functional limitation reporting, as discussed in Chapter 3.

Description of the Interventions Provided

What treatment was provided

The Objective data may include information about the treatment parameters, sets and repetitions of exercises, or other tests and measurements that can be recorded. The interventions may be described in the daily note, recorded on a flow chart, or described on a separate form elsewhere in the medical record (with a note referring the reader to the separate location). In addition, this information may be a combination of narrative progress notes and checklists. In addition to being recorded in the medical record, often the interventions are detailed on a cardex located in the physical therapy department. The PTA should follow the protocol for the specific facility in which he or she works.

Intervention details must be complete and thorough so that the intervention can be duplicated when the patient is being treated by another therapist. The following information should be included for the intervention description to be reproducible:

1. The modality, exercise, or activity
2. Dosage, number of repetitions, and distance
3. The exact piece of equipment, when applicable
4. Settings of dials or programs on equipment
5. Target tissue or treatment area
6. Purpose of the treatment
7. Patient positioning
8. Duration, frequency, and rest breaks
9. Other information that the therapist needs to be aware of that is outside standard procedure or protocol (e.g., a cane is adjusted higher than the height determined by standard procedure because the increased height provided greater assistance to the patient for ambulation)
10. Anything that is unique to the treatment of that particular patient (e.g., complicating factors, such as taking the patient's pulse rate every 5 minutes or oxygen saturation levels prior to and following the treatment sessions)

Appendix D provides guidelines for documenting specific interventions.

The intervention description should include or be combined with a description of the patient's response to the intervention. For example: "Decreased muscle spasm (decreased muscle tone) was palpable following ice massage, due to numbing response (7 min), paraspinal mms, L3–5, with pt. prone over one pillow."

The details of the intervention can also be included to describe function. For example: "Following instructions regarding appropriate step length and posture control, pt. safely walked using axillary crutches, non weightt.-bearing (NWB) on Ⓛ foot, from bed to dining room (50 ft) on tiled level surface with standby assist (SBA) for support for loss of balance (LOB) recovery 2X."

In these two examples, a reader untrained in physical therapy can visualize the patient's performance, and another PTA could duplicate the interventions.

A copy of any written instructions or information provided to the patient, as part of the treatment session, should be placed in the medical record. Frequently, the PTA gives the patient or a caregiver written instructions for exercises or activities that were taught during the treatment session, such as a home exercise program (HEP). This is noted in the Objective data, and the reader is informed that a copy is in the chart. When the reader can reproduce the intervention by following the written instructions on the handout, it is not necessary to describe the exercises in the progress note. Figure 11–2 illustrates the objective documentation of a treatment session that includes instructing the patient in a home exercise program. In the Objective data section, any equipment that was given, lent, or sold to the patient should be noted.

> **O:** Following verbal instructions and demonstrations, pt. accurately performed home exercise program designed to strengthen Ⓡ hip abductors, extensors, and quadriceps, 5 reps of each ex. today. Pt. provided written instructions, refer to copy in chart.
>
> **O:** Pt. accurately demonstrated set-up of home cervical polyaxial traction unit; gave self 10-min intermittent traction,15 lb, approximately 5 sec on, 3 sec off, supine. Pt. provided written instructions, see copy in chart.

Figure 11—2 Objective documentation of a treatment session that included instructing the patient in a home exercise program.

PTA's Objective Patient Observations

A description of what the PTA sees or feels (visual and tactile observations) constitutes objective data if it is an observation that another PT or PTA with the same training would also make or if the observation could be duplicated or confirmed by another PT or PTA. Two examples of objective observations are (1) describing reddened skin over a bony area after application of hot packs, such as "a nickel-size, reddened area noted over inferior angle of left scapular after hot pack treatment," and (2) describing the patient's gait pattern or how the patient walks, such as "client walks with an antalgic gait; trunk held in a slightly forward-leaning posture, minimal arm swing, no pelvic rotation, uneven step length, and shortened stance time on compared with Ⓛ."

Proof of the Necessity for Skilled Physical Therapy Services

Anyone who reads the daily note must come to the conclusion that the physical therapy services that the patient received required the unique skills of physical therapy–trained personnel. With this in mind, the PTA should constantly be asking him- or herself, "Could someone not trained in physical therapy do what I have just described?" If the instructions presented in this chapter are being followed, the PTA is well on the way to writing the Objective data so they describe the need for skilled services. Comparing the Objective data in the daily note with the Objective data in the initial evaluation is one way of proving that skilled services are needed.

Careful selection of terms is also important. For example, PTs and PTAs do not *walk, ambulate,* or *transfer* their patients; they *teach, educate,* or *train* their patients in proper gait patterns or appropriate transfers. Therefore, the intervention described in the daily note should be listed as gait training or transfer training, not simply ambulation. The note should describe the patient's response to the training or indicate whether the patient understood the instructions or learned the skill or technique (e.g., "During gait training, patient ambulated with axillary crutches, NWB on Ⓛ, needing contact guard assist [CGA] for security when recovering from occasional LOB, 30 ft on carpeting, 5X, responding to vc for correct posture and proper step-through pattern but needing frequent cueing first 2X and improving to needing one cue by 5X."). When the patient is taught something, such as exercises, body mechanics, or posture, the note should document either that the patient gave a correct and independent return demonstration of what was taught or that the patient needed additional instructions. Again, the note should use words to paint a picture of the patient's treatment session, provide enough information for another therapist to reproduce the therapy session, and provide appropriate progress within the POC to ensure continuity in care for the third-party payer.

It is not appropriate to ask a patient about his or her exercise program or what he or she has been doing with another therapist. The treating therapist should have enough information from the initial evaluation or previous notes to have a good idea of what the patient is doing, where he or she is functioning, and how much progress he or she has made within the POC. If not, the therapist who wrote the notes did not provide appropriate documentation! Again, any patient education that was performed during the treatment session should be included in the Objective section.

Record of Treatment Sessions

The PTA should keep track of the patient's attendance by recording the number of treatment sessions that have been provided in the daily note. "Documenting attendance reflects the patient's compliance and participation in rehabilitation."[6] The note should also identify appointments that the patient did not keep and the reason for not attending. When a third-party payer has limited the number of treatment sessions that a patient may receive, the daily note can be a method for tracking the number of sessions for discharge planning. The Objective data section can report the number of times the patient has been treated, and the information in the Plan section of the note can state how many more treatment sessions are scheduled.

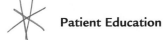

Patient Education

Patient education should also be included in this section. Patient education is related to teaching the patient exercises that will be included in the home exercise program and his or her ability to perform a correct and independent return demonstration of those exercises to the PTA. This allows the PTA to document that the patient received instruction in the home exercise program and that he or she was competent to perform it in a safe and appropriate manner when doing those exercises in the home setting.

Common Mistakes Students Make When Documenting Objective Data

The major mistake that PTA students make when writing Objective data, especially when documenting the interventions provided, is reporting what they did and not how the patient responded or performed—for example, "Instructed pt. in crutch walking, NWB Ⓡ." This statement refers to what the therapist did. However, it does not give the reader a picture of the patient's performance. The Objective section of the progress note is about the patient—it should describe the patient's response to the interventions. Examples of progress notes written by students describing what they did are found in Figure 11–3. Figure 11–4 shows those notes rewritten to include information about the patient's response.

When first learning to document, students tend to include information that is not relevant to the treatment. Organizing the information according to topics prevents rambling. Figure 11–5 is an example of an unorganized Objective section of a progress note. Figure 11–6 shows the same note with the information now grouped by topic.

For additional information regarding documentation specifics and support from APTA for appropriate documentation, see the documentation section on the APTA website.[7] You may want to review this website as you continue to review each section of the SOAP notes in subsequent chapters.

5-31-17: **PT Dx:** Sciatic nerve pain limiting sitting tolerance due to disc protrusion L4–5.
 S: Pt. stated he has pain extending down back of Ⓡ leg, and it came on "all of a sudden" while moving his TV set. He wished he could sit long enough to watch his son's hockey games. After traction and treatment, pt. reported pain no longer in leg but located in low back.
 O: Pt. demonstrated frequent wt. shifting and position changing while sitting for 15 min prior to tx. Gave mech. static lumbar traction to L4–5 area, 10 min, 90 lb, pt. prone over 1 pillow, table split, to decrease protrusion and pressure on nerve to decrease pain. Instructed pt. in ADL body mechanics, how to maintain lumbar lordosis at all times, and explained the process of a protruded disc. Instructed how to get on/off bed. Gave home instructions of McKenzie extension exercises.
 A: _____
 P: _____
 _____ Bayana Student, SPTA/Marisol Therapist, PT Lic #4321

11-11-17: **PT Dx:** Flexed posture, shuffling gait due to Parkinson's disease.
 S: Pt. states his legs feel stiff and he stumbles frequently. Feels he needs to hold on to something when he walks.
 O: Pt. observed using shuffling gait with hips, knees, and trunk in slight flexion. Min. knee flexion during pre-swing and initial swing. Instructed pt. how to walk with front-wheeled rolling walker, instructed heel to toe. Did reciprocal inhibition to quads to relax quads and increase knee flexion.
 A: _____
 P: _____
 _____ Bayana Student, SPTA/Marisol Therapist, PTA Lic #4321

Figure 11—3 Examples of a common mistake students make: writing the Objective section of the progress note in terms of what they did.

5-31-17: PT Dx: Sciatic nerve pain limiting sitting tolerance due to disc protrusion L4–5.
   S: Pt. states he has pain extending down back of Ⓡ leg, and it came on "all of a sudden" while moving his TV set. He wishes he could sit long enough to watch his son's hockey games. After traction & treatment, pt. reports pain no longer in leg but is located in low back.
   O: Pt. demonstrated frequent wt. shifting and position changing while sitting for 15 min prior to tx. tx: mech. static lumbar traction to L4–5 area, 10 min, 90 lb, prone over 1 pillow, table split, to decrease protrusion and pressure on nerve to decrease pain. Pt. demonstrated an understanding of spine and disc anatomy education, as well as instructions in maintaining a lumbar lordosis and correct body mechanics for ADLs by giving correct return demonstrations of lifting/reaching/bending/pushing/pulling body mechanics, by maintaining his lumbar lordosis when getting up off of the traction table, and by sitting without wt. shifts for 15 min using lumbar cushion. Pt. correctly performed McKenzie extension exercises per written instructions (see copy in chart).
   A: _____
   P: _____
   _____ Bayana Student, SPA/Marisol Therapist, PT Lic. #4321

11-11-17: PT Dx: Flexed posture, shuffling gait due to Parkinson's disease.
   S: Pt. states his legs feel stiff and he stumbles frequently. Feels he needs to hold on to something when he walks.
   O: Pt. observed using shuffling gait with hips, and trunk in slight flexion. Min. knee flexion during pre-swing and initial swing. After 3 reps, reciprocal inhibition exercise to quads bil, sitting, to relax the muscles and encourage knee flexion; pt. demonstrated improved knee flexion during the swing phase of gait. Pt. ambulated with a front-wheeled rolling walker, 100 ft in PT depart. on tiled floor, 3X with SBA, 1X for frequent verbal cues for heel–toe gait pattern and knee flexion. Pt. demonstrated erect posture with walker.
   A: _____
   P: _____
   _____ Bayana Student, SPA/Marisol Therapist, PT Lic. #4321

Figure 11—4   The notes in Figure 11-3 rewritten in terms of what the patient did.

5-3-17: PT Dx: No knee extension during gait due to biceps femoris tendon tear.
   S: Pt. states she feels more comfortable walking after US tx.
   O: Direct contact US/1 MHz/0.7 w/cm^2/5 min/CW/mild heat, prone to biceps femoris insertion to increase circulation, and promote healing of tendon. Working on increasing Ⓡ knee extension for initial contact. Quadriceps, hip flexors F+ strength (F in initial eval.). Ⓡ knee AROM before tx, 20–100°, after tx 15–100°. Manual resistance strengthening exercise to quadriceps and hip flexors with isometric contractions at end of range, 10X each, 6-sec hold. Instructed in home exercises (see chart). Assessed FWB gait, no Ⓡ heel contact. Pt. correctly demonstrated home exercises.
   A: _____
   P: _____
   _____ Jesus Jiminez, SPTA/Takahiro Sun, PT Lic #1006

Figure 11—5   A disorganized Objective section of the progress note in which the information rambles.

5-3-17: PT Dx: No knee extension during gait due to right biceps femoris tendon tear.
   S: Pt. states she feels more comfortable walking after US tx.
   O: Pt. demonstrated FWB gait but does not fully extend right knee at initial contact. After US and exercise treatment, pt. was able consciously to improve knee extension at initial contact. Direct contact US/1MHz/0.7w/cm^2/CW/mild heat, prone to right biceps femoris insertion to increase circulation, promote healing of tendon, and gain knee extension for initial contact in gait. Right quadriceps, hip flexors F+ strength (F in initial eval). Manual resistance strengthening exercise to right quads and hip flexors with isometric contractions at end of range, sitting, 10X each, 6-sec hold. Pt. correctly demonstrated home exercises to strengthen quads and hip flexors and gentle stretching exercises for hamstrings to gain knee extension during gait (see copy of written instructions in chart). Ⓡ knee AROM before tx 20–100°, after tx 15-100°.
   A: _____
   P: _____
   _____ Jesus Jiminez, SPTA/Takahiro Sun, PT Lic #1006

Figure 11—6   The note in Figure 11-5 rewritten with the information organized.

SUMMARY The objective data included in the progress note provide proof of interventions performed, their effectiveness, and the extent of patient progress, if any. This content must be measurable and reproducible. Objective data include intervention details, a comparison of the results of current measurements and tests with previous results, visual and tactile observations made by the PTA, and descriptions of the patient's functional abilities. The Objective section should be written so the words paint a picture of the patient and the treatment session, allowing the reader to visualize how the patient is functioning. The Objective data must be relevant to the chief complaint, the goals or functional outcomes, and the reason for the provision of skilled physical therapy services. PTs and PTAs need to ensure they are writing Objective data about the patient's actions, not the actions of the PT or PTA, during the patient's treatment session.

REFERENCES

1. Objective. (2011). In *Merriam-Webster's online dictionary*. Retrieved from http://www.merriam-webster.com/dictionary/objective
2. Tinetti Assessment Tool. (n.d.). Retrieved from http://www.bhps.org.uk/falls/documents/TinettiBalance-Assessment.pdf
3. The Peabody Developmental Motor Scales—2nd Edition (PDMS-2). (n.d.). Retrieved from http://www.proedinc.com/customer/productView.aspx?ID=1783
4. The Barthel Index. (n.d.). Retrieved from http://www.strokecenter.org/wp-content/uploads/2011/08/barthel.pdf
5. Functional Independence Measure (FIM). (n.d.). Retrieved from http://www.rehabmeasures.org/Lists/RehabMeasures/DispForm.aspx?ID=889
6. Baeten, A. M., Moran, M. L., & Phillippi, L. M. (1999). *Documenting physical therapy: The reviewer perspective*. Boston, MA: Butterworth-Heinemann.
7. American Physical Therapy Association. (2010). Defensible documentation for patient/client management. Retrieved from http://www.apta.org/Documentation/DefensibleDocumentation

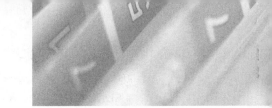

Review Exercises

1. **Describe** the **criteria** for information to be considered objective data.

2. List the **types** of information included in the Objective section of the SOAP note.

3. **Describe** how the results of tests and measurements are documented.

4. **Explain** what information should be included when describing the patient's function.

5. **Describe** what information needs to be included for the interventions to be **reproducible.**

6. Describe the **two** most common mistakes that students make when documenting objective data.

PRACTICE EXERCISES

Practice Exercise 1 ➤ *Write "Pr" next to the problem or PT diagnosis statements, "S" next to the subjective data statements, "O" next to the objective data statements, and "N/A" if none of the above applies.*

S _____ 1. Pt. complained of pain with prolonged sitting.

O _____ 2. Decubitus ulcer on sacrum measures 3 cm from Ⓛ outer edge to Ⓡ outer edge.

O _____ 3. Pt. ambulates with ataxic gait, 10 ft max. (A) to prevent loss of balance and to prevent falls.

O _____ 4. Knee flexion PROM 30°–90°.

O _____ 5. Walks c̄ standard walker, partial weight-bearing from bed to bathroom (20 ft), tiled surface, min. (A) 1X for balance.

S _____ 6. Pt. states he is fearful of crutch walking.

A _____ 7. Limited ROM in Ⓡ shoulder secondary to fractured greater tubercle of humerus and unable to put on winter coat without help.

S _____ 8. Complained of itching in scar Ⓛ knee.

O _____ 9. Transfers: supine ↔ sit c̄ min. (A) of 1 for strength.

A _____ 10. Unable to feed self with Ⓡ hand because of limited elbow ROM secondary to fracture of the Ⓡ olecranon process.

O _____ 11. Active range of motion is within normal limits (WNL), Ⓑ lower extremities.

_____ 12. Pt. demonstrated adequate knee flexion during initial swing c̄ vc p̄ hamstring exercises. *ICK!*

A _____ 13. Dependent in bed mobility due to dislocated Ⓛ hip.

S _____ 14. Expresses concern over lack of progress.

O _____ 15. Ⓛ shoulder flexion passive range of motion (PROM) 0°–100°, lateral rotation, PROM 0°–40°.

_____ 16. Kirsten reports PTA courses are easy.

O _____ 17. Pt. pivot transfers, non-weight-bearing (NWB) Ⓡ, bed ↔ w/c, max. (A) 2X for strength, balance, NWB cueing.

S _____ 18. Pt. rates Ⓡ knee pain 5/10 when going up stairs.

O _____ 19. BP 125/80 mm Hg, pulse 78 BPM, regular, strong.

Practice Exercise 2 ➤   *For this practice exercise, please follow the instructions listed below:*

1. For each of the statements in Practice Exercise 1 marked "Pr," <u>underline</u> the impairment and ⟨circle⟩ the functional limitation.

2. For each of the statements in Practice Exercise 1 marked "S," <u>underline</u> the key verb that led you to determine it was an "S" statement.

3. For each of the statements in Practice Exercise 1 marked "O," <u>underline</u> the key information that led you to determine it was an "O" statement.

4. List the medical diagnoses you can find in the statements in Practice Exercise 1.

_____

_____

_____

_____

_____

_____

_____

_____

_____

Practice Exercise 3 ➤   *Review each of the following statements documenting the results of a test or measurement. Write what, if anything, is missing or incorrect in the documentation. If the statement is fine, write "N/A" in the comment section. An example follows:*

The patient was able to walk 20 feet today.
    Comment: This statement tells the therapist how far the patient was able to walk but does not say anything about the patient's dependence level, equipment used, type of

surface, etc. A more appropriate statement would be: "Today the patient, with a Ⓛ CVA, was able to walk 20 ft, 2X, with CGA and the use of a FWW on an even surface c̄ Ⓡ step length ½ that of Ⓛ step length despite vc."

1. Mrs. Sawyer was able to use a stand-pivot transfer from the bed to the wheelchair, independently with SBA and verbal cueing.

    Comment: _____

    _____

    _____

    _____

    _____

2. The patient, with an L1 SCI, was able to move from the floor to the mat.

    Comment: _____

    _____

    _____

    _____

    _____

3. Pt. in sitting, Ⓛ knee flexion measured 0°–63° PROM today (0°–55° in initial evaluation).

    Comment: _____

    _____

    _____

    _____

    _____

4. Hip ROM 75°.

    Comment: _____

    _____

    _____

    _____

    _____

5. Hip abductor strength G– (good minus), 3/5 in initial evaluation.

Comment: _____

_____

_____

_____

_____

6. Left hip hyperextension with anterior pelvic tilt, prone, 20°.

Comment: _____

_____

_____

_____

_____

7. Circumference at Ⓡ olecranon process 4 inches, upper arm 6 inches, lower arm 3 inches.

Comment: _____

_____

_____

_____

_____

8. Blood pressure of 120/70, pulse 72.

Comment: _____

_____

_____

_____

_____

9. Circumference Ⓡ wrist, supine, upper extremity elevated 45°, 3rd metacarpal head 8 inches, 2 inches superior to 3rd metacarpal head 8 inches, superior edge of ulnar styloid process 7 cm, taken along superior border of marks.

Comment: _____

_____

_____

_____

_____

10. Resting respiratory rate of 12 breaths per minute, relaxed, quiet, sitting position.

Comment: _____

_____

_____

_____

_____

11. Left shoulder flex 100°, abd 100°, external rotation 60°, internal rotation 40°.

Comment: _____

_____

_____

_____

_____

12. Left knee flex PROM, prone with towel under thigh, 20°–110° (30°–90° initial evaluation).

Comment: _____

_____

_____

_____

_____

13. Right leg 1 inch longer than left.

Comment: _____

_____

_____

_____

_____

14. Trunk forward bend 20%.

Comment: _____

_____

_____

_____

_____

15. Trunk side bend greater on right than left.

Comment: _____

_____

_____

_____

_____

16. Cervical rotation to right 0°–25°, aligned with nose, sitting position, shoulders stabilized.

Comment: _____

_____

_____

_____

_____

Practice Exercise 4 ➤ *Write each of the following objective statements more succinctly using the approved abbreviations in Appendix A. The first one has been done for you.*

1. Today, the patient's blood pressure in sitting, prior to treatment was 120/70, halfway through the treatment, while walking, his blood pressure was 130/80, and following the treatment, sitting, his blood pressure was 125/75 mm Hg.

   Revision: Pt. sitting BP $\bar{a}$ ex 120/70 mm Hg, during ex (walking) BP was 130/80 mm Hg, and $\bar{p}$ ex – pt. sitting BP was 125/75 mm Hg to monitor BP for abnormal increases $\bar{c}$ ex.

2. Patient lacked 20° of full active knee extension on the Ⓡ leg.

   Revision: _____

   _____

   _____

3. The patient moved from sitting in her w/c to standing in the // bars with the PTA giving the patient max (A).

   Revision: _____

   _____

   _____

4. The patient was instructed in ascending and descending 4 steps with the axillary crutches with the handrail on the Ⓛ side going ↑ and the Ⓡ side going ↓. The patient successfully ascended and descended the 4 steps with only vc from the PTA.

   Revision: _____

   _____

   _____

5. The patient was placed in a side-lying position on his Ⓛ side with a pillow behind his back so that US (1 MHz/1 W/cm²) could be applied for 7 min to Ⓡ shoulder.

   Revision: _____

   _____

   _____

Practice Exercise 5 ➤   *Rewrite the following notes so that the information given fits in either the "S" or "O" sections of a SOAP note and use the abbreviations in Appendix A. Write "N/A" in any section not used.*

Example:

The pt. stated his pain in his left hip decreased to 3/10 after last treatment. However, after driving home from the last treatment session, his pain increased to 5/10.

S: Pt. stated his pain was 3/10 p̄ the last Tx session but it ↑ to 5/10 by the time he had driven 40 minutes to his home.

O: N/A

1. Pt. is a 52-year-old female with a grade 1 medial collateral sprain on her Ⓡ side that occurred while she was skiing.

    S _____

    O _____

2. The patient reported that she wore her knee-immobilizing brace on the Ⓛ side to come to the clinic today because it felt unstable.

    S _____

    O _____

3. Patient, in sitting, was able to perform 3 sets of 15 ankle pumps on the Ⓡ side.

    S _____

    O _____

4. The patient said that she cannot bend her Ⓡ knee all the way yet because it is still very painful, with pain rated on a verbal rating scale (VRS) of 6/10.

    S _____

    O _____

5. Patient in supine was able to perform 3 sets of 10 isometric quadriceps sets on the Ⓡ side.

    S _____

    O _____

6. Patient, in supine, was able to perform 3 sets of 10 straight-leg raises on the Ⓡ side but complained of increased pain and needed a 3-minute rest period after completion.

    S _____

    O _____

7. The patient's motor vehicle accident occurred 5 days ago.

    S _____

    O _____

8. Patient said pain was 5 on verbal rating pain scale of 0–10 today when she arrived at the clinic.

S _____

O _____

9. Patient was positioned in a supine position with a pillow under her knee and given ice massage for 15 minutes to the Ⓡ knee following exercises today.

S _____

O _____

10. The patient said that she and her doctor do not want to do a surgical repair unless it is absolutely necessary.

S _____

O _____

11. The patient's active range of motion in the right knee is –10 to 100 degrees.

S _____

O _____

12. The patient reported she will see the orthopedic surgeon on September 2, 2017.

S _____

O _____

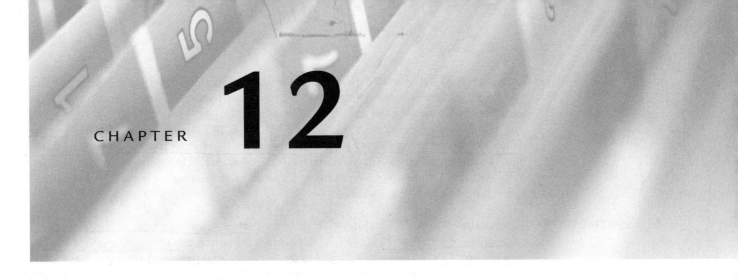

CHAPTER 12

What Are Assessment Data and Why Are They Important?

LEARNING OBJECTIVES	SUMMARY
INTRODUCTION	REFERENCES
ASSESSMENT DATA	REVIEW EXERCISES
ORGANIZING ASSESSMENT DATA	PRACTICE EXERCISES
WRITING ASSESSMENT DATA	
INTERPRETATION OF THE DATA IN THE	
DAILY NOTE	

LEARNING OBJECTIVES

After studying this chapter, the student will be able to:

☐ Identify assessment data

☐ Organize assessment data for easy reading and understanding

☐ Demonstrate adherence to recommended guidelines for documenting assessment data

☐ Document the patient's functional abilities to provide the reader with a picture of the patient's functional level and rate of progression

☐ Document interventions so they are reproducible by another PTA or a PT

☐ Document assessment data consistent with the data in the PT's initial examination

☐ Identify common mistakes students typically make when documenting assessment data

☐ Explain the differences among subjective, objective, and assessment information

INTRODUCTION

Merriam-Webster's Online Dictionary defines the word *assessment* as "the act of making a judgment about something; the act of assessing something."[1] In the Assessment section of the SOAP note, identified by the letter "A," the PT summarizes the subjective and objective information and answers the question, "What does it mean?" The PT also interprets, makes a clinical judgment, and sets functional outcomes and goals on the basis of the information in the Subjective and Objective sections. In the daily note, the PTA summarizes the information in the Subjective and Objective sections and reports the progress being made toward accomplishing the goals in the Assessment section for the patient's current visit. The PTA's summary also answers the "What does it mean?" question for each treatment session. This information ties into the initial and subsequent information to provide a timeline of continuity of care for the patient as he or she is progressing through the treatment process.

After reviewing subjective and objective data—the informative facts—whoever is reading the medical record may ask, "What does this information mean?" Readers of the record who are not trained in physical therapy (e.g., insurance representatives, lawyers, physicians) may not understand the subjective and objective data unless they are interpreted. The interpretation and significance of the subjective and objective data are reflected in the initial evaluation that had been completed by the PT as well as in the physical therapy diagnosis, the treatment plan and goals, and the treatment outcomes and effectiveness. These elements of the record support the necessity for the physical therapy treatment.

The PTA documents the significance of the data in the daily note by <u>describing the patient's response to the treatment plan</u> and the patient's <u>progress toward accomplishing the goals</u>. For ease of discussion in this chapter, this information will be referred to as interpretation of the data content. Interpretation of the data content is more complex in the PT's initial evaluation than in the PTA's daily notes.

ASSESSMENT DATA

Assessment data consist of information about the <u>patient's progress, treatment effectiveness, completion of goals</u> set by the PT in the initial evaluation, <u>changes recommended in the plan of care (POC)</u>, and <u>goals completed for the individual treatment sessions</u>. The PTA is responsible for communicating any recommended changes in the POC, completion of skills within the goals set by the PT, changes within the POC, and recommendations for discharge. Figure 12–1 provides information about data that supports the PTA's conclusion about the patient's progress toward the goal, including the patient's pain rating prior to and following the treatment session, correct demonstration of the home exercise program (HEP) by the patient, progress toward the outcome of safe stair use without a railing, and reciprocal step pattern at 0% this visit.

Goals or Functional Outcomes

INITIAL EVALUATION. Goals or functional outcomes are set by the patient and PT during the initial evaluation.

DAILY NOTE. Goals may need to be modified as the patient and the PTA become better acquainted and the PTA learns more about the patient's needs and desires. For example:

> Sam told the PT that he needs to be able to climb only two steps to get into his house; the rest of his house is on one floor. They set a stair-climbing goal: "To be able to climb two steps independently using the railing on the left and be able to ascend and descend a curb independently with no ambulation device." One week later, during a treatment session, Sam tells the PTA, Jesús, about his cabin on a nearby lake and how anxious he is to go to the cabin and go fishing. Sam casually mentions that there are six wooden steps down to the dock. Jesús makes a mental

---

6-15-17 PT Dx: Anterior rotation of right ilium limiting sitting and stair climbing tolerance.
Patient states she has been doing her home exercises regularly, can sit 45 minutes now, but still has pain when attempting to step up with her right leg. Reports feeling unsafe when carrying her 18-month-old daughter up the stairs. Rates her pain 7/10 before and after treatment. Pt. has been seen for three sessions. Direct contact US/1 MHz/vigorous heat/10 min/prone/right PSIS/to relax muscle spasms and prepare ligaments for mobilization. Pt. correctly performed muscle energy self-mobilization techniques to move ilium posteriorly. (See copy of instructions in chart.) Equal leg length observed supine and long sitting after US & mobilization, uneven leg length during same test before tx. Unable to palpate muscle spasms or level of PSIS due to patient's obesity. Patient correctly demonstrated her home exercises (see copy in chart), and used correct body mechanics to minimize right hip flexion when reviewing safe technique for picking up her baby. Ambulates with an antalgic limp, shorter step length and stance time on the right. Unable to step up on 7-inch stair with right leg, due to reporting too much pain. Sat with good posture, relaxed, minimal weight shifting 45 minutes watching nutrition video and waiting for her "ride." As patient was leaving the clinic, observed her climbing into her pick-up truck by stepping up with her right leg and using smooth, quick movements. This looked like it required approximately 80–90° hip flexion. Goal of 45-minute sitting tolerance met. Progress toward outcome of safe stair climbing without railing and using step-over-step pattern appears 0% in the clinic. Performance in the clinic of good sitting tolerance but poor stair climbing tolerance is inconsistent with patient's pain rating, equal leg length test, and observed performance outside the clinic. Will consult PT as to what should be done next treatment session. Pt. has two more treatment sessions scheduled. Kayla McLaughlin, PTA Lic. #439

Figure 12—1 Evidence in the data that supports the PTA's conclusion about progress toward the goal.

note to share this information with the PT. Jesús will suggest that the PT modify the goal set for household stair use to also include the use of stairs at the patient's cabin. Jesús also documents this information in the patient's medical record.

Response to Treatment

DAILY NOTE. Reporting the patient's ability to perform the prescribed treatment documents the effectiveness of the treatment program and influences future treatment plans. For example:

PTA Brenna treats Roberto, who has a mild lumbar disc protrusion and complains of waking up often at night with tingling in his left leg. During yesterday's treatment session, Brenna showed Roberto how to use pillows and a rolled towel to support his spine and maintain proper positioning while sleeping. Today, Roberto reports that he awoke only three times the previous night because of back soreness and did not have any tingling in his leg when he used the pillows for support. Brenna makes a mental note to quote Roberto in the subjective section of the daily note to provide evidence that her instructions in sleeping positions were effective and to report the information to the supervising PT to adapt the treatment plan to reflect goals toward strengthening and increased range of motion.

Level of Function in the Initial Evaluation

INITIAL EVALUATION. The initial evaluation describes the patient's functional level at the time of the examination.

DAILY NOTE. The patient's description of his or her functional level provided in the initial evaluation may help the PTA assess the patient's progress or response to treatment. For example:

PTA Maelee is treating Mr. Juarez, who had an acute flare-up of osteoarthritis in his hands. His chief complaint during the initial evaluation was an inability to get dressed, stating he had difficulty especially handling buttons and snaps because of the pain. Following the initial evaluation and some tips from the PT to help with this issue, the patient arrived for treatment today wearing a sweater. He said that he buttoned his sweater without needing to ask for help because he has been doing what the PT asked him to do to help with his range of motion. Maelee documents this fact in the daily note as possible evidence that Mr. Juarez has met a goal or outcome.

ORGANIZING ASSESSMENT DATA

The Assessment information in the initial evaluation may be more complex and detailed than the Assessment information in the daily notes. The PT may organize this information into subcategories, such as

- Active and passive range of motion (AROM and PROM)
- Strength
- Alignment
- Presence of any abnormal reflexes or responses
- Muscle tone
- Quality of movement
- Automatic reactions and balance responses
- Functional capabilities (e.g., transition in and out of different positions, ability to ambulate on even and uneven surfaces, ability to ascend and descend steps)
- The patient's functional outcomes for improvement in activity
- The function and reduction of any perceived pain
- The patient's ability to communicate and comprehend
- The patient's use of any adaptive equipment that may be used for mobility

Organizing content in this way helps the PT confine the data to only the categories that are relevant. Organizing the content makes it easy to read and to locate information. In Figure 12–2, the note presents Assessment information that does not include goals. The example in Figure 12–3 presents assessment data that are not necessarily supported by the Subjective and Objective portions of the note. For additional clarification regarding

---

6-15-17   Dx: ®̶ UE lymphedema 2° mastectomy.

PT Dx: Edema ®̶ UE limiting elbow ROM with inability to feed self and groom hair using ®̶ UE. Pt. states she is able to move her arm and use it more to help dress herself and to adjust her bed covers. Measurements taken before and after (I)CP/1 hr/50 lb/30 sec on 10 sec off/supine/®̶ UE elevated 45° to reduce edema. _____

	Before	After	3-4-16
Superior edge olecranon process	13"	12"	14"
3" above edge olecranon process	13.5"	12.5"	14.5"
3" below edge olecranon process	12.5"	11.5"	13.5"

All measurements read at superior edge of mark. Elbow flexion 0–95° today compared with 0–85° on 3-4-17. Observed pt. feeding self today using long-handled spoon in ®̶ hand. ICP effective in reducing edema and allowing increased ROM in elbow flexion. Pt. making progress toward goal of decreased edema and increased elbow room so pt. wil be independent in feeding and grooming hair without needing assistive devices. Will continue ICP treatment per PT initial plan.

Aaron Chapman, SPTA/Tamika Wright, PT Lic #1063

Figure 12—2 A daily note that does not mention the goals but confines comments to only the data that measure the impairment severity level and the treatment procedures.

A. Situation: Patient had stroke (CVA) 2 weeks ago and is now home, receiving physical therapy 3 times a week through a home health agency. His wife is the caregiver.

Dx: ®̶ CVA.

PT Dx: Ⓛ hemiparesis with dependent mobility in all aspects.

Expected functional outcomes: At anticipated discharge date in 1 month.
1. Patient will ambulate with an assistive device and minimal assist for balance to the bathroom and to meals in 3 weeks.
2. Patient will be able to manage two steps with an assistive device and a railing as well as car transfers for next visit to the doctor in 4 weeks.

Anticipated goals:
1. Pt. will consistently move up and down in bed and roll from side to side with SBA in 2 weeks.
2. Pt. will consistently roll to Ⓛ side and reach for telephone and call bell with SBA in 3 weeks.
3. Pt. will consistently move from supine to sitting on edge of bed and return to supine position with minimal assist to help swing Ⓛ leg into bed in 1 week.
4. Pt. will consistently move from sitting to standing and back to sitting from bed, toilet, wheelchair, and standard chair with minimum assist for balance, control, and even weight-bearing cueing in 2 weeks.
5. Using a quad cane, pt. will consistently ambulate bed to bathroom, and to meals with moderate assist for balance control and gait posture cueing in 1 week.

B. Situation: Patient is 1 week postoperation for total hip replacement and is in a subacute rehabilitation unit. Patient is receiving physical therapy 2X/day with plans to be discharged to home.

Dx: Ⓛ total hip replacement

PT Dx: Weakened hip musculature and dependent in rising from sit to stand and ambulation.

Expected functional outcomes: At anticipated discharge in 20 days, patient will transfer and ambulate independently for return to home.
1. Patient will independently and consistently move from sit to stand and stand to sit using elevated toilet seat, and all other surfaces no lower than 18 inches.
2. Patient will independently and consistently walk with a straight cane on all surfaces and in the community.

Anticipated goals:
1. Pt. will consistently be able to sit to stand and return with SBA if boost is needed from edge of bed, elevated toilet seat, wheelchair, and standard dining room chair in 10 days.
2. Pt. will consistently be able to ambulate using a straight cane for balance on tiled and carpeted level surfaces, to bathroom and dining room for meals with SBA for balance control in 10 days.

Figure 12—3 Daily note with assessment statements that are not supported by information in the subjective or objective data.

---

information that should be included in the Assessment section of the SOAP note, the reader can review the SOAP note rubric included in Appendix C.

WRITING ASSESSMENT DATA

APTA's "Guidelines for Physical Therapy Documentation" states that the evaluation report should include the physical therapy diagnosis or problem and the goals to be accomplished.[2] As noted previously, when organizing the evaluation information in SOAP format, the PT places this information in the "A" section. This section contains the PT's interpretation of the signs and symptoms, test results, and observations made during the evaluation, as well as a conclusion or judgment about the meaning or relevance of the information. The physical therapy diagnoses are based on this interpretation. Desired functional outcomes and anticipated goals are based on the problems. Thus, the subjective and objective information is summarized, and the "What does it mean?" question is answered in the Assessment section of the SOAP note.

It is important to note that any assessment information provided must be compared with the initial evaluation or with a previous treatment session to show progress, if any occurs (e.g., "The pt. was able to complete 3/5 trials of sitting with upright posture for 30 seconds compared with 1/5 trials for 10 seconds at the initial evaluation."). Such a statement not only provides a progression statement for the third-party payer but also delineates how much progress the patient has made compared with another point in time.

The Physical Therapy Diagnosis/Problem   The first conclusion the PT reaches after evaluating the data is the identification of the physical therapy diagnosis or problem (see Chapter 5). It is necessary to determine this information to develop an appropriate POC that addresses the patient's decreased level of function and restores the patient to the highest level of function possible following skilled therapeutic intervention.

Outcomes and Goals   The PT and the patient (or a representative of the patient) collaborate to establish the expected functional outcomes and anticipated goals for the duration of the physical therapy treatment. The APTA *Guide to Physical Therapist Practice* indicates that outcomes must relate to the patient's functional limitations or the reason he or she is receiving skilled therapy, and the goals should address current impairments.[3]

Expected Functional Outcomes   The statement of expected functional outcomes is a broad statement describing the functional abilities necessary for the patient to discontinue skilled physical therapy services and to be able to return to his or her prior level of function, if possible. Functional abilities are the abilities to perform activities or tasks that support the individual's physical, social, and psychological well-being, creating a personal sense of meaningful living.[3] When these abilities are regained, the patient's functional limitations and the disability identified in the physical therapy diagnosis or problem will be eliminated or decreased in severity. This is the criterion for the conclusion of the episode of skilled physical therapy care. The *Guide to Physical Therapist Practice* defines an episode of physical therapy care as "all physical therapy services that are (1) provided by a physical therapist or under the direction and supervision of a physical therapist, (2) provided in an unbroken sequence, and (3) related to the physical therapy interventions for a given condition or problem."[3] Again, such interventions must be skilled interventions provided by a licensed PT or PTA.

During a patient's episode of care, he or she may transfer to another facility (perhaps more than once) to stay on a continuum of skilled physical therapy services. Outcomes may be developed that describe the functional abilities that the patient will need to accomplish to be discharged from one facility and transferred to the next. These short-term outcomes are steps that must be completed to accomplish the overall expected functional outcome.

For example, a patient who has undergone total knee replacement surgery desires to return to independence in walking throughout her home and in the community. This becomes one of the expected functional outcomes for this patient's episode of physical therapy care. The hospital physical therapist works toward the short-term outcome of independent ambulation with a walker in the patient's room and bathroom and for short distances in the facility's hallways. When the patient accomplishes the functional outcomes within the hospital setting and is transferred to a rehabilitation facility, then physical therapy is directed toward the short-term outcome of independent ambulation with an appropriate ambulation device for longer distances and on even and uneven surfaces (e.g., carpeting, grass, gravel, stairs, and ramps).

When this goal is accomplished, the patient is discharged and transferred to the home setting where the home health-care or outpatient therapist works toward the overall expected functional outcome for this episode of care, which is independent ambulation without an ambulation device in the home and community.

Anticipated Goals

Anticipated goals describe the changes in the impairments necessary for the patient's function to improve. They are the steps for accomplishing the outcomes and thus should relate to the outcomes. For example, goals may describe the desired strength gain and improvement in range of motion and balance needed for the outcome to be accomplished. They may describe the progression of the quality of the movement, the efficiency of the task, and the assistance needed to eventually accomplish the functional outcome.

Writing the Functional Outcomes and Goals

While the supervising PT develops the actual short- and long-term goals, the PTA addresses these outcomes and goals in his or her daily notes. The outcomes and goals developed by the PT must be written to include (1) the action or performance (e.g., "was instructed to ambulate"), (2) measurable criteria that determine whether a task has been accomplished (e.g., "ambulated from bedroom to kitchen for a distance of 50 feet"), and (3) a time period within which it is expected the outcome or goal will be met (e.g., "in 1 week"). Then the PTA will follow these goals by addressing the measurable criteria as the patient progresses through those goals. Measurable criteria are the most important parts of the outcomes and goals. An action or performance can be measured in a variety of ways. A few examples of measurable criteria include the following:

- Strength grade
- Degrees of joint motion
- Scores on standardized tests
- Time of exercises or activities in seconds and minutes
- Description of the quality of the movement
- Proper posture and body mechanics
- Correct techniques
- Amount of assistance needed
- Assistive equipment needed
- Pain rating

When goals address specific impairments, they should also describe how the desired change in the impairment relates to the desired change in the functional limitation. A description of the change in function becomes another method of measuring the accomplishment of the goal and the best measurement to ensure third-party reimbursement. Examples of expected functional outcomes and anticipated goals are provided in Figure 12–4. Writing the outcomes and goals in this manner gives the PTA direction for planning treatment sessions that include activities enabling the patient's progression toward the goal, methods for measuring the patient's progress, and standards for determining when to recommend discharge from the treatment program.

Examples of goals relating to the desired change in the impairments and functional limitations include the following:

- ROM for left shoulder flexion will improve from 0° to 110° so patient can reach top of head for grooming in 2 weeks.

10-25-17   **Dx:** Ⓡ CVA.
    PT Dx: Ⓛ hemiparesis with dependent mobility in all aspects.
Pt. has been receiving PT twice a day for 3 days. Pt. able to lift buttocks with smooth motion 5X & scoot up and down in bed, roll 5X independently to Ⓛ side, roll to Ⓡ side with minimum assist to bring Ⓛ shoulder over 5X. Pt. practiced 3X moving from sitting on edge of bed to sidelying on three pillows and returned to sitting with minimum assist to initiate sidelying to sit 1X. Able to move from sit to stand and to return to sit from edge of bed with bed raised to highest level, SBA for cueing for even wt. bearing, 3X. Pt. ambulated from bed to bathroom to bed 3X using quad cane and moderate assist for balance and assist in advancing Ⓛ leg 2X. Pt. circumducts Ⓛ leg due to inability to flex knee during pre-swing. Pt. making progress toward goals of independent bed mobility, sit to stand with SBA and ambulation with quad cane and minimum assist. Will consult with PT about adding exercises for knee flexion with hip extended to improve gait next session. Jemma Ramunto, PTA Lic. #2961

Figure 12–4   Examples of expected functional outcomes and anticipated goals.

- Strength of right gluteus medius will increase to 4/5 so patient will no longer demonstrate a significant trunk shift to the right during stance phase of ambulation in 4 weeks.
- Amount of edema will decrease so girth measurements of right upper arm will be within 1 inch of left upper arm, and patient's right arm will fit into the sleeves of her clothing in 1 week.

In the first goal, the action or performance is left shoulder flexion, the measurable criteria are ROM from 0° to 110° and the patient's ability to reach the top of his or her head, and the time period is 2 weeks. In the second goal, the action or performance is increased strength, the measurable criteria are strength grade of 4/5 and no demonstration of a significant trunk shift to the right, and the time period is 4 weeks. The reader should determine whether the third goal is properly written. (The answer is provided at the end of the next paragraph.)

The PTA helping the patient to accomplish the first goal sees that the desired improvement in flexion needs to be met in 2 weeks. The PTA then plans each treatment session, based on the POC developed by the PT, to include appropriate exercises and activities that will increase the flexion range of motion. The PTA guides the exercises accordingly, monitoring progress by measuring the range of motion and observing the patient's attempts to touch the top of his head. At 2 weeks, the projected goal is for the patient to be able to perform left shoulder flexion through the range of motion from 0° to 110° and reach the top of his or her head. The PTA reports to the PT and records achievement of this goal in the daily note. Note: The third goal is appropriately written and addresses the ability of the patient to be able to wear her clothing without restriction.

The anticipated goals shown in Figure 12–4 also demonstrate proper formulation and writing. Some of the performance goals are scooting up and down in bed, rolling from side to side, and moving from sit to stand. The measurable criterion is standby assist, and the time period is 2 weeks. In this case, the PTA can structure the treatment sessions to include instructions and practice in bed mobility, rolling, and moving from sit to stand. The PTA will help the patient progress by decreasing the amount of assistance provided until the patient can perform these movements with only standby assist. One goal requires the PTA to work with the patient to improve the patient's ability to move from supine to a sitting position on the edge of the bed (action). The PTA will help the patient progress by decreasing the level of assistance provided, until only minimal assist is needed (measurable criterion). The PTA may choose to spend most of the treatment session time on this activity during the first week because the time period for meeting this goal is just 1 week. These goals describe functional tasks and do not include other impairments so a description of the patient performing the tasks with standby assist is the only measurable criterion needed. Goals could be written to include the quality or speed of the movements as other measurable criteria for these functional tasks.

Although the PTA does not determine the functional outcomes or the anticipated goals, he or she can work with the PT by offering suggestions, notifying the PT when goals are met, and recognizing when the PT needs to modify or change goals. A PTA may write goals for each individual treatment session, within the POC, to help the PTA stay focused on the patient's progress toward accomplishing the overall anticipated goals and the functional outcomes. The treatment session goals are the steps to accomplish the overall anticipated goals set by the physical therapist in the POC.

The PTA knows the patient's evaluation results and refers to the goals listed in the evaluation when writing the interpretation of the daily note data. This coordination of the goals outlined in the initial evaluation and those addressed in each daily note provides written proof of the PT–PTA team approach and communication related to the patient's care, thus enabling whoever reads the chart to determine the quality of care being provided.

INTERPRETATION OF THE DATA IN THE DAILY NOTE

Interpretation of the data is the PTA's summary of the daily note data with comments about the relevance and meaning of the information, and it is the most important section of the daily note. Most readers of the medical record look for this information first because it tells the reader whether skilled physical therapy services are necessary, are helping the patient progress within the prescribed POC, and are increasing the patient's functional abilities. It informs the reader of the patient's overall response within the POC. This is in contrast to the Objective section, which records the patient's response to each intervention. The reader of the daily note is told whether the patient is making progress toward accomplishing the outcomes and goals. Any comment made by the PTA must be supported by the subjective and/or objective information. The comments should be grouped or organized so the information is easy to follow and understand.

Change in the Impairment

A summary of the meaning of measurements and test results or observations recorded in the Objective data can describe a change in the severity of the impairment when this information is compared with the status of the patient at the initial evaluation. For example, if the Objective data include girth measurements of the patient's arm that are less than previous measurements and the patient's elbow flexion measurements show greater range of motion, then the PTA can comment that the intervention has been effective in decreasing swelling and thus improving the elbow's ability to move (decreasing the severity of the impairment) compared with the patient's condition at the initial evaluation. See the example daily note in Figure 12–2.

Progress Toward Functional Outcomes and Goals

The PTA informs the reader about the patient's progress through comments about improvement in functional abilities and progress toward, or accomplishment of, the expected functional outcomes and anticipated goals. A statement about whether an outcome or goal has been met is documented in the Assessment section. The reader also can find a description of the patient's functioning in the Objective data, which provide evidence to support the PTA's conclusion about progress toward the outcome or goal (Fig. 12–4).

Lack of Progress Toward Goals

Lack of progress or ineffectiveness of an intervention in the treatment plan is acknowledged, and comments are made about complicating factors. The PTA may offer suggestions and indicate the need to consult the supervising PT. Again, there should be subjective or objective information to substantiate the PTA's conclusion or opinion and evidence of communication with the supervising PT that describes the lack of progress. Figure 12–5 provides an example of a progress note reporting lack of progress and offering recommendations.

Inconsistency in the Data

Sometimes there is an inconsistency between the subjective information and the objective information. The PTA calls the reader's attention to this in the interpretation of the data content. For example, a patient may report a pain rating of 9/10 on a verbal rating scale (VRS) of 1 to 10, with 10 meaning excruciating pain. Then the PTA may observe the patient moving about in a relaxed manner and using smooth movements, with no demonstration of increased pain behaviors or mannerisms that would be consistent with the higher pain level rated previously. This inconsistency is noted, and the PTA may want to include possible suggestions on what to do. Again, this is a good place for consultation with the supervising PT (Fig. 12–1). The PTA should be cautious when documenting inconsistencies because this information may be interpreted as accusing the patient of lying or faking the injury or illness. The Subjective and Objective data

---

2-17-17   **PT Dx:** Decreased walking tolerance due to Ⓡ quad tendon repair.
        S: Pt. states eager to walk with cane, no c/o.
        O: tx: Respond E-stim./distal end Ⓡ quad/supine/15 min/motor response/for muscle
           re-education. Pt. performed three sets of 15 reps of each of following strengthening exercises
           in supine: quad sets, terminal knee extensions, AROM hip abd./add., SLR. Pt. ambulated
           150 ft from bed down hall, tiled level surface, with single end cane in Ⓛ UE, contact guard
           assist for sense of balance and security.
        A: Decreased quad strength, decreased control with knee extension ex. Concern with problem of
           no superior excursion with max. attempt of quad set. At max. attempt, patella is able to be
           shifted med. & lat. Suspicion of scarring & adhesion on Ⓡ quad tendon.
        P: More balance work with SEC. Cont. tx 3X/week. Will consult PT about patella concerns.
           Pt. will see physician at 1st of next week. Maelee Son, PTA Lic. #346

Figure 12—5   An example of a daily note in which lack of progress is reported and recommendations are made.

should indicate clearly that something "isn't right." The PTA also should confirm the inconsistency when interpreting the data. The inconsistency may indicate that the patient should be referred to another health-care provider or have the treatment plan revised. For example, the patient comes to the clinic for the treatment sessions with the PTA and reports (R) shoulder pain, prior to treatment, at 8/10. The patient's facial features, body language, or use of the (R) shoulder do not match the pain level reported by the patient. The PTA notes the patient is able to reach above his or her head to hang his or her coat on the coat hook without any grimace of pain, limited active range of motion, or use of the other arm to help reach up. Because of these differences, the PTA is concerned the patient may not understand the pain rating given.

Common Mistakes Students Make When Documenting the Interpretation of the Data Content

Comments such as "pt. tolerated treatment well" and "pt. was cooperative and motivated" are commonly found in documentation. These types of comments do not provide objective information related to the patient or his or her progress. They are to be avoided unless they are relevant to the content of the entire daily note and are supported by the subjective and objective data. If they are relevant and supported by the data, this information is better presented through descriptions and measurements of the patient's response and functional abilities. For example, instead of stating "pt. tolerated treatment well," the PTA should write, for instance, "pt. was able to complete 10 minutes of stabilized sitting on edge of bed without loss of balance, compared with 5 minutes in yesterday's session, demonstrating an increase in tolerance to sitting."

In addition, students commonly comment about something that is not mentioned previously in the note. Sometimes a topic is documented that appears to "come out of nowhere." Again, evidence in the Subjective or Objective data must be present to support the interpretation of the data. Figure 12–3 is an example of a note with information that is not supported by data in the note.

It is not unusual to see students' notes that do not mention the goals or provide any comments about whether the patient is accomplishing the outcomes or goals. Comments tend to include only data that measure the impairment severity level and about the treatment procedures. Figure 12–2 illustrates this type of mistake.

SUMMARY

Interpretation of the data is completed in the Assessment portion of the PTA daily note, and it provides a summary of the Subjective and Objective information, thereby making the data meaningful. Comments are made about the patient's progress and the effectiveness of the treatment plan. This section must always contain statements describing the patient's progress toward accomplishing the outcomes and goals listed in the initial evaluation. It coordinates the initial evaluation with the daily notes to demonstrate PT–PTA communication, teamwork, and continuum of skilled care. The PTA may make suggestions and report information that should be brought to the PT's attention when changes occur within the prescribed POC.

All statements in the Assessment section must be supported by the Subjective or Objective information. The same rules discussed in previous chapters about Subjective and Objective content also apply here. Topics in this section should be organized and easy to read. All information must be relevant to the treatment plan and the patient's problem. It is also imperative that the PTA provide progress statements related to the initial evaluation or previous treatment sessions to further delineate the type of progress being made toward completion of the goals outlined in the POC. Statements that do not provide a comparison are not helpful in the assessment process. For example, today the patient was able to perform 10 repetitions and two sets of (R) knee flexion with a 2-pound weight, in sitting, as compared with 10 repetitions and one set of (R) knee flexion with no weight used, in sitting, 1 week ago.

REFERENCES

1. Assessment. (2016). In *Merriam-Webster's online dictionary*. Retrieved from http://www.learnersdictionary.com/search/assessment
2. American Physical Therapy Association. (2003). Guidelines for physical therapy documentation. In *Guide to physical therapist practice* (2nd ed.). Alexandria, VA: Author.
3. American Physical Therapy Association. (2003). Documentation for physical therapist patient/client management. In *Guide to physical therapist practice* (2nd ed.). Alexandria, VA: Author.

Review Exercises

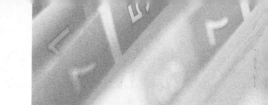

1. **Define** assessment data.

2. Discuss the **type** of assessment data relevant to the patient that the PTA should include in the daily note.

3. **Describe** the organization of assessment data.

4. **Who** is involved in the establishment of the expected functional outcomes and anticipated goals of the PT treatment?

5. Explain **why** information about range of motion is included as assessment data.

6. Discuss **two mistakes** students often make when writing assessment data.

PRACTICE EXERCISES

Practice Exercise 1 ➤ *Write "Pr" next to statements that describe the physical therapy problem or diagnosis, "S" next to statements that fit the subjective data category, "O" next to the statements that fit the objective data category, and "A" next to the statements that fit the assessment data category. Write "N/A" for statements that do not fall into any of these categories.*

1. _____ Pt. states she has a clear understanding of her disease and her prognosis.

2. _____ Pt. expresses surprise that the ice massage relaxed her muscle spasm.

3. _____ Muscle spasms Ⓛ lumbar paraspinals with sitting tolerance limited to 10 min.

4. _____ Pt. describes tingling pain down back of Ⓡ leg to heel.

5. _____ Dependent in ADLs because of flaccid paralysis in Ⓡ upper and lower extremities.

6. _____ Sue states her Ⓛ ear hurts.

7. _____ Pt. able to reach above head to comb hair Ⓘ with return of full AROM in shoulder following last session.

8. _____ Reports he must be able to return to work as a welder.

9. _____ Patient, in sitting, completed 3 reps/3 sets of Ⓑ elbow flex c̄ 3 lb wt. Ⓘ.

10. _____ Paraplegic 2° SCI T12 and dependent in w/c transfers.

11. _____ States Hx of RA since 2010.

12. _____ Pt. denies pain c̄ cough.

13. _____ States injury occurred December 30, 2016.

14. _____ Student PTA c/o he has to sit for 2 hours in the PTA lectures.

15. _____ Pt. grip strength has increased and she is now able to turn all doorknobs independently compared with initial evaluation.

16. _____ Pt. in side-lying completed 10x/2 sets of Ⓛ hip abd. c̄ verbal cues to Ⓛ keep knee straight.

17. _____ Unable to sit because of decubitus ulcer over sacrum.

18. _____ Unable to feed self because of limited elbow flexion due to Ⓛ olecranon fracture.

19. _____ Pt. rates her pain a 4 on an ascending scale of 0–10.

20. _____ States able to sit through a 2-hour movie last night.

Practice Exercise 2 ➤   *For this practice exercise, please follow the instructions listed below.*

1. For each of the statements in Practice Exercise 1 marked "Pr," <u>underline</u> the impairment and (circle) the functional limitation.

2. For each of the statements in Practice Exercise 1 marked "S," <u>underline</u> the key verb that led you to write "S."

3. For each of the statements in Practice Exercise 1 marked "O," <u>underline</u> the portion of the statement that led you to write "O."

4. List the medical diagnoses you can find in the statements.

5. Identify any statements that are assessments of the patient by writing an "A" next to the statement number.

_____

_____

_____

_____

_____

Practice Exercise 3 ➤   *You are treating Namrata, who has been diagnosed as having a mild disc protrusion at L4, 5 with spasms in the right lumbar paraspinal muscles. You read in the PT initial evaluation that she reported pain in the right lower back and buttock areas of 7/10, and you see the areas marked on a body drawing. The spasms and pain have interfered with Namrata's ability to sit; she is unable to tolerate sitting longer than 15 minutes and unable to sleep more than 2 hours at a time. She also reports having difficulty with bathing and dressing activities. Namrata works as a nursing assistant at the local hospital and has been unable to perform her job tasks. The desired functional outcomes for Namrata are to be able to sit 30 minutes, sleep 5 hours, achieve independence in bathing and dressing, and return to her work as a nursing assistant. The treatment plan and objectives are to include massage to the lumbar paraspinal muscles to relax the spasms, static pelvic traction for 10 minutes to encourage receding of the disc protrusion, stretching and relaxing the lumbar paraspinal muscles, patient education in a home exercise program (HEP) for lumbar extension and control of the disc protrusion, and instructions* *on posture and body mechanics for correct and safe sitting, sleeping, bathing, dressing, and performance of work tasks. You have written this daily note:*

| **6-3-17: Dx:** | Disc protrusion L4, 5. | **PT Dx:** | Muscle spasms lumbar paraspinals with limited sitting, sleeping tolerance, difficulty with ADLs, and unable to perform work tasks. |

Patient states she was able to sit through 30 minutes of her favorite television show yesterday. Rates her pain a 5 on a VRS of 0–10. Patient has received 4 treatment sessions. Decrease in muscle tone palpable after 10-minute massage to right lumbar paraspinal muscles, prone position over one thin pillow. Unable to tolerate lying propped on elbows because of pain before traction, able to lie propped on elbows 5 minutes following 10 minutes prone, static pelvic traction, 70 pounds. No pain in buttock area. Correctly performed lumbar extension exercises 1, 2, and 3 of the home exercise program (see copy in chart) and observed consistently using correct sitting posture with lumbar roll. Patient required frequent verbal cueing for correct body mechanics while performing 10 repetitions (3 reps in initial evaluation) of circuit of job simulation activities consisting of bed making, rolling, and moving 30 pounds (10 pounds in initial evaluation) dummy "patient" in bed, pivot transferring the dummy, and wheelchair handling. She did 10 back arches between each task without reminders. Patient has reached 30-minute sitting tolerance outcome, is independent with home exercise program, and compliant with techniques for controlling the protrusion. Progress toward outcome of return to work is 60% with more consistent use of correct body mechanics and ability to lift 50-pound dummy required. Patient to continue treatment sessions 3X/week for 2 more weeks per PT's initial plan. Will notify PT that interim evaluation is scheduled for 6-7-17.

—Madi Noni, PTA, License #35871

This note is not written correctly, making it difficult to read. Rewrite this note in the correct SOAP note format.

_____

_____

_____

_____

_____

_____

_____

_____

_____

_____

_____

Practice Exercise 4 ➤   *Write "Yes" next to relevant assessment data statements and "No" next to those that are not relevant.*

_____ 1. Client stated her dog was hit by a car last night and she buried him under her flower bed.

_____ 2. Client reported he increased his exercises to 50 push-ups yesterday.

_____ 3. Patient was able to ambulate independently, 50 ft with FWW walker.

_____ 4. Patient states he does not like the hospital food and is hungry for some ice cream.

_____ 5. Patient was able to lift 5 lb in shoulder flexion 10X, 3 sets, today compared with 0 lb, 3x/1 set at initial evaluation.

_____ 6. Patient now able to reach the second shelf of her kitchen cupboard to reach for a glass compared with IE when she could not reach the first shelf.

_____ 7. Patient was able to walk 100 ft, independently, 2X compared with last session of 50 ft 2x.

_____ 8. Client experienced an aching in his "elbow bone" after the ultrasound treatment yesterday.

_____ 9. Patient says she has 10 grandchildren and four great grandchildren.

_____ 10. Client states she forgot to tell the PT that she loves to bowl.

_____ 11. Patient was able to move from sit to stand, independently, with good balance, 4X today compared with IE with mod A and fair balance.

_____ 12. Client reports he sat in his fishing boat for 3 hours and caught a 7-pound northern pike this weekend.

_____ 13. Client states he played golf yesterday for the first time since his back injury.

_____ 14. Patient ambulated 25 ft with FWW and SBA compared with last session of 10 ft.

_____ 15. Client states she cannot turn her head to look over her shoulder to back the car out of the garage following her MVA last week.

_____ 16. Patient's mother wants to know when her son will come out of the coma and return to his PLOF.

_____ 17. Patient in supine, lifted 20 lb wt. in hip flexion, 10X, 2 sets compared with initial evaluation of 5x/1 set.

_____ 18. Patient reported he must go up a flight of stairs with ten steps, a landing, and then five more steps with the railing on the right when going up to get into his apartment.

_____ 19. Patient ascended and descended four steps with the use of a single point cane and one rail on Ⓡ to get in and out of her apartment with CGA compared with 1 step last week.

_____ 20. Patient states, "I'm going to Macy's to shop and have lunch today." (Patient is 89 years old and is a resident in a long-term-care facility in a small town in Ohio. She has been placed on some new medication.)

Practice Exercise 5 ➤   *The daily notes in Figure 11–4 in Chapter 11 are incomplete. Finish the notes by writing the assessment sections, stating how the patient has progressed in the goals within the POC compared with the initial evaluation or a previous treatment session, whether there has been regression, and whether the patient can follow the HEP with a correct return demonstration given. Remember, this section should summarize the subjective and objective sections of the note.*

_____

_____

_____

_____

_____

_____

_____

_____

Practice Exercise 6 ➤   *The daily note in Figure 11–6 in Chapter 11 is incomplete. Finish the note by writing the assessment section, stating how the patient has progressed in the goals within the POC compared with the initial evaluation or a previous treatment session, whether there has been regression, and whether the patient can follow the HEP with a correct return demonstration given. Remember, this section should summarize the subjective and objective sections of the note.*

_____

_____

_____

_____

_____

_____

_____

Practice Exercise 7 ➤   *Read the goals listed below. Circle the activity or intervention and underline the measurable information. Then provide the frequencies and durations (time periods) for each objective on the blank lines.*

Example: (Ultrasound) to ℝ trochanteric bursa, moderate heating effect, to <u>increase circulation</u> and <u>decrease inflammation and discomfort.</u>

1. Increase ambulation to 90 feet, 4 trials, rolling walker, stand-by assist in 2 weeks.

   _____

   _____

2. Improve left shoulder flexion to 0°–110° with active reaching.

   _____

   _____

3. Pivot transfer wheelchair to bed, min A, 3 repetitions/2 sets.

   _____

   _____

4. Increase right ankle dorsiflexion PROM to 0°–15° in 4 weeks.

   _____

   _____

5. Ascend and descend stairs with single point cane and use of left handrail.

   _____

   _____

6. Increase strength in left gluteus medius from 3/5 to 4/5 in 3 weeks.

   _____

   _____

7. Transfer from wheelchair to floor 3/5X in 6 weeks.

   _____

   _____

8. Ambulate independently with forearm crutches from bed to dining room for all meals in 3 weeks.

   _____

   _____

9. Lift 35-lb boxes from floor to shelf in 4 weeks.

_____

_____

10. Able to perform 3 sets of 10 repetitions of leg presses with 150 lb, consistently controlling the movement so the knees do not hyperextend and the weight plates do not clang.

_____

_____

Practice Exercise 8 ➤   *Look at Figure 12–3. It illustrates documentation of information not mentioned in the subjective or objective sections in the A section of this SOAP-organized note. There is more in this note that does not constitute quality documentation. Critique the "A" section and rewrite it to make this a well-written daily note.*

Practice Exercise 9 ➤   *You are on your last clinical affiliation at Happy Rehabilitation Center, where they use the SOAP format for documentation. Your patient is Seth, who has quadriplegia as a result of a spinal cord injury from a snowmobile accident. When he tries to sit, he faints because blood pools in his paralyzed legs, causing his blood pressure to drop (orthostatic hypotension). You have been working on a tilt-table treatment to overcome the orthostatic hypotension and to accomplish the anticipated goal of tolerating the upright position for 30 minutes. The functional outcome is for Seth to be able to sit for 2 hours (with breaks every 30 minutes). It is Friday afternoon, and you are writing your daily notes from the past week.*
Interpret the subjective and objective data in the "A" section of this incomplete note.

1-20-17 Dx: Orthostatic hypotension 2° SCI C7.

_____

PT Dx: Unable to tolerate upright sitting.

_____

S: Pt. continues to c/o dizziness when he attempts sitting.

O: Pt. has had 3 sessions on the tilt table to develop tolerance for upright sitting. First session blood pressure dropped from 130/80 mm Hg to 90/50 mm Hg p̄ 10 min at 40° elevation. Today's blood pressure dropped from 130/80 mm Hg ā treatment to 100/60 mm Hg p̄ 15 min on tilt table at 50°. Blood pressure was 125/75 mm Hg 5 min p̄ pt. returned to supine position.

A:

_____

_____

_____

_____

_____

Practice Exercise 10 ➤   *You are on your second clinical affiliation at Saint Mary's Hospital and have been working with Tamika, who burned her Ⓛ hip. You give her whirlpool treatments daily so the moving water will debride (i.e., clean out) the wound, and you use sterile technique to change the dressing. The goal is to promote healing of the wound so she will be able to sit properly and begin walking. You are writing your daily note following today's treatment session. Write the interpretation of the data portion of this incomplete note.*

11-2-17 PT Dx: Open wound due to 2nd-degree burn on Ⓛ gluteus medius, not able to sit with even wt.-bearing.

Pt. reports itching around edge of wound. Pt. sat in whirlpool 100°F, 20 min, for wound debridement and to increase circulation for healing, sterile technique dressing change. No eschar, edges pink, 1 tsp drainage, clear, odorless. Diameter Ⓡ outer edge to Ⓛ outer edge: 4 cm today compared with 4-3/4 cm 10-31-17. Pt. sat in whirlpool with even weight-bearing on pelvis and taking support from arms on edge of whirlpool.

_____

_____

_____

_____

_____

Practice Exercise 11 ➤   *Write the assessment of the data portion of this note.*

Dx: Subacromial bursitis Ⓡ shoulder.

PT Dx: Pain c/o, ROM deficit in all shoulder motions, and strength deficit in anterior and middle deltoid, limiting ability to load luggage into trunk of taxi and work as a taxi driver.

Expected Functional Outcome: Able to consistently load luggage into the trunk of the taxi with 0–3/10 pain rating in 10 days.

Anticipated Goals:

Pain rating reduced from 8/10 to 5/10 with shoulder movements for lifting and carrying objects in 5 days.

Consistent use of proper body mechanics using legs and minimizing shoulder motion for lifting, reaching, and carrying in 5 days. AROM of all movements of the shoulder will increase by 50% of the AROM measured in the initial examination for lifting, reaching, and carrying in 5 days.

Subjective and objective information from your treatment session.

4-18-17   Pt. reported he was able to lift a passenger's briefcase today with no pain, guessed the briefcase weighed about 15 lb; rated his pain with shoulder flexion 6/10 before ultrasound and 4/10 after the ultrasound treatment. Pt. has not missed any appointments. This is the 4th visit. Direct US/subacromial bursa/sitting with shoulder extended/forearm resting on pillow/1 w/cm2/8 min/to increase circulation and decrease inflammation. Pt. correctly followed home exercise instructions for AAROM "wand" exercises for Ⓡ shoulder using a cane (see copy in chart). AROM shoulder flexion 0°–120° (0°–80° initial evaluation). Initiated body mechanics training for reaching into trunk of car, needed frequent verbal cues to keep arms close to body and weight shift with legs. Consistently demonstrated proper form for squatting and lifting, no verbal cueing needed (verbal cues needed last visit for keeping head and shoulders up). Able to lift 30 lb from floor 5X (20 lb 5X last visit).

A. What would you write next in the interpretation of the data section?

B. Are the subjective and objective data recorded correctly?

C. Are the goals written correctly?

_____

_____

_____

_____

_____

_____

_____

Practice Exercise 12 ➤   *Write the assessment portion for the following patient's SOAP note:*

Dx: 4 weeks status post-surgery for herniated disc C4–C5.

PT Dx: ROM deficit in all cervical motions, limiting ability to look around and over shoulders for safe driving.

Expected Functional Outcome: Able to return to safely driving in 2 months

Anticipated Goals:

Ⓑ AROM cervical rotation will improve 0°–45° to be able to see objects at shoulder level in 2 weeks.

Independent in performing home exercise program (HEP) of cervical AROM exercises to be able to look over shoulders in 1 week.

S: Pt. reports having difficulty with chin tuck exercises at home, notices she can see more items on the wall in the garage when she tries to look over her shoulder.

O: Pt. has been seen three times. Passive manual stretching, all cervical motions, 30-sec hold, 5 reps, supine, to increase ROM. Pt. gave correct demonstration of all exercises in home exercise program (see copy in chart) but needed correction and cueing to pull occiput toward ceiling with chin tuck exercises. Quality of the exercise improved after 10 reps. Bilateral cervical AROM rotation 0°–30° before stretching, 0°–35° after stretching (0°–20° initially).

A:

_____

_____

_____

_____

Practice Exercise 13 ➤ _Write the assessment portion for the following patient's SOAP note:_

Dx: Ⓛ lower extremity bone cancer with above-knee amputation.

PT Dx: Ⓛ hip flexion/extension ROM deficit, hip abductor strength deficit limiting ability to walk safely with prosthesis.

Expected Functional Outcome: Independent ambulation in home and community with prosthesis and appropriate ambulation aid in 1 month.

Anticipated Goals:

Hip flexion/extension PROM 0°–110°, hip hyperextension 0°–10°. Ⓛ hip abductor strength increase to lift 10 lb, 3 sets of 10 reps in 1 month. Ambulation with cane on carpet, grass, steps in 2 weeks.
Pt. states he is able to lie prone with one thin pillow under abdomen instead of two pillows for 1 hour. Missed yesterday's session because of the flu. This is pt.'s 5th session. Hot pack to Ⓛ iliopsoas/20 min/to increase elasticity to prepare for stretching. Hip flexion PROM 15°–110° before hot pack, 10°–110° after hot pack. Contract-relax active stretching/Ⓛ hip flexors/5X prone/to gain hip extension ROM. PROM hip flexion 5°–110° after stretching (20°–110° initial exam). Required frequent reminders to breathe while performing 10 repetitions active extension exercises, prone over one pillow. Exercise performed with effort, movements not smooth. Required some verbal cueing to maintain Ⓛ leg in midline while performing Ⓛ hip abduction strengthening exercises, side-lying, using 4-lb cuff weight (up from 3-lb last visit), 3 sets of 10 repetitions (reps), exerting effort last 3 reps and tending to hold breath. Provided written instructions (see copy in chart) and 4-lb cuff weight for this exercise to be continued at home. Gait training on grass with quad cane on Ⓡ (walker initial exam) requiring contact guard assist for safety with uncertain balance due to slight hip-flexed posture, uneven strides with shorter stance time on Ⓛ.

A. Write the assessment of the data information next.

B. Are the subjective and objective data written correctly? If not, put them in SOAP note format.

C. Are the goals written correctly?

_____

_____

_____

CHAPTER 13

What Is the Plan and Why Is It Important?

LEARNING OBJECTIVES	REFERENCES
INTRODUCTION	REVIEW EXERCISES
TREATMENT PLAN CONTENT	PRACTICE EXERCISES
SUMMARY	

LEARNING OBJECTIVES

After studying this chapter, the student will be able to:

☐ Compare and contrast the Plan content in the PT's evaluation with the Plan content in the PTA's daily note

☐ Discuss how the Plan section incorporates the PT–PTA team approach to patient care

☐ Incorporate the plan into the rest of the SOAP note or daily note

INTRODUCTION

Merriam-Webster's Online Dictionary defines the word *plan* as "a detailed program (as for payment or the provision of some service)."[1] In the SOAP note format, the Plan is identified by the letter "P." The information in this section describes the next step for the patient in the plan of care (POC). The PT's treatment plan is outlined in this section of the evaluation report. In the daily note, the PTA describes what he or she may need to do before and during the next treatment session.

The previous chapters have shown how the initial evaluation and daily note tell a story about the patient's physical therapy episode. First, the patient's subjective thoughts or contribution to the information is presented. Then, the objective facts are gathered and documented. Next, the information is summed up and assessed. Finally, a plan is outlined to describe what interventions are proposed for the patient.

TREATMENT PLAN CONTENT

The Plan section in the PT's initial evaluation is more detailed than the Plan content in the daily notes that the PTA completes. APTA's "Guidelines for Physical Therapy Documentation" states that treatment plans "shall be related to goals and expected functional outcomes, should include the frequency and duration to achieve the stated goals."[2]

Plan Content in the Evaluation Report

The PT outlines the treatment plan designed to accomplish the expected goals and functional outcomes. The plan is documented in the Plan section of the initial evaluation. The treatment is directed toward the physical therapy diagnosis and includes two parts: (1) physical therapy activities or interventions that treat the impairments contributing to the patient's functional limitations, and (2) training in the functional tasks described in the goals and outcomes. The PT's Plan includes treatment objectives. Written the same way as goals, treatment objectives contain action words (verbs), are measurable, and have a time frame. They document the rationale for each activity or intervention listed in the plan. Figure 13–1 provides three examples of intervention plans.

INTERVENTION PLAN #1

Dx: Ⓡ hip trochanteric bursitis.

PT Dx: Hip abductor muscle weakness and discomfort limiting tolerance for walking and stair climbing required at work.

Expected Functional Outcome: To be able to walk from car in parking lot to office and to climb two flights of stairs without using a railing in 4 weeks for return to work.

Anticipated Goals:

1. To be able to walk equivalent of two blocks with minimal hip abductor limp and 3/10 pain rating in 3 weeks.
2. To be able to climb one flight of stairs using railing and with 3/10 pain rating in 3 weeks.
3. To be able to increase hip abductor muscle strength to 5/5 in 4 weeks.

Intervention:

1. Ultrasound to Ⓡ trochanteric bursa, moderate heating effect, to increase circulation to decrease inflammation and discomfort.
2. Exercises, including home program, for hip abductor muscles to strengthen to grade 5/5.
3. Home program of structured, progressive walking and stair climbing activities to increase tolerance to the activities without aggravating the bursitis.

US and exercise 3X/week for 2 weeks, then 2X/week for 2 weeks with emphasis on self-management and monitoring of home programs and discontinuation of US. Pt. has appointment with physician in one month. Rehab potential is good.

INTERVENTION PLAN #2

Dx: Fractures of Ⓛ olecranon process and Ⓛ hip.

PT Dx: Immobility required to allow healing causing patient to be dependent in ADLs, transfers, and ambulation so is unable to return to home.

Expected Functional Outcome: At discharge time, patient will be able to transfer and ambulate with support for return to home.

Short-term Functional Outcomes:

1. To be able to transfer from bed <--> chair <--> toilet with SBA in 2 weeks.
2. To ambulate with platform walker for support on Ⓛ from bed to bathroom, and 200 ft to be able to ambulate required distances in the home with SBA in 2 weeks.
3. To be able to ascend one step using walker and SBA to enter home in 2 weeks.

Intervention Plan:

1. Exercises to strengthen all extremities to aid transfers and ambulation. Exercise plan to include home program.
2. Training and practice for transfers from all types of surfaces as required in the home.
3. Gait training with platform walker on level tiled and carpeted surfaces and one step as required in the home.
4. Home assessment visit to clarify needs for transfer and gait training planning.
5. Educate patient and family on hip protection and safety precautions for safe functioning in the home.

Pt. to be treated bid for 2 weeks with discharge to home with support and continued physical therapy through home health agency. Rehab potential good.

INTERVENTION PLAN #3

Dx: 4 weeks post fractures of Ⓛ olecranon process and hip with healing in process.

PT Dx: Limited ROM and strength in Ⓛ elbow and hip causing patient to be confined to ADLs within her home and requiring SBA.

Expected Functional Outcome: Discharge plan is for patient to be able to transfer and ambulate independently in her home environment, and to join family for summer activities in motor home on lake.

Short-term Functional Outcomes:

1. To ambulate independently using single-end cane within the home in 3 weeks.
2. To ascend and descend stairs using single-end cane and the railing independently in 2 weeks.
3. To walk to the end of the dock using single-end cane and SBA to sit and fish in 3 weeks.
4. To climb steps into motor home using single-end cane and SBA in 3 weeks.
5. To perform home exercise program independently and accurately in 1 week.

Intervention Plan:

1. Home program of exercises to increase ROM and strength of Ⓛ elbow and hip in preparation for ambulation with cane and independent ADLs.
2. Transfer and ambulation training with progression of assistive devices appropriate for safe change from platform walker to goal of single-end cane.
3. Ambulation training on grass and dock using assistive device.
4. Stair climbing training with assistive device and railing in home and into motor home.

Home health physical therapy 3X/week for 2 weeks and decrease to 2X/week for 1 week. Rehab potential is good.

Figure 13–1   Three examples of intervention plan documentation.

As the patient's status changes and goals are met, only the PT may modify or change the treatment plan. These changes are documented in the interim evaluations. The PTA may not modify the treatment plan without consulting the PT, but he or she may communicate the completion of goals and make suggestions for additional activities or recommend discharge, if the goals have been met. Discharge evaluations contain the plan for any follow-up or further treatment that may be required. When goals, functional outcomes, and treatment objectives are written correctly, the PTA can easily follow them to plan treatment sessions and measure treatment effectiveness, related to the patient's progress toward meeting the goals. (See Chapter 12 for more information.)

Plan Content in the Daily Note

The Plan content in the PTA's daily note contains brief statements about the following:

1. What will be done in the next session to enable the patient to progress toward meeting the goals presented in the initial POC
2. When the patient's next session will be scheduled
3. What PT consultation or involvement is needed and when the next supervisory visit is scheduled (it is helpful for the PTA to list an actual date or an approximate visit schedule for the supervisory visit)
4. Any equipment or information that needs to be ordered or prepared before the next treatment session
5. The number of treatment sessions the patient has remaining before being re-evaluated by the supervising PT or before being discharged. The treating PTA must word any reference to the discharge process carefully. The PTA should not make statements such as:
   • Patient is ready for discharge
   • Patient is noncompliant and will be discharged
   • Patient has met all goals except . . . and is ready for discharge
   Such statements denote the patient is ready for immediate discharge and further skilled visits are not necessary. Because the discharge process is outside the scope of practice for the PTA, more appropriate statements might be:
   • Patient has met all short-term and long-term goals within the POC, and PTA will discuss re-evaluation of pt.'s functional level with supervising PT.
   • Pt. is noncompliant with HEP and therapy sessions. PTA will communicate difficulty with supervising PT for further direction.
   • Patient has met all goals within the POC except . . PTA will discuss re-evaluation of patient with supervising PT.
   PTAs should follow the protocols of the facility and state within which they complete their clinical externship or are employed.
6. Whether consultation is needed with another health-care provider, such as the primary care physician, OT, SLP, or nutritionist
7. Anything that the patient or caregiver may need to do prior to the next treatment session (e.g., purchasing shoes with greater support and stability, removing physical obstacles from the home)
   These statements typically contain verbs in the future tense. The verbs describe what will happen between the time of writing and the next treatment session or what will happen at the next session. For example:
   • "Pt. will make an appointment with the orthopedic physician to re-evaluate the date the pt. will return to work."
   • "Pt. will be referred to OT services for evaluation of Ⓛ UE use in ADLs."
   • "Pt. needs to see orthotist for reassessment of AFO due to continued skin breakdown; pt. will make appt. before next PT session."
   • "Pt. will be seen for PT supervisory visit on 12-5-17 and will discuss progression within POC with PT."

don't agree c̄ some of these

Comments about something specific the PTA wants to be sure to do at the next session also go in the Plan section. These written comments serve as self-reminders for the PTA (e.g., "Will update written home exercise instructions next visit," or "Will check skin over lateral malleolus this p.m. after patient has worn new AFO 6 hours"). It is also a way to tell another therapist, who may be treating the patient at his or her next session, what should be accomplished.

When commenting elsewhere in the note about concerns, suggestions, or something that must be brought to the PT's attention, a statement is written in the Plan section to indicate that the PT will be consulted or contacted (e.g., "Will consult PT about referring the patient to social services"). This ensures follow-through, quality continuum of care, and PT–PTA communication. When the PTA writes the daily note, the inclusion of such a statement in the Plan section provides evidence of PT–PTA teamwork and communication. When the situation does not require consultation or immediate communication with the PT, the PTA demonstrates PT–PTA teamwork by referring to the PT's goals or plan in the evaluation (e.g., "Will gait train patient on grass and curbs this p.m. per PT's goal in initial eval to gait train pt. on uneven surfaces"). The PTA can also address PT–PTA teamwork in the "A" section of the SOAP note by stating that the patient is progressing toward the goals established in the PT evaluation and subsequent POC.

When the daily note is used as the method for keeping track of the number of treatment sessions the patient is receiving, the number of sessions to be scheduled is reported in the Plan section. The Objective data may state, "Pt. has been seen for physical therapy 3X." The Plan portion of the note may read, "Pt. to receive 3 more treatment sessions before re-evaluation for possible discharge," "Pt. has 2 more approved visits scheduled before reevaluation by supervising PT," or "Pt. will return on 2-16-17 and 2-23-17, working toward completion of the goals outlined within the POC by 3-1-17."

Additional examples of Plan content statements in a PTA's daily notes may include the following:

- "Will increase weights from 2 lb to 5 lb, in PRE strengthening exercises next session, to improve pt. strength in UEs."
- "Will discuss with PT patient's noncompliance with exercise program and possible re-evaluation."
- "Will consult with PT about adding ultrasound to treatment plan to increase PROM in Ⓡ Ⓡ knee from 100° of flex. to 120° of flex."
- "Will notify PT that patient is ready for re-evaluation as patient has met all short- and long-term goals in POC."
- "PT will see patient next session for re-evaluation as all goals have been met."
- "Will instruct pt. in gait-training on stairs this p.m. for increased endurance and stability using reciprocal gait pattern to ascend and marking time to descend six steps."
- "Will order standard walker to be available for treatment session on 8-4-17 to progress patient in gait training with appropriate step length."
- "Will have blueprints for constructing a standing table for increasing core stability ready for home visit on 9-10-17 so father can begin construction of table."
- "Pt.'s spouse will remove all throw rugs from the home to make the environment safe and to decrease fall risk before pt. is discharged from the hospital."
- "Pt. will discuss side effects of the medication with PCP at a later appt. today to decrease dizziness and fall risk."

Remember, simply stating that the current POC will continue is not enough. You must have specific parameters to outline what will be done within the POC.

For additional clarification regarding information that should be included in the Plan section of the SOAP note, review the SOAP note rubric included in Appendix C.

SUMMARY   The Plan section of physical therapy documentation addresses what will happen during the patient's subsequent treatment sessions or in future treatment sessions. The evaluation contains a treatment plan and objectives designed by the PT to accomplish expected goals and expected functional outcomes. The PTA carries out the treatment plan designed by the PT and contacts the PT when the plan needs to be changed or modified. The PTA designs activities to help the patient progress within the guidelines described in the plan.

In the Plan content of the daily notes, the PTA documents what is planned for the patient at the next session(s), describing generally how the patient will make progress toward the goals. The Plan section may also include (1) a reminder to do something specific, (2) statements of intent to consult with the PT regarding any concerns or suggestions that were mentioned elsewhere in the daily note, (3) the number of treatment sessions yet to be completed, and (4) when the next PT supervisory visit is scheduled. A statement in the Plan section that mentions communication with the PT reinforces and demonstrates the PT–PTA team approach to patient care and the policy that the PTA follows the supervising PT's POC.

REFERENCES   1. Plan. (2011). In *Merriam-Webster's online dictionary*. Retrieved from http://www.merriam-webster.com/dictionary/plan
2. American Physical Therapy Association. (2003). Guidelines for physical therapy documentation. In *Guide to physical therapist practice* (2nd ed.). Alexandria, VA: Author.

Review Exercises

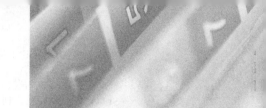

1. **Discuss** what the reader will find in the Plan section of the PT's evaluation.

2. **Describe** the PTA's role in designing the intervention plan.

3. **Describe** the **content** of the Plan section of a PTA's daily note.

4. **Explain** how the Plan section of the daily note can **support** the PT–PTA approach to patient care.

5. **Describe** the **difference** between an expected outcome or goal that is desired for the patient and what is listed in the Plan section of a daily note.

PRACTICE EXERCISES

Practice Exercise 1 ➤ *The daily note dated 5-31-17 in Figure 11–4 in Chapter 11 is incomplete. Finish the note by writing the plan section, stating what you will do next.*

_____

_____

_____

_____

Practice Exercise 2 ➤ *Write "S" next to the subjective data statements, "O" next to the objective data statements, "A" next to the assessment data statements, and "P" next to the plan statements.*

_____ 1. Pt. complained of pain with prolonged sitting over 15 minutes.

_____ 2. Decubitus ulcer on heel measure 1 cm from Ⓛ outer edge to Ⓡ outer edge.

_____ 3. Pt. ambulates with ataxic gait, 10 ft max. A, on even tiled floor, using front wheeled walker, to prevent loss of balance.

_____ 4. Pt. will see orthopedic surgeon tomorrow for follow-up visit.

_____ 5. Pt. ambulates c̄ standard walker, partial weight-bearing on Ⓛ lower extremity, bed to bathroom (20 ft), tiled surface, min. A 1X for balance, vc for appropriate reciprocal, heel-toe gait pattern.

_____ 6. Pt. states he is fearful of crutch walking and falling.

_____ 7. Pt. continues to have limited AROM in Ⓛ shoulder flex and abd and cannot put on his shirt or winter coat without mod. A, following exercises today.

_____ 8. Pt. c/o itching in Ⓡ knee scar, over the weekend.

_____ 9. Pt. transferred from supine to sit c̄ min. A and 3 reps today without any pain compared with last session with pain at 3/10.

_____ 10. AROM is limited in elbow flexion –10° today, compared with IE of –30°.

_____ 11. AROM WNL Ⓑ LEs.

_____ 12. Pt. demonstrated adequate knee flexion during initial swing c̄ vc p̄ hamstring exercises with gait training on even, tiled surface.

_____ 13. Pt. remains dependent in bed mobility and was unable to perform a transfer from bed to chair with max. A due to continued flaccidity this session.

_____ 14. Pt. reported he will see the doctor tomorrow and tell him his pain level is decreasing with exercise from 6/10 at IE to 3/10, following treatment today.

_____ 15. Pt. had increased strength in Ⓛ shoulder flexion from 3/5 to 4/5 from last week. Pt. would like to talk to the social worker and he was given the phone number.

_____ 16. Will discuss completion of goals with PT after next visit as pt's AROM in shld has improved by another 20°.

_____ 17. Pt. pivot transfers, non-weight-bearing (NWB) Ⓡ lower extremity, bed ↔ w/c, max. A 2X for strength, balance, NWB cueing, compared with 1x last session.

_____ 18. Pt. rates Ⓛ knee pain 5/10 when going up six steps using nonreciprocal gait pattern.

_____ 19. Ⓛ upper extremity circumference at 3 cm superior to olecranon process is 12 cm compared with 14 cm at initial evaluation.

_____ 20. Blood pressure of 125/80 mm Hg, pulse 78 beats per minute, regular, strong following exercise today.

Practice Exercise 3 ➤   _Complete the plan section of the note from Figure 11–5 in Chapter 11 dated 5-3-17._

1. _____

_____

_____

_____

2. _____

_____

_____

_____

Practice Exercise 4 ➤   _Complete the plan section from Figure 11–6 in Chapter 11._

Example:
The patient will be referred to OT for evaluation of fine motor skills. SV with PT will be on 5-3-17.
    Pt. has met all goals outlined in initial POC and PT will be notified to complete reevaluation by 7-7-17.

1. _____

_____

_____

_____

2. _____

_____

_____

_____

Practice Exercise 5 ➤ *The following are treatment scenarios in which you are the PTA working on functional activities with your patients. Paint a picture of each patient's functioning as if it is being recorded in the Subjective, Objective, Assessment, and Plan sections of your daily note. Mentally reproduce the treatment session and write the plan for each scenario.*

1. You instructed Mrs. Soto, who had severely sprained her Ⓡ ankle, in crutch walking using a NWB gait pattern. Her ankle has been casted, and she is not allowed to bear weight on the Ⓡ LE for 2 weeks. You fitted her with axillary crutches and taught her how to walk 100 ft on tiled and carpeted level surfaces; how to sit down and get up from bed, chair, and toilet; how to climb a flight of stairs with the railing on the right going up and on the left going down; how to manage curbs and two steps without using a railing; and how to get in and out of her car. Mrs. Soto safely ambulated and required only verbal cueing from you to climb the stairs, going up with the uninvolved leg. You gave her written crutch-walking instructions. Mrs. Soto stated that she is concerned because her sister had an allergic reaction to the pain medication that the doctor had prescribed to her. She also said that there are two steps into her living room at home. The PT's expected outcomes for this patient are to be able to walk independently throughout her home and at work, in a safe and timely manner, following the doctor's prescribed decrease in non–weight-bearing restrictions. She will be seen again by the PT in 14 days for a re-evaluation, when her weight-bearing restrictions will change.

   P: _____

   _____

   _____

   _____

   _____

2. You supervised Jack while practicing his circuit of job-simulation activities using correct body mechanics for 20 minutes, 15 repetitions. Jack has had back surgery (laminectomy L4, 5) and is preparing to return to work as a bricklayer. You observed that he consistently maintained his correct lumbar curve when squatting to lift bricks and shifting weight to spread the mortar. He did need vc to maintain proper body mechanics when he lifted the wheelbarrow handle and while wheeling the wheelbarrow, especially for turns. He tended to bend from the waist to reach the handles and to twist his trunk when turning the wheelbarrow. Jack complained of increased back pain after pushing the wheelbarrow 25 ft with 35 lb of weight in it, but he stated that he forgot to take his pain medication until 5 minutes before the treatment session today. The PT's expected goals for this patient are to return to work as a bricklayer, which involves full ROM of back and trunk and the ability to lift 50 lb and push a wheelbarrow weighing 75 lb at least 50 ft.

   P: _____

   _____

   _____

   _____

   _____

3. You taught Shelby, a patient with paraplegia from a spinal cord injury, how to transfer from her wheelchair to the toilet by using a sliding board. Shelby stated that she really did not see the point of learning this activity because she wished she had died in the accident that paralyzed her. She required constant instructions and cueing regarding safety precautions, and you needed to help push her across the board. The first two times that you attempted it, you felt as though you did most of the work. The third time she tried, she was able to slide herself from the chair to the toilet with only a little boost from you. However, when going from the toilet to the chair, it felt as though you and Shelby had exerted equal effort. You decided that you should talk to the social worker at the rehabilitation hospital about Shelby's comment and inform your supervising PT. The PT's expected goals for this patient are to be able to complete all activities of daily living as independently as possible.

(Hint: max. assist means the therapist does most of the work; mod. assist means the therapist and patient exerts about equal effort; min. assist means the patient does most of the work.)

P: _____

_____

_____

_____

_____

4. You instructed Mr. Okuda in gait training to learn to walk with a wide-base quad cane (WBQC) in his left hand. He had a stroke and has Ⓡ UE and LE weakness. You ambulated with him from his bed into the bathroom, to the bedroom window, out into the hall area in front of the door, and back to his wheelchair next to the bed. He walked this circuit five times, with a 2-minute rest in the wheelchair between each trip. You needed to hold his gait belt and to help him shift his weight to his right leg. He stumbled three times (LOB), but he was able to recover his balance without your help. During the fourth and fifth trips, he was able to shift his weight to the right appropriately without your help. Prior to treatment, the nurse informed you that Mr. Okuda was started on an antacid medication last night and that he has an appointment for an MRI later this afternoon (you were planning on seeing the patient again today but now will be able to see him only once).

P: _____

_____

_____

_____

Practice Exercise 6 ➤   *Decide whether the following statements are expected goals for a patient or whether they should be included in the P section of the SOAP note. Place a "G" next to the statements that are goals for the patient and a "P" next to the statements that should be in the P section of the SOAP note.*

1. _____ Pt. will be instructed in independent donning and doffing of AFO at next session.

2. _____ Pt. will walk independently with WBQC on uneven surfaces up to 30 ft. in 2 min by the second week of treatment.

3. _____ Pt.'s mother will call the PCP to ask about supplemental feedings.

4. _____ Pt. will be seen 1X/wk at home by PTA to work on independent amb. skills without an AD.

5. _____ Pt. will be able to reach overhead with Ⓑ UEs to comb hair and wash face independently prior to discharge.

6. _____ Pt. will be seen at BS to work on independent bed mobility skills 2X/day by PTA.

7. _____ Pt. will be Ⓘ in bed mobility skills, including rolling, moving up/down in bed, and moving from lying down to sitting, by the end of the week, for increased core stability for Ⓘ sitting balance.

8. _____ PTA will discuss adding use of the paraffin bath to the pt. HEP, with PT.

9. _____ Pt. will be scheduled for re-evaluation by PT after 3 more visits.

10. _____ Pt. will receive TENS 3X/wk to decrease pain as per PT's POC.

11. _____ Pt. will report a decrease in pain of 8/10 to 4/10 on a descending pain scale following exercise sessions, by the end of the week.

12. _____ Pt. will be instructed in home use of TENS unit by PTA at next treatment session.

13. _____ Pt. will be discharged from inpatient PT care and transferred to home health-care facility on Friday per PT re-evaluation.

14. _____ PTA will contact primary care physician (PCP) to find out about pt.'s weight-bearing status and report it to the PT for update in POC.

15. _____ Next treatment session will be a joint visit with the OT to help pt. learn to dress himself while maintaining Ⓘ sitting balance.

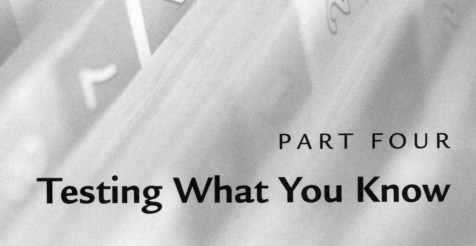

PART FOUR

Testing What You Know

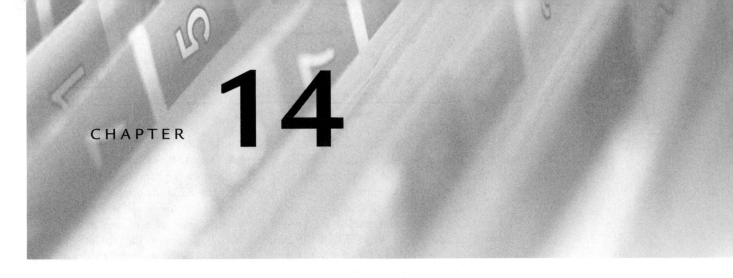

CHAPTER 14

Putting the Pieces Together

LEARNING OBJECTIVES
INTRODUCTION
REVIEW OF THE SOAP NOTE
AN EXAMPLE OF A COMPLETED SOAP
    NOTE

SUMMARY
REFERENCES
REVIEW EXERCISES
PRACTICE EXERCISES

**LEARNING
OBJECTIVES**

After studying this chapter, the student will be able to:

☐ Compare and contrast all parts of the SOAP note, including the Subjective, Objective, Assessment, and Plan sections

☐ Select relevant subjective, objective, assessment, and plan information to document the patient's physical therapy diagnosis and treatment

☐ Organize subjective, objective, assessment, and plan information for easy reading and understanding

☐ Use the SOAP note rubric to assess the complete note

INTRODUCTION

In the preceding 13 chapters, we reviewed important information about the development of appropriate documentation and the parts that should be included in documentation, specifically using a SOAP note format. Now you should have a basic idea about the type of information to include in each of the four sections of a SOAP note, be able to identify information that is not appropriate, and be able to provide information that will make the treatment session reproducible for another therapist who may assume responsibility for the patient's care. As with any new skill, it will take a new therapist some time to be able to organize data in a SOAP note format, maintain organization of the overall note, and remember to put into the note the information that will ensure reimbursement, that covers how the sessions are following the PT's plan of care (POC), and that outlines how continuing care meets the goals outlined in the POC. See APTA's *Guide to Physical Therapist Practice*[1] for further clarification.

In addition, it is necessary for the PTA to complete a thorough review of the patient's chart, especially the section that includes the PT's evaluation of the patient's function. The PT should also have provided short- and long-term goals for the patient's POC. If the PTA was not present at the initial evaluation, this review of the patient's chart is critical for providing appropriate care within the PTA's scope of practice as dictated by the state where the PTA practices. It is also important that the PTA discuss any questions or concerns with the supervising PT to ensure that the PTA correctly follows the POC developed by the PT.

As previously reviewed, it is essential that any information related to the patient's care and treatment be documented appropriately in the SOAP note by the treating PTA. The PTA must review the short- and long-term goals set by the PT and make any necessary referrals for the patient's care. The PTA must communicate all of this information to the supervising PT on a regular basis (the exact reporting requirements vary by facility), and it is also the PTA's responsibility to ensure that the required supervisory visits/re-evaluations are completed per the guidelines of the state in which the PTA practices.

REVIEW OF THE SOAP NOTE

Prior to reviewing each of the sections of the SOAP note, it is important for the PTA to be able to organize a note and to address the parameters that should be included in each section. This ensures that the PTA is reviewing the initial evaluation appropriately, following the POC, presenting the patient for discharge to the supervising PT at the appropriate time, and maintaining communication throughout the entire process. As discussed in Chapter 9, the PTA must organize data related to the patient treatment session in a manageable fashion. This provides the supervising PT with the ability to accurately review the patient's progress within the prescribed POC. Using a SOAP note rubric can help the student PTA organize all of these data (see Appendix C).

Subjective

The "S" section of the SOAP note contains the information that the patient or a family member tells the therapist. Remember, the patient, a family member, or another interested party must provide the subjective information to you. (Refer to Appendix C for a review of the Subjective section of the SOAP note rubric.) Any information you are given that you place in the medical record must be relevant to the patient's care and should not include any other type of information, such as personal statements, information regarding another family member that is not relevant to the patient's care, or any other inappropriate comments (e.g., "patient reported her husband was tired last night," "patient's husband states he went golfing yesterday," "patient's friend stated that the patient went to the movies with her and had popcorn").

For this section of the SOAP note, it is vital that the PTA address any changes in the patient's description of his or her pain level or level of function, poor responses to previous interventions or treatment sessions, and any changes in the patient's condition. Common mistakes to avoid when writing subjective information include the following:

- Not providing pain level changes (e.g., not stating the current pain level of 7/10 in the ℝ shoulder as compared with a pain level of 9/10 from the previous treatment session. A statement may also be made in the Assessment section that compares pre- and post-treatment pain levels.
- Not providing enough detail related to the Subjective information (e.g., the location of the pain given, activities that might increase/decrease pain levels at home)
- Providing information not related to the patient's care (e.g., patient went shopping, sister is making pies for a party, has a brother who has the same job)
- Providing information that violates guidelines of the Health Insurance Portability and Accountability Act (HIPAA) (e.g., responding to a neighbor's questions regarding the patient's program without the patient's written consent)
- Erasing any mistakes made in the note—to correct an error, the PTA should instead draw one line through the mistake, write his or her initials (and possibly the date, depending on the facility's protocol) above the error, and write the correct information or complete an addendum if in an EHR

The following are examples of Subjective information written incorrectly and then correctly:

1. S: written INCORRECTLY: The patient stated that his pain level today was an 8 in the right shoulder.
   - S: written CORRECTLY: The patient reported that his pain level was an 8/10 today in the ℝ shoulder, prior to Tx.
2. S: WRITTEN INCORRECTLY: The patient watched football last night and was not happy with the outcome.
   - S: written CORRECTLY: The patient stated he was able to sit up for more than 1 hour while watching TV last night without increased pain.

3. S: written INCORRECTLY: The patient's neighbor wanted to know what was wrong with her friend.
   - S: written CORRECTLY: This would not be an appropriate statement for a patient's note; the documentation could include the fact that the neighbor accompanied the patient to treatment.
4. S: written INCORRECTLY: The patient's pain level was written as 6/10 today but was really reported as 8/10.
   - S: written CORRECTLY: Because the pain level was actually 8/10, the PTA needs to draw a single line through the incorrect pain level of 6/10 and put his or her initials and that day's date above the mistake. Then the PTA should rewrite the pain level correctly to reflect an 8/10 pain level. The PTA also needs to state where the pain is located ®️ shld). Any type of error in the note would require this type of notation.

Objective

The "O" section of the SOAP note contains objective data—that is, data that can be reproduced or confirmed by another professional with the same training as the person originally gathering the objective information. It must include measurable or reproducible tests and observations. (Refer to Appendix C for a review of the Objective section of the SOAP note rubric.) Therefore, information reported to or by the PTA must meet these guidelines. This section provides the signs of the patient's pathology and describes how it has influenced the patient's function. Some examples include measurable range of motion, measurable strength, number of repetitions or sets in an exercise pattern, and the distance the patient can ambulate.

In the Objective section, the PTA is responsible for performing and documenting objective tests and measures, during every treatment session, to determine changes in the patient's strength, function, and/or range of motion within the POC and then communicating such information to the PT. It is important that any measurable information is included in this section. Patient education—teaching the patient exercises that are included in the home exercise program and confirming that he or she can perform a correct return demonstration of those exercises—also should be documented in this section. Common mistakes to avoid when writing Objective information include the following (note that these statements are not complete in order to emphasize only the mistake being identified):

- Not providing a complete statement of the activity performed (e.g., "the patient was able to complete 10 reps/1 set of the bilateral upper extremity exercises, all planes of motion, in a seated position with a 5 pound weight today" instead of " the patient was able to complete 10 reps of the arm exercises today")
- Not addressing expected goals for length or type of surface when ambulating (e.g., "the patient was instructed to walk today" instead of "the patient was instructed to walk 20 feet today on an even, tiled surface")
- Not providing the amount and/or type of assistance necessary, or what portion of the task needed assistance (e.g., contact guard, moderate assist during w/c to mat transfers) during the treatment session (e.g., "the patient was able to transfer from the bed to the w/c today" instead of "the patient was able to transfer from the bed to the w/c with minimal assistance today")
- Not providing the type of assistive device used by the patient (e.g., "the patient was able to ambulate up a ramp" instead of "the pt. was able to amb up a 5-ft ramp using a FWW, c̄ SBA, on even surface, with vc to maintain upright posture and core stability p̄ LOB 2x")
- Erasing any mistakes made in the note—to correct an error, the PTA should instead draw one line through the mistake, write his or her initials (and possibly the date, depending on the facility's protocol) above the error, and write the correct information, or complete an addendum if in an EHR
- Not providing the specific parameters of the treatment procedure, including type of modality, specific settings used, time frame of treatment, side of body treated, position of patient, distance covered by patient, type of surface (e.g., "patient ambulated

using a reciprocal gait pattern for 50 ft using a FWW on an even, tiled floor in 5 min. without LOB or SOB")

■ Not providing appropriate patient education (e.g., "PTA reviewed HEP exercises with patient and patient was able to perform a correct return demonstration of all ex. Pt. verbalized understanding of all ex")

The following are examples of Objective information written incorrectly and then correctly:

1. O: written INCORRECTLY: The patient ambulated 50 feet today.
   • O: written CORRECTLY: The patient was instructed to ambulate 50 feet using a FWW $\bar{c}$ standby assist 2X today on an even tiled surface with vc to pick up both feet using a stepping gait pattern to decrease fall risk and LOB.
2. O: written INCORRECTLY: The patient was able to transfer from the bed to the wheelchair today.
   • O: written CORRECTLY: The patient was instructed to transfer from the bed to the wheelchair using a stand pivot procedure, $\bar{c}$ vc to maintain equal weight on Ⓑ LE $\bar{c}$ contact guard assist 3X before she experienced fatigue and needed a 5 min. rest period to return to normal vital signs.
3. O: written INCORRECTLY: The patient was able to complete knee extension exercises with a 5-lb weight.
   • O: written CORRECTLY: The patient was able to complete Ⓡ knee extension exercises to 180° in a sitting position using a 5-lb weight, Ⓘ. The patient completed 10 repetitions and 3 sets without fatigue.

Assessment   The "A" stands for assessment. In this section of the SOAP note, the PT or PTA summarizes the "S" and "O" information and answers the question, "What does it mean?" In the Assessment section, the PT (not the PTA) interprets the information in the Subjective and Objective sections, makes a clinical judgment, and sets functional outcomes and goals based on that information. (Refer to Appendix C for a review of the Assessment section of the SOAP note rubric.) Again, the Assessment section must include the short- and long-term goals. While both the short- and long-term goals are developed by the PT, the PTA should address both of these goals in the treatment session and the daily notes to show progress within the POC.

This section is often confusing for PTAs, and many PTAs tend to put objective information in this section by mistake. This section should address the patient's progress within the POC, suggest changes to the POC, and address any completed short- or long-term goals. Common mistakes to avoid when writing Assessment information include the following:

■ Putting objective information in this section (e.g., "patient sitting, completed 10 reps/3 sets of knee extension independently")
■ Changing the POC (this can be done only by the PT)
■ Changing the short- or long-term goals (this can be done only by the PT)
■ Adding any new information that was not mentioned in the "S" or "O" sections
■ Erasing any mistakes made in the note—to correct an error, the PTA should instead draw one line through the mistake, write his or her initials (and possibly the date, depending on the facility's protocol) above the error, and write the correct information, or complete an addendum if in an EHR

The following are examples of Assessment information written incorrectly and then correctly:

1. A: written INCORRECTLY: The patient completed all her short-term goals and new ones were added.
   • A: WRITTEN CORRECTLY: The patient was able to complete all of her short-term goals without fatigue today and within the POC. The PTA will communicate with the PT to re-evaluate the pt. and discuss making changes to the POC, and the PTA will follow the new goals.

2. A: written INCORRECTLY: The patient has completed all his goals and will be discharged tomorrow.
   - A: written CORRECTLY: The patient has completed all the goals set within the initial PT POC, and the PTA will discuss a re-evaluation or suggest possible discharge with the PT today.
3. A: written INCORRECTLY: The patient did not tolerate the treatment session so the POC was changed.
   - A: written CORRECTLY: The patient did not tolerate the treatment session today and became very fatigued following three reps of knee extension with a 5-lb weight. This is a decrease in strength from the last session of five reps. The PTA will discuss this change with the PT and follow any changes to the POC.
4. A: written INCORRECTLY: The patient's ®️ shoulder AROM was 120°.
   - A: written CORRECTLY: The patient's ®️ shoulder AROM was 120° today compared with 90° at the IE, with the patient now able to reach into cupboards above her head.

Plan   The "P" stands for plan. In this section of the SOAP note, the treating therapist includes information about any referrals necessary for additional medical treatments, when the next session will be, how many sessions there are until discharge, how many sessions there are until a supervisory session will occur and/or when the date of the supervisory visit will occur, referrals for other services that might be needed (e.g., OT, Speech), and recommendations for any equipment or home services before or upon discharge. This section should not include the expected goals for the patient's POC. (Refer to Appendix C for a review of the Plan section of the SOAP note rubric.)

This information is communicated to the supervising PT to ensure the POC is being followed. Common mistakes to avoid when writing Plan information include the following:

- Not stating the number of treatment sessions left (e.g., "the patient will be seen next week" instead of "the patient will be seen for 3 more visits before re-evaluation by the PT on 12-6-17")
- Not providing referrals as necessary (e.g., "the patient should see an OT" instead of "the patient will be referred for an OT evaluation")
- Not specifying equipment needs (e.g., "the patient needs an assistive device" instead of "a quad cane will be ordered for the patient")
- Not setting up the supervisory visit (SV) with the PT (e.g., "the PT will see the patient" instead of "the SV with the PT will occur on the next treatment session on 1-12-17")
- Erasing any mistakes made in the note—to correct an error, the PTA should instead draw one line through the mistake, write his or her initials (and possibly the date, depending on the facility's protocol) above the error, and write the correct information or complete an addendum if in an EHR

Here are examples of Plan information written incorrectly and then correctly:

1. P: written INCORRECTLY: The patient will be seen again.
   - P: written CORRECTLY: The patient has six more treatments before a re-evaluation for insurance purposes needs to be completed by PT. The patient continues to be seen 2X/week.
2. P: written INCORRECTLY: The patient is having fine motor problems.
   - P: written CORRECTLY: The patient will be referred to the occupational therapist tomorrow because of problems with dressing and shaving.
3. P: written INCORRECTLY: The patient needs a wheelchair.
   - P: written CORRECTLY: The patient will need a manual wheelchair for pending discharge to home next week. Will communicate with the PT regarding type of wheelchair and projected date of discharge.
4. P: written INCORRECTLY: The PT will see the patient soon.
   - P: written CORRECTLY: The PT will see pt. for a supervisory visit on 1-20-17.

In addition, it is important for the PTA to complete the note with a proper signature (e.g., "Linda Jones, PTA," with the date and time of the note), and if there is empty space following the signature, a line is drawn through it so that additional information cannot be added to the note.

AN EXAMPLE OF A COMPLETED SOAP NOTE

The importance of accurate and complete documentation for the practicing PTA has been detailed, and now a completed SOAP note will be provided. This note will include a brief example of the PT evaluation, the patient's physical therapy diagnosis, and several functional outcomes delineated by the supervising PT. This completed SOAP note is provided for review, and additional notes will be provided in the Practice Exercises at the end of the chapter.

Patient With Cerebral Vascular Accident (seen in hospital setting)

SDX: I63.01-cerebral infarction due to thrombosis of (R) cerebral artery; I69.354-hemiplegia and hemiparesis following cerebral infarction affecting left, non-dominant side

PT DX: I69.354-hemiplegia and hemiparesis following cerebral infarction affecting left, non-dominant side; G81.94-hemiplegia, unspecified affecting (L) non-dominant side; R26.89: other abnormalities of gait and mobility.

BACKGROUND: The pt. is a 75-year-old male who experienced a right-sided vertebral artery CVA 2 days ago. He was brought to the ER, evaluated by the attending physician, and given tPA to break up his clot. He was admitted to the hospital for a few days of observation and follow-up evaluations. The pt. presents to the PT with mild left-sided paralysis and wants to go home. (R) side AROM and muscle strength are WFL with (L) UE and LE PROM, WNL. Pt. has overall grade 3+/5 muscle strength in the (L) LE and 4/5 muscle strength in the (R) LE. Sensation on the (L) side is WNL. The PT performed an evaluation and determined that the pt. is unable to roll in bed, cannot sit @ bedside without LOB, and cannot walk to the bathroom without CGA and use of FWW. You will follow up with this pt. 2x/day. The following functional outcomes were listed in the evaluation:

PT GOALS: within 4 days the pt. will be able to:

1. Walk to and from the hospital bathroom, on tiled floor, using a FWW, appropriate reciprocal gait pattern, with SBA.
2. Get in and out of bed (I), using his (R) UE for support, and with assistance of his (L) UE, from side-lying to sit.
3. Sit @ EOB, (I), for 10-15 minutes, without LOB, feet flat on floor.

Daily Note: 01/09/2017, 0809:

S: Pt. stated he was tired this a.m. but felt his (L) arm and leg were "coming back." He stated that his wife spent the night with him and wanted to know where she could take a shower. He reported that he wanted to go home today and go to OP therapy. Pt. did not report any pain today.

O: The pt. was instructed in rolling safely to the side of bed by pushing up on his (R) UE to sit @ EOB. He performed 2 trials using (R) UE with complete (I). He was then assisted on the (L) side, with min support @ the elbow to maintain ext. as well. The pt. was able to perform 2 additional trials to the (L) side. The FWW was appropriately fitted for the pts. height and the pt. was instructed in the use of a FWW, for moving forward and for making turns, using both hands to grasp the handles. The pt. pushed the walker to the bathroom, turned it around, and walked back to bedside with CGA, 1x using both hands to grasp the handles. Pt. sat (I) @ EOB, after needing SBA, to get into the position from (R) side-lying. Pt. was able to sit for 5 minutes, with some LOB, with no challenges in any direction.

A: Pt was able to complete 4 trials moving from side-lying to sit @ EOB with min assist @ elbow when using (B) UEs. Also, the pt. was instructed in the safe use of the FWW, following appropriate adjustment for his height, and was allowed to use FWW to go to the bathroom. The pt. was able to make one trip to the bathroom, with CGA. Pt. was able to sit (I) @ EOB for 5 minutes, upon return from bathroom, with feet flat on floor, min LOB, but without challenges in any direction. He reported being tired following the 30-minute session. The pt. did not report any pain following the tx session. Discussed the timeline for possible DC with the pt. and his wife, dependent on his progress within the PT POC.

P: The pt. will be seen this afternoon to continue his PT treatments 2x/day, with instructions given to his wife for assistance with beginning ADLs.

—Kayla, PTA, License #A1294

SUMMARY The SOAP note format divides the patient treatment information into four specific sections, thereby providing an organized report of the patient's treatment and progress. This type of reporting provides the student or new therapist with the means to determine and report what happened during the treatment session, allows another therapist to replicate the next session, documents progress within the POC, and moves the patient toward discharge and return to the individual's highest functional level.

REFERENCE 1. American Physical Therapy Association. (2014). Guidelines for physical therapy documentation. In *Guide to physical therapist practice* (3rd ed.). Alexandria, VA: Author.

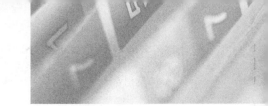

Review Exercises

1. **Describe** the **importance** of each section of the SOAP note. Give an example of information you would find in each section.

2. List **one appropriate** statement for the Subjective section and **one inappropriate** statement for the Subjective section.

3. List **three activities** that could be included in the **Objective** section of the SOAP note.

4. **What** is the purpose of the goals in the Assessment section?

5. What **role** does the PTA play in the patient's discharge process?

PRACTICE EXERCISES

Practice Exercise 1 ➤

Write "S" next to statements that fit the subjective data category, "O" next to the statements that fit the objective data category, "A" next to the statements that fit the assessment category, "P" next to the statements that fit the plan category, and "N/A" next to the statements that would be inappropriate to include in any section within the SOAP note.

_____ 1. Pt. was able to complete an additional five repetitions of the exercise program today compared with three repetitions at the initial evaluation.

_____ 2. Will refer pt. to OT for evaluation of hand function before next week.

_____ 3. Will set up supervisory visit with PT by 3/15/17.

_____ 4. Pt. ambulated 50 feet/1x with FWW and SBA on uneven grass.

_____ 5. Pt. stated she went to the store last night.

_____ 6. Pt. referred to social worker for preparation for discharge on 3/15/17, per PT.

_____ 7. Pt. stated she had pain relief of 8/10 for several hours after last treatment session.

_____ 8. Pt. able to walk 150 ft independently without AD compared with use of SPC last week.

_____ 9. Pt. will be able to ascend four steps independently with one handrail and rec. gait by next visit.

_____ 10. Pt. able to accept increased weights for shld. abd ex. from 5-lb to 20-lb with reps unchanged today compared with initial evaluation.

_____ 11. Will recommend SLP referral before next visit and communicate referral to PT.

_____ 12. Pt. prone, PROM in SLR measured at 165°, 5 reps/2 sets.

_____ 13. Pt.'s husband stated she had a fever last night after session was completed.

_____ 14. Pt. had increased pain in Ⓛ ankle, from 4/10 to 6/10, following stretching and strengthening program today.

_____ 15. Pt. tolerated Ⓛ knee flexion to 98° on CPM for two 60-minute sessions, without increased pain/swelling.

_____ 16. Pt. states the session went well last visit with no increase in pain and just a mild increase in swelling to ankle.

_____ 17. Will continue seeing pt. for therapy session 3X/week.

_____ 18. Will increase pt. ambulation from mat exercises, independently, 100 ft with crutches, on even surfaces, next visit.

Practice Exercise 2 ➤   *Organize the following information into the SOAP note format and* (circle) *statements that can be reproduced or confirmed by another professional:*

Increase wts. in hip extension from 2-lb to 3-lb by the end of the session; reviewed home ex. program with pt., and pt. was able to complete an appropriate and safe return demo; pt. states that pain has decreased from 9/10 to 7/10 with strengthening exercises in shld. horiz. abd with yellow theraband and 10 reps/3 set done once a day at home; will refer patient to OT for eval of wrist range and strength; refer pt. to neurologist for eval of arm tingling and pain; pt. PROM in shld. flex. measured 90° before exercise session and 110° following ex. with no complaint of increased pain; Padma is a 40-year-old patient with tenderness in the bicipital groove during active shld. flex. and horiz. abd; will speak with PT about next supervisory visit on 4/5/17; pt. questions home exercise of shld. horiz. abd because it hurts to do it and it did not hurt during the last treatment session; pt's overall UE strength was 4/5 following the treatment session today.

_____

_____

_____

_____

_____

_____

_____

_____

_____

_____

_____

_____

_____

_____

_____

Practice Exercise 3 ➤   *Organize the following information into a SOAP note format, use approved abbreviations, and* (circle) *statements that can be reproduced or confirmed by another professional:*

This is the first patient you are seeing this morning. Anthony is a 65-year-old male who underwent thoracic surgery to remove a cancerous section of his left upper lobe yesterday.

Your supervising PT completed the evaluation last night. The patient completed shoulder ROM exercise on the left side today, shoulder flexion to 45° and shoulder abduction to 45°, 10 repetitions each. The patient is sitting with the head of the bed elevated to 45° when you enter his hospital room. The patient states that he knew the pain would be bad, but he didn't realize it would hurt as much as it does. He rated his pain as a 9/10 on a verbal rating scale. You demonstrate to him, again, how to produce the most effective cough by bracing a pillow over his chest, and he then accurately demonstrates it back to you. You will see this patient for a second visit later this afternoon. You inform the patient that when he is lying down, he should keep the head of the bed at 30° with his hips and knees slightly flexed to reduce pressure on his chest and decrease his pain. He has a posterior lateral incision. The patient states that he tried to cough last night holding a pillow over his chest like the PT showed him, but he does not know if he is doing it right. He completes 3 sets of 10 reps of ankle pumps with each side and did 5 SAQ with each leg. You decide that you should ask the PT when the patient will be allowed to get out of bed and start ambulating. The patient was able to cough by bracing with the pillow 3X during the treatment session. The PT goals are to increase total lung volume by teaching the patient to have an effective cough, managing his pain, preventing DVT, and restoring normal active and passive ROM in his left shoulder to return to his prior level of function (PLOF).

_____

_____

_____

_____

_____

_____

_____

_____

_____

Practice Exercise 4 ➤   *Place a check mark next to the statements that are written correctly, and rewrite any statement that is written incorrectly.*

1. _____ Increase Ⓛ ankle ROM to 25° of plantarflexion.

2. _____ Will discuss with PT the pt.'s noncompliance with home exercise program.

3. _____ Ultrasound to Ⓡ gluteal area.

4. _____ Pt. able to walk 30 ft in 2 min today, 4 min yesterday.

5. _____ Pt. demonstrated decrease in Ⓛ LE strength.

6. _____ Pt. complained of hip pain.

7. _____ Pt. will perform UE PNF patterns diagonally.

8. _____ Pt. stated he was able to ambulate to the end of his driveway and pick up his newspaper this a.m. for the first time since treatment began.

9. _____ NWB Ⓡ UE.

10. _____ Ⓡ shld. not assessed.

11. _____ Diameter of wound Ⓡ outer edge to Ⓛ outer edge: 5.5 cm at eval. last Tuesday, 4.0 cm today.

12. _____ LE strength is within normal limits at knee and hip.

13. _____ Pt. is left-handed.

14. _____ ROM good (G) in Ⓑ UEs.

15. _____ Pt. will receive US to Ⓡ upper trapezius at 1.0 W/cm^2 for 7 min.

Practice Exercise 5 ➤   *Review the following SOAP note and complete the "A" and "P" sections:*

Patient with Spinal Cord injury (seen in inpatient rehabilitation hospital setting)

DX: M43.27-lumbar-sacral fusion

PT DX: M43.27-LS fusion; R53.81-debility; R26.89: other abnormalities of gait and mobility; M62.81-muscle weakness

---

Background: The pt. is a 34 y/o female who was involved in a head-on collision approximately 3 weeks ago. The pt. is s/p decompression @ L1-L2, a laminectomy and fusion from L3-L4, L5-S1. The pt. sustained an incomplete L1-2 spinal cord injury. The pt. has full use of her UEs, full strength in (B) hip flexion and knee extensors, with sensation in the groin area.

The PT's POC includes monitoring the pts. responses to positional changes and instructing caregiver/family with donning/doffing the custom TLSO. The TLSO is to be worn with all out of bed activities. The TLSO is to be applied in supine following all spinal precautions. TX is ordered 1-2x/day, 7x/wk.

PT GOALS: within 4 weeks the pt. will be able to:

1. Perform rolling side to side, using a log roll technique, with less than mod assist, 5x/3 sets, in bed, or in the gym using the mat table.
2. Demonstrate AROM in (B) UEs for 10 x/3 sets in supine and sit, in shoulder abd, add, flex, and ext using a 2 lb weight for each exercise position with SBA.
3. Sit on EOB for 10 min, without LOB, with SBA, 2 sets.

Note: The pts. caregiver and family members will be instructed in applying the custom TLSO, in supine using a log roll technique, following all spinal precautions, with SBA.

Daily Note: 1/18/17, 1000:

S: The pt. was transferred to the rehab facility several days ago and the PT evaluation was completed yesterday. The pt. reports that she has some (L) shld pain and rated it @ 4/10 with activity. She reports that she and her family continue to have difficulty putting on the TLSO and she continues to get dizzy when sitting up. The pt.'s husband is concerned that he will not be able to care for his wife once she comes home.

O: The pt. was instructed how to move her body from side to side in a log roll technique, with assist @ hips and using trunk musculature with TLSO applied. Both the pt. and the family members were instructed to apply the TLSO in a supine position, observing all spinal precautions. The family members were able to appropriately demonstrate how to don and doff the TLSO, but the pt. was only able to do so with max assist. The pt. was able to sit @ the edge of the mat table, with SBA, and perform AROM using no weights, in (B) shld abd, add, flex and ext, for 5x/2 sets, with CGA. She maintained sitting @ the edge of the mat for 5 minutes, resting for 1 minute and performed 2 sets with SBA.

A: _____

_____

_____

_____

P: _____

_____

_____

Practice Exercise 6 ➤   *Review the following SOAP note and complete the "A" and "P" sections:*
Patient with Total Knee replacement (seen in outpatient setting)

DX: M17.11: unilateral primary osteoarthritis, right knee; Z96.651: Presence of right artificial knee joint; Z47.1: aftercare following joint replacement surgery

PT DX: Z96.651: Presence of right artificial knee joint; Z47.1: aftercare following joint replacement surgery: M25.561: pain in right knee; M25.661: stiffness of right knee, not elsewhere classified; M25.461: effusion, right knee; R26.89: other abnormalities of gait and mobility

Background: The pt. is a 55 y/o female s/p (R) med compartment knee replacement on 5/16/17, secondary to severe OA. She was seen through a home health agency for five visits and discharged to OP PT, with last HH visit on 5/31/17. Pt. is currently limited in normal activities and has (R) knee pain. She presents with a mild antalgic gait pattern with a decrease in heel strike secondary to knee flexion and limited knee extension. She is able to walk up to a mile without an AD, but with difficulty due to ↑ knee pain. (R) knee ROM is (-10° to 75°) prior to treatment. Pt. negotiates steps using a one step gait pattern and a handrail for support. Strength is 3-/5, hindering ADL functions and gait. Pt. reports (R) med knee pain @ best 2-3/10 and @ worst 4/10, using 1/2 pain pill as needed. There is significant swelling in the (R) knee, which could contribute to her loss of range and ↑ pain. Pt. completed an LEFS with a score of 61/80 = 76%, indicating a moderate disability. Pt. will be seen 2x/wk for 6 weeks.

PT GOALS: within 6 weeks the pt. will be able to:

1. Improve (R) knee ROM (0° to 120°) with improved ability to transition in/out of chairs, etc., and to ambulate on stairs using a reciprocal gait pattern.
2. Demonstrate improved (R) knee strength to 4/5 with ↑ ADL function and gait.
3. Improve the LEFS Score to 65-79/80, indicating a minimal disability, with improvement in >4 functional categories.
4. Be (I) and compliant with ther ex and written HEP (copy in pt. file), with pt. able to perform a correct return demo of all exs.

Daily Note: 6/16/17, 1100:

S: Pt. reported (R) knee pain @ 4/10 today, prior to tx. She reports she walked yesterday for several blocks and when she returned home, her knee had ↑ swelling with less motion, noted. She reported that she did ice it afterward, and the swelling decreased.

O: Manual E-stim was applied with pt. in a supine position, with knee extended. IFC on H/S @ intensity of 15 mA to (R) knee with electrodes in a x-pattern with a CP for 12 min. Pt. performed ther ex in the gym setting (see exercise card for detail) with pt. review of ex. and a correct return demo of all exs.

A: _____

_____

_____

_____

P: _____

_____

_____

Practice Exercise 7 ➤   *Review the following SOAP note and complete the "A" and "P" sections:*
Patient with Spastic Diplegic Cerebral Palsy (seen in a school setting)

DX: G80.1-Spastic Diplegic cerebral palsy

PT DX: G81.10-(R) spastic hemiplegia, unspecified dominance; P94.2-congenital hypotonic; M62.81-muscle weakness; R26.89-other abnormalities of gait and mobility

Background: The student is a 7 y/o female, with spastic Diplegic Cerebral Palsy in the LEs. The (R) LE is more hypertonic than the (L) LE. Postural tremors were observed when the (R) LE is positioned in extension for more than 5 minutes. The trunk musculature is hypotonic with a forward lean in standing, sitting, or when walking. Weakness of (B) LEs exist with the R (3/5) > L (4/5).

Background: The student is able to roll side↔side, supine↔prone, and sit supported with mod assist. She is able to hold a cup with a lid in her hands and roll a ball. She participates in conversation with 1 or 2 simple word responses, with delayed responses. Ambulation requires min assist from her family. She demonstrates a gait pattern with min toe walking and (B) LEs fully extended with a waddling walk. The student has a manual w/c for sitting at her desk and for mobility in the school environment.

The PT's POC includes treatment 3 x/wk. Treatment will include positioning to decrease tone of the extremities, increase balance with sitting and standing activities, increasing strength of the trunk musculature and instruction to school staff for all activities.

PT GOALS: within 6 weeks the pt. will be able to:

1. Maintain midline posture (I) in sitting for 15 minutes/1 set, using vc and SBA, feet flat on floor, to work on school projects.
2. Participate in AAROM with stretching of (B) LEs to WFL to stand with extended LEs and appropriate posture while working at the classroom counter and maintaining balance, with SBA, 15 minutes, 2x/2sets/day, without tremors.

3. ↑ strength on (R) LE to a 4/5 and the (L) LE to 4+/5, to transition from sit to stand/stand to sit, SBA, 10 x/2 sets for ↑ mobility in the classroom.
4. Increase walking 30' w/o LOB and with SBA, on tiled and carpeted surfaces, vc for ↑ use of her knees in a marching pattern, wearing (B) articulating AFO and shoes.

Daily Note: 4/20/17, 0920:

S: The teacher reports that it has been difficult getting the student to sit at the desk to work on school projects and perform transfers, without using her w/c.

O: Instructed school aide in positioning student in armchair with feet flat on floor and pillow behind back for upright posture, 3-5 minutes/2 sets. Instructed school aide for appropriate placement in standing frame to increase (B) WB in stand with support for 5-10 minutes or until tremors begin, provide rest period for 1–2 minutes and repeat positioning in standing frame for an additional 5-10 minutes. Instructed school aide in transition from sit to stand and stand to sit, using gait belt for safety and blocking knees, to increase (B) WB with vc to student throughout the transitions.

A: _____

_____

_____

_____

P: _____

_____

_____

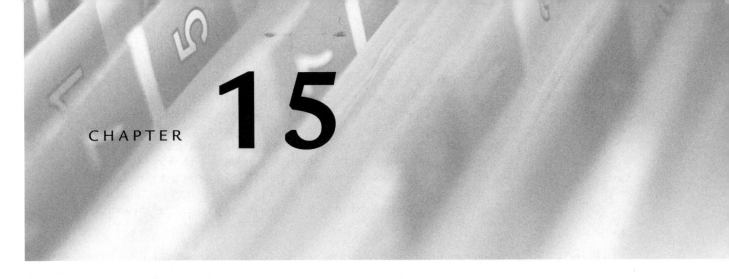

CHAPTER **15**

Do You Know Enough?

LEARNING OBJECTIVES

After studying this chapter, the student will be able to:

☐ Further practice comparing and contrasting all parts of the SOAP note, including the Subjective, Objective, Assessment, and Plan sections

☐ Further practice selecting relevant information for each section of the SOAP note to document the patient's physical therapy diagnosis and treatment

☐ Further practice organizing information for each section of the SOAP note for easy reading and understanding

☐ Understand the implications for and necessity of telerehabilitation/telehealth

INTRODUCTION

As a student and a clinical practitioner, you will provide documentation that can mean the difference between payment for therapy services rendered and denial of those services. Proper documentation is also important to help protect the patient, the medical facility for which the PTA works, and ultimately, the PTA and supervising PT. In addition, appropriate documentation ensures that the patient receives the correct care given the skill level of the practitioner. The PTA is bound by the standards of ethical conduct to ensure that the patient is safe and that the PTA meets the scope of practice requirements for the state in which he or she is licensed to practice.[1] It is the responsibility of every PTA to know that scope of practice and to abide by those rules and regulations.

LICENSING EXAMINATION QUESTIONS

Usually questions on the national licensing exam related to SOAP notes are very generic and nonspecific. The questions test the student's ability to think through a scenario critically, to determine what types of comments and measurements should be included in each section, and to make the patient's next session reproducible by another therapist. The examination is structured such that, if the student, as a practicing clinician, can meet those requirements, he or she will have a firm grasp on the appropriate information to include in a SOAP note and the methods necessary to ensure the note can be followed by another therapist for continuity in the patient's care. There are multiple methods to study for the licensing exam, and many companies provide practice exams for students. One of the best sources for review exams is the Federation for State Boards of Physical Therapy Practice (FSBPT). The FSBPT is the board responsible for providing the national licensing exam for physical therapists and physical therapist assistants and provides two practices exams, for a fee, on their website. For more information, visit www.fsbpt.org,

THE PTA'S RESPONSIBILITIES

As a student, you are required to provide appropriate documentation of patient care. This documentation should ensure that any other therapist providing care to the patient can follow the plan of care (POC), progress the patient within the POC, and make recommendations for continued therapy, discharge, or referral to other services. All of this information must be provided in the patient note whenever the PTA treats a patient! The PTA remains responsible for the patient's care until the patient is discharged from therapy services by the supervising PT.[1] Also, the PTA is responsible for providing ethical and appropriate care that falls within his or her scope of practice in the state in which he or she is licensed. That way, the patient receives appropriate and consistent care when receiving physical therapy services throughout the continuum of care.

LICENSURE REQUIREMENTS FOR PTAs

Following graduation from an accredited physical therapist assistant program, the PTA will continue to have responsibilities for lifelong learning, accumulation of continuing education units as prescribed within the state in which he or she practices, and the responsibility to ensure he or she maintains a license by following the requirements of that state. The PTA who chooses to practice in more than one state must be cognizant of all of the requirements in each of those states as they may not be the same.

Practicing PTAs are responsible for ensuring that any continuing education they obtain will meet the guidelines of the state in which they practice before they complete such a course. All states have rules and regulations that should be followed in the safe practice for physical therapy, and it would be helpful for the practicing PTA to review such guidelines on an annual basis.

TELEREHABILITATION/ TELEHEALTH ISSUES

Along with the many changes that will occur with the ACA, insurance coverage, and coding, the need for telerehabilitation/telehealth also will increase because of the inability to provide on-site PT services to some patients. Telerehabilitation/telehealth includes interactive audio, video, or other electronic media to deliver health care to a patient in a different physical location. It includes the use of electronic media for diagnosis, consultation, treatment, transfer of health or medical data, and continuing education, dependent on each state's practice act.[2,3] It is important that a PT/PTA practicing through this type of process ensure that the patient's health care coverage will pay for such services and that full disclosure has been made for such services, prior to their implementation.

The increased need for telerehabilitation/telehealth has developed owing to the rural nature of the living situation for many patients or the inability to hire licensed personnel to provide such services in a particular region. Alaska is one state that has provided physical therapy services in rural areas without the presence of a licensed physical therapist on-site. Through an interactive telecommunication system, such services are provided on-site with the patient, while the PT provides verbal instructions for an initial evaluation. The PT develops the POC that then is followed by the PTA or patient, dependent on the practice act requirements. Not all states have such procedures in their practice acts to date, but this will become more widespread as patients' needs expand. Based on the states that do have some form of telerehabilitation/ telehealth services in their state, here is a list of considerations that must be made prior to the implementation of such services (based on the individual state practice acts for physical therapists and physical therapist assistants):

- The PT/PTA must ensure that informed consent of the patient, or another appropriate person with authority to make the health-care treatment decision for the patient, is obtained before services are provided through telerehabilitation/telehealth.
- The PT/PTA must be physically present in the state while performing telerehabilitation/ telehealth and follow the practice act for that state.
- The PT/PTA must interact with the patient, maintaining the same ethical conduct and integrity as for a patient who is on-site as required under the practice act for that state.
- The PTA must comply with the requirements of the state law for any licensed physical therapist assistant providing services in that state.

- The PT may conduct one-on-one consultations, including initial evaluation, under the state law.
- The PT/PTA must provide and ensure appropriate client confidentiality and HIPAA compliance, establish secure connections, activate firewalls, and encrypt confidential information.[2, 3]

SUMMARY

As seen in previous chapters, the importance of appropriate documentation is the "bread and butter" of reimbursement for services provided for a patient's treatment and progress within the PT POC. The PTA, as a partner in that POC, must be held responsible for following the POC per state practice guidelines within the state where the PTA practices. He or she is also responsible for appropriate communication with the supervising PT.

As part of that responsibility, completion of the requirements following graduation, passing the national licensing exam, and meeting the requirements of the state in which the PTA practices will ensure the PTA remains a professional member of the physical therapy field. This ensures appropriate patient care as prescribed within the guidelines of ethical behavior for PTs and PTAs.

In addition to proper documentation in the on-site clinical setting, with the implementation of telerehabiliation/telehealth, documentation will be even more important to ensure appropriate patient care, adherence to the PT POC, progression through the POC, and final discharge for the patient receiving this type of physical therapy. Many states will have to address this issue as this type of intervention becomes more prolific.

REFERENCES

1. American Physical Therapy Association. (2014). Guidelines for physical therapy documentation. In *Guide to physical therapist practice* (3rd ed., Chapter 1). Alexandria, VA: Author.
2. State of Alaska. (2016, January). *Statutes and regulations for physical therapy and occupational therapy. Standards for practice of telerehabilitation by physical therapy.* 12 AAC 54.530. Retrieved from https://www.commerce.alaska.gov/web/portals/5/pub/pt-otstatutes.pdf
3. State of Kentucky. (2016). *Statutes and regulations for physical therapy practice utilizing telehealth.* KRS 327 200. Retrieved from http://www.lrc.ky.gov/Statutes/statute.aspx?id=31724

The following multiple-choice questions review all sections of a SOAP note and help prepare a student for questions that he or she might see on the national licensing examination. They also review how a SOAP note can help protect a student or clinical practitioner from litigation.

Practice Exercise 1 ➤ *Identify the statement that **would** be placed in the **Subjective** section of a SOAP note.*

A. AROM has ↑ to 90° in the Ⓛ LE knee extension compared with 70° at the initial evaluation.

B. The patient stated her pain is 9/10 in her low back today when she arrived at the clinic.

C. Harry was able to walk with CGA 50 ft using a quad cane on the right side.

D. The patient demonstrated a correct HEP following the session today.

Practice Exercise 2 ➤ *Identify the statement that **would** be placed in the **Objective** section of a SOAP note.*

A. Shoulder flexion measures 120° AROM, an increase of 10° from the initial evaluation.

B. The patient will be referred to OT for an evaluation.

C. The patient increased ambulation from 50 ft to 100 ft during today's session.

D. The patient stated she did not sleep well last night.

Practice Exercise 3 ➤ *Identify the statement that **would** be placed in the **Assessment** section of the SOAP note.*

A. The patient stated that her husband drank too much last night.

B. The patient, in sit, has completed the short-term goal of 10 reps/3 sets of shld. flex.

C. The patient will see the orthopedic surgeon next week.

D. The patient was able to walk to his mailbox yesterday.

Practice Exercise 4 ➤ *Identify the statement that **would** be placed in the **Plan** section of the SOAP note.*

A. The patient has stopped taking her pain medication because it makes her sick.

B. The patient demonstrated home exercises properly today.

C. The patient will return to the surgeon for a follow-up appointment.

D. The patient's family wants her to come home.

Practice Exercise 5 ➤ *Identify the statement that should **not** be in the **Subjective** section of a SOAP note.*

A. The patient complained of increased pain (from 5/10 to 8/10) with hip abduction.

B. The patient's mother states that he is difficult to listen to during her TV show.

C. The patient stated that the swelling has decreased in the left knee.

D. The patient will make an appointment with the physician next week.

Practice Exercise 6 ➤ *Identify the statement that should **not** be in the **Objective** section of a SOAP note.*

A. The patient's Ⓛ UE abd AROM has ↑ 15° since the last treatment session.

B. The patient took her pain pill 30 minutes before the treatment session today.

C. The patient has met the short-term goal of Ⓘ sitting.

D. Active shld. flex. is 150°.

Practice Exercise 7 ➤ *Identify the sentence that is **not** an **assessment** statement.*

A. The patient was able to ascend four steps with a reciprocal gait pattern today compared with one step at the initial evaluation.

B. The patient completed 9/10 reps and 3 sets of her exercises today compared with the last session of 3/10 reps/1 set.

C. The patient complained that her husband is not helping around the house.

D. The patient complained of increased swelling in her neck following the treatment session today.

Practice Exercise 8 ➤ *Identify the statement that should **not** be in the **Plan** section of a SOAP note.*

A. The patient reported his pain was 9/10 when he arrived today for his therapy session.

B. The patient complained of increased tightness in shld. ext. after yesterday's session, and PTA will communicate with PT regarding a change in the exercises.

C. Will discuss the referral of pt. to SLP for evaluation in team meeting.

D. Physical therapy will continue 2X/week with a reevaluation on 7-9-17.

Practice Exercise 9 ➤ *Identify the statement that **should** be included in the **Subjective** section of a SOAP note.*

A. The patient completed 3 reps/2 sets of the exercise program today.

B. The patient stated his pain was 5/10 in the Ⓡ knee prior to exercising.

C. The patient's mother stated they were going on a 3-month cruise.

D. The patient reported he wanted to commit suicide.

Practice Exercise 10 ➤ *Identify the statement that **should** be included in the **Objective** section of a SOAP note.*

A. The patient completed 10 reps/3 sets for hip flex against max. resistance today.

B. The patient will be referred to OT for an evaluation.

C. The patient will return for one more visit before the SV.

D. The PT has ↑ the sessions for next week from 2X/week to 3X/week.

Practice Exercise 11 ➤   *Identify the statement that **should** be included in the **Assessment** section of a SOAP note.*

A. The patient stated that the exercises were too difficult and pain ↑.

B. The patient will see the orthopedic physician next week.

C. The patient completed all of his short-term goals.

D. The patient will be referred for a speech evaluation.

Practice Exercise 12 ➤   *Identify the statement that **should** be included in the **Plan** section of the SOAP note.*

A. The patient requested that the spouse not be involved in the therapy session.

B. The patient stated that she is able to complete all exercises and wants to ↑ them.

C. The patient completed Ⓘ COG wheel exercises without pain.

D. The patient was able to complete all reps and sets of her exercises today.

Practice Exercise 13 ➤   *Identify the statement that **should** be included in the **Subjective** section of a SOAP note.*

A. The patient's father stated that she did not sleep well last night.

B. The patient stated that her pain, prior to exercising, was 5/10 in the Ⓛ hip on the VRS.

C. The patient was able to increase the weights for hip flex from 3-lb to 5-lb during the treatment session today.

D. The patient stated that she was able to walk to her car today.

Practice Exercise 14 ➤   *Place an "**S**," "**O**," "**A**," or "**P**" next to each statement to represent the section of the SOAP note in which the statement would be placed. If the statement is inappropriate for a SOAP note, write "**N/A**."*

1. _____ The patient's daughter said that she is going to buy him a shower chair when he is discharged from the hospital so he can take a shower by himself.

2. _____ The patient's daughter said she is going to buy him some new towels when he is discharged from the rehab center.

3. _____ The patient was able to stand Ⓘ next to the sink to brush his teeth (~10 minutes) following treatment.

4. _____ The patient became agitated during the treatment session and refused to finish his exercises.

5. _____ Patient's Ⓡ UE shld. flex. = 120°.

6. _____ Patient ↑ Ⓡ UE shld. flex. since last treatment session by 10°.

7. _____ Patient now able to reach items on highest kitchen shelf.

8. _____ Patient will walk Ⓘ 3 yards by Thursday.

9. _____ Patient will be seen by nutritionist on Monday.

10. _____ Patient will have her son bring her to therapy on Friday.

*In the following note, some of the statements are **incorrect** or **incomplete**. Identify them and provide a correction in the space below.*

Dx: 6-year-old male with type II spinal muscular atrophy.

S: Pt.'s parents state that they would like their son to have the best life possible. Pt.'s parents also state that they want him to be included in all the same activities as the other children his age.

O: ROM: all within normal limits. Strength: 1–2/5 in some muscle groups, right is stronger than the Ⓛ UE. Tone: flaccid. Alignment: not tested. Quality of movement: Pt. is dependent in all movement while in the bed or in a seated position. Pt. is unable to roll or sit without max assist. Pt. is unable to use the joystick on his power wheelchair. Automatic reactions: not tested. Functional skills: not tested. Adaptive equipment: pw w/c, padded wooden adjustment chair, TV pillow, jogging stroller, lap desk for eating, laptop computer, bath chair, custom-made table for w/c, wooden ramp, seatbelt, light plastic cup.

A: Pt. will benefit from skilled physical therapy to improve his quality of life.

P: Cont. skilled physical therapy 3X/wk for 6 wk for ROM training and hand-eye coordination training for ↑ ADL function.

—Andrew, PTA, License #453

_____

_____

_____

_____

_____

_____

_____

_____

Practice Exercise 16 ➤   *Write a SOAP note based on the following information. Use today's date. This is a daily progress note.*

Pt. name: Joaquin Simon, age 81

_____

Dx: ESRD, vision loss, ⒧ BKA, CHF, and depression.

_____

YOUR SUPERVISING PT told you that she did a supervisory visit with Mr. Simon this morning, and she wants you, the PTA, to see him twice a day in his hospital room to maintain his ROM and ↑ his ⒝ UE strength. The PT wants you to end each session by getting the patient into his w/c so the nurse's aide can wheel him down the hall and into a small courtyard outside.

You walk into Mr. Simon's room and find him asleep, so you gently shake his shoulder to wake him up. You tell him that you are there for his PT, and he says he will try to do it but he is very tired today.

You begin the treatment session by asking Mr. Simon whether you can raise the head of his bed so that he will be in a sitting position, and he says okay. After you have him sitting up, you ask him to raise both of his arms up above his head. He raises his arms, but his elbows are still bent at a 90° angle. You have him repeat this five times. Then you ask him whether he can hold both arms straight out in front of him while you count to five. He does it three times, but the last two times he could hold it for only 3 seconds. You then have him hold his arms in front of him again and ask him to do biceps curls on each side, 10 times. He still lacks about 20° of full elbow extension. You ask him to straighten out his elbows, but he can't do so. You do PROM to get him to full extension and hold it for 45 seconds, repeating it five times.

You perform a foot check of his ⒭ LE and see that everything looks good and healthy. You hold on to his foot and ask him to bring it up toward his bottom. He does it 10 times. You then ask Mr. Simon whether he can sit up at the edge of the bed (you have been working with him on this skill). He again states that he is very tired but that he will try. He moves his bottom over to the edge of the bed and puts his leg over the edge. He then sits there for about 30 seconds to catch his breath. You already have the w/c next to the bed with the brakes on, so you tell him where it is and that you will help him get into it. He stands on his ⒭ leg and puts about 50% of his weight on your shoulders. You then do a pivot transfer and lower him into the chair. At this time, the nurse's aide walks into the room to take Mr. Simon to the courtyard.

As the three of you are walking out of the room, you tell Mr. Simon that he did well and that you will be back in the afternoon to see him again. The nurse's aide states that Mr. Simon will be having his dialysis early today because a specialist is coming to see him at 4:00 p.m. You make a note in the chart regarding this visit and realize that you will not be able to see Mr. Simon again today because you are scheduled to attend an in-service training being led by a student PTA right after lunch.

_____

_____

_____

_____

_____

_____

_____

_____

_____

_____

Practice Exercise 17 ➤   *Write two separate SOAP notes based on the following evaluation information and **first** and **second** treatment sessions:*

Evaluation Notes

Name: *Petra Bunson*   **Age:** *48 yrs. old*

Past Med. Hx: *Three years ago, pt. had three seizures and was dx'd with a brain tumor. Pt. reported that he had chemotherapy and radiation and had been monitored for 2 years. A year ago, the tumor returned, and he had surgery to remove it. Pt. had a second surgery 2 months ago to remove necrotic tissue following radiation.*
    Pt. told PT and PTA the following information during the initial evaluation:

1. He had physical therapy after the first surgery and had been able to start jogging.

2. He had inpatient physical therapy after the second surgery for 2 weeks but did not continue it in an outpatient setting when released from the hospital.

3. Complains of left-sided weakness.

4. He has intermittent MRIs to monitor his brain for additional tumors.

5. His condition has limited his ADLs, such as working on his car, driving, hunting, fishing, doing laundry, and cleaning his house.

6. He can dress, bathe, brush his teeth, shave, and feed himself independently.

7. No complaints of pain.

8. He does fall frequently, about 2X/month.

9. He has three steps into his house, which he can do independently with a quad cane. However, someone must hold the screen door open for him.

10. Pt. lives with his 20-year-old daughter, who helps with ADLs when needed.

11. He has been receiving chemotherapy for the past year for 5 days every 2 months. Pt. reported that this causes him to become very fatigued. He said that the doctor told him the chemotherapy will have to be continued for the next 1–2 years, depending on his blood work.

12. He is on two different seizure meds and takes oxycodone as needed for pain.

13. Pt. reported that his goals are to increase his function, to be able to drive and work on his car, to be able to perform activities such as doing the dishes, and to achieve increased independence in ADLs.

You Observed the Following During the Treatment Session:

1. Pt. uses a quad cane on the (R) side.

2. Pt. has a slow gait pattern with decreased arm swing on the (L) side.

3. Pt. demonstrates increased (L) hip flexion, knee flexion, and dorsiflexion during gait with (L) lower extremity externally rotated and decreased toe clearance on the (L) during swing phase.

4. ROM: LEs: Demonstrated full passive range of motion in (B) hips and knees. (L) ankle AROM dorsiflexion is 110° and PROM dorsiflexion is 120°.

   UEs: (R) upper extremity is within normal limits (WNL); (L) upper extremity is as follows:

   shld. flex. = 65°   shld. abd = 75°

   elbow flex. = 135°   elbow ext. = −5°

   Pt. demonstrated no active movement in the (L) wrist or hand.

5. Strength:

Hip flex.	R = 3+/5	L = 3/5
Hip abd	R = 4+/5	L = 3–/5
Knee ext.	R = WNL	L = 4/5
Knee flex.	R = WNL	L = 3–/5
Dorsiflexion	R = WNL	L = 1/5
Plantar flexion	R = WNL	L = 1/5
Ankle inversion	R = WNL	L = WNL
Eversion	R = WNL	L = 0/5
Shld. flex.	R = WNL	L = 2/5
Abduction	R = WNL	L = WNL
Shld. shrug	R = WNL	L = 3–/5
Elbow ext.	R = WNL	L = 5/5
Elbow flex.	R = WNL	L = 4–/5
Wrist flexion	R = WNL	L = 1/5
Wrist ext.	R = WNL	L = 1/5

Here are some goals your PT told you to include in the POC.

STGs: *To be completed in 2 weeks:*

1. Increase wrist and ankle strength from 3/5 to 4/5.

2. Instruct pt. in HEP for increased strength and ROM with pt. performing correct return demo of all exercises.

3. Increase Ⓛ ankle PROM to 90° of dorsiflexion.

LTGs: *To be completed in 4 weeks:*

1. Increase Ⓛ UE and LE strength to 5/5.

2. Increase Ⓛ ankle dorsiflexion AROM to functional range.

3. Increase Ⓛ shld. AROM in flex. and abd to 100°.

4. Pt. will report no falls during the certification period.

5. Pt. will be able to ascend three steps into his house and open the screen door independently 100% of the time.

6. Pt. will be able to do dishes using both hands to wash and dry.

7. Pt. will walk 50 ft independently without an assistive device using a heel to toe gait pattern with equal weight-bearing and a normal swing pattern on an even surface.

The PT informs you that the pt. will be seen 1 to 2X/week for 2.5 months.

Notes From 1st Treatment Session:

Pt. stated that he has been doing the HEP (copy in chart) he had been given after his initial evaluation. He stated that he can move his left ankle independently more now and has less stiffness in his left hand. During the first treatment session, you perform the following:

1. AROM ex. with Ⓛ wrist and ankle, pt. demonstrated some independent extension in Ⓛ wrist increased by 2° and increased PROM of dorsiflexion to –15°.

2. You also performed some resistance training in the Ⓛ upper extremity with a 1-lb. weight. Pt. was able to perform 5 shoulder shrugs c̄ flexion and abduction motions.

3. You did short arc quads on the Ⓛ side with a 2-lb ankle weight; the pt. was able to complete eight repetitions.

4. You finished with soft-tissue massage to the Ⓛ upper extremity.

5. You decide that you will talk to the PT about ordering a spasticity splint for the pt.'s Ⓛ hand.

Write a SOAP Note Based on the First Treatment Session.

_____

_____

_____

_____

_____

_____

_____

_____

_____

_____

_____

_____

Notes From 2nd Treatment Session:

1. Told the pt. that the PT has ordered a special splint for his Ⓛ hand and that it should arrive before his next treatment session.

2. AROM ex. to Ⓛ upper and lower extremity. Pt. demonstrated increased AROM in dorsi-flexion and was able to flex his wrist about 15°.

3. Resistance training to upper and lower extremities using same amount of weight as first treatment session, but this time he did 10 shoulder shrugs, five each of shoulder flexion and extension, and 10 short arc quads (SAQ).

4. Pt. was able to ambulate about five steps without his quad cane 2X today.

5. Session was completed with friction massage to Ⓛ UE.

Write a SOAP Note Based on the Second Treatment Session.

_____

_____

_____

_____

_____

_____

_____

_____

_____

_____

_____

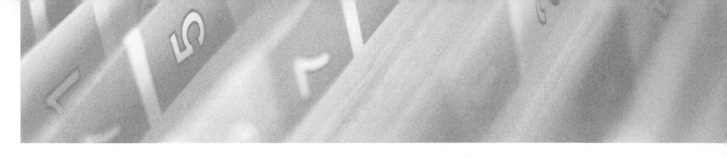

Bibliography

CHAPTER ONE

1. Document and documentation. (2016). In *Merriam-Webster's online dictionary*. Retrieved from http://www. merriam-webster.com/dictionary
2. Signing of AB 1000 concludes busy legislative year for California chapter. (2013). *PT in Motion News.* Retrieved from http://www.apta.org/PTinMotion/NewsNow/2013/10/11/CA/
3. American Physical Therapy Association. (2016). *A summary of direct access language in state physical therapy acts.* Retrieved from http://www.apta.org/StateIssues/DirectAccess
4. Healthcare Finance Administration (HCFA), minimal data set (MDS), regulations, HCFA/AMA documentation guidelines, home health regulations. Retrieved from http://www.ncbi.nlm.nih.gov/pmc/articles/PMC2232246/
5. Nagi, S. Z. (1969). *Disability and rehabilitation.* Columbus: Ohio State University Press.
6. World Health Organization. (1980). *International classification of impairments, disabilities, and handicaps.* Geneva, Switzerland: Author.
7. World Health Organization. (2001). *International classification of functioning, disability and health.* Geneva, Switzerland: Author.
8. Center for an Accessible Society. (n.d.). *Research on definitions of disability from NIDRR.* Retrieved from http://www.accessiblesociety.org/topics/demographics-identity/nidrr-lrp-defs.htm.
9. American Physical Therapy Association. (2014). Content, development and concepts. In *Guide to physical therapist practice* (3rd ed., Chapter 1). Alexandria, VA: Author.
10. American Physical Therapy Association. (2014). Standards of practice for physical therapy and the criteria. In *Guide to physical therapist practice* (3rd ed., Chapters 1 and 2). Alexandria, VA: Author.
11. American Physical Therapy Association. (2012). Defensible documentation for patient/client management. Retrieved from http://www.apta.org/Documentation/DefensibleDocumentation/
12. The Joint Commission on Accreditation of Healthcare Organizations. (1996). *Comprehensive accreditation manual for hospitals.* Oakbrook Terrace, IL: Author.
13. Commission on Accreditation for Rehabilitation Facilities. Retrieved from http://www.carf.org
14. Commission on Accreditation in Physical Therapy Education. Retrieved from http://www.capteonline.org/home.aspx

CHAPTER TWO

1. Madden, R., Sykes, & C., Bedirhan Ustun, T. (n.d.). *World Health Organization Family of International Classifications: Definition, scope and purpose.* Retrieved from World Health Organization http://www.who.int/classifications/en/FamilyDocument2007.pdf
2. World Health Organization. (n.d.). *International classification of functioning, disability, and health (ICF).* Retrieved from http://www.who.int/classifications/icf/en
3. American Physical Therapy Association. (2008, July 10). APTA endorses World Health Organization ICF model. *Medical News Today.* Retrieved from http://www.medicalnewstoday.com/releases/114422.php
4. The World Conference for Physical Therapy (WCPT). (2015). *Policy statement: standards of physical therapy practice.* Retrieved from http://www.wcpt.org/policy/ps-standards
5. World Health Organization. (2001). *International classification of functioning, disability, and health.* Geneva, Switzerland: Author.
6. Centers for Disease Control and Prevention. (2016). *The ICF model.* Retrieved from https://www.cdc.gov/nchs/data/icd/icfoverview_finalforwho10sept.pdf

CHAPTER THREE

1. Hansell, A. (2016). *Speaking in code: documentation to support the ICD-10 code set.* Combined sections presentation, American Physical Therapy Association, Anaheim, California.
2. Gawenda, R. (2016). *The ABC's of ICD-10 for physical therapists.* Combined sections presentation, American Physical Therapy Association, Anaheim, California.
3. Healthcare IT News. (2010). Why move to ICD-10, if ICD-11 is on the horizon? Retrieved from http://www.icd10watch.com/headline/why-move-icd-10-if-icd-11-horizon
4. WebPT. (2015). *The physical therapist's crunch-time guide to ICD-10.* Retrieved from https://www.webpt.com/resources/download/the-physical-therapists-crunch-time-guide-to-icd-10.
5. e-Meds Blog. (2015). ICD-9 vs ICD-10: Use of exclusions. Retrieved from http://www.e-mds.com/icd-9-vs-icd-10-use-exclusions
6. Medicare Learning Network. (2012). Preparing for therapy required functional reporting implementation in CY 2013. Retrieved from https://www.cms.gov/Outreach-and-Education/Outreach/NPC/Downloads/FunctionalReportingNPC.pdf
7. Medicare Quick Guide. (2014). *8-minute rule.* Retrieved from https://www.webpt.com/8-minute-rule
8. WebPT. (2016). PQRS 2016 FAQ [Web log post]. Retrieved from https://www.webpt.com/blog/post/pqrs-2016-faq
9. CMS. (2016). *2016 speciality measure sets.* Retrieved from https://www.cms.gov/Medicare/Quality-Initiatives-Patient-Assessment-Instruments/PQRS/MeasuresCodes.html

10. WebPT. (2016). Understanding the new evaluation codes for 2017. Rick Gawenda, PT, Author. Retrieved from https://www.webpt.com/ascend/files/handouts/Day%202_Understanding%20the%20New%20Evaluation%20Codes%20for%202017_handout.pdf?__hstc=194109170.e06eef88364d86cb0b0b60d28d2d97b6.1473811200109.1473811200111.1473811200112.2&__hssc=194109170.1.1473811200112&__hsfp=1773666937

CHAPTER FOUR

1. Bihari, M. (2016, April 21). HMOs vs. PPOs—What are the differences between HMOs and PPOs? About.com. Retrieved from https://www.verywell.com/what-are-the-differences-between-hmos-and-ppos-1739063
2. Rural Assistance Center. (n.d.). Medicare frequently asked questions: Who is covered by Medicare? Retrieved from https://www.ruralhealthinfo.org/topics/medicare#faqs
3. Bihari, M. (2014, June 19). Health reform and the doctor shortage in the U.S.: Availability of primary care physicians—the Massachusetts experience. Retrieved from http://healthinsurance.about.com/od/reform/a/PCP_shortage.htm
4. Rittenhouse, D. R., & Shortell, S. M. (2009). The patient-centered medical home: Will it stand the test of health reform? *JAMA, 301*(19), 2038–2040. Retrieved from http://jama.jamanetwork.com/article.aspx?articleid=183908
5. Centers for Medicare & Medicaid Services. (n.d.). Regulations, guidance, and standards. Retrieved from https://www.cms.gov/home/regsguidance.asp
6. Medicare. (2011). Understanding Medicare enrollment periods: How do I get Medicare Part A and Part B? Retrieved from http://www.medicare.gov/Publications/Pubs/pdf/11219.pdf
7. Centers for Medicare & Medicaid Services. (n.d.). Medicare program—general information. Retrieved from http://www.cms.gov/MedicareGenInfo/
8. Medicare Consumer Guide. (2012). Medicare advantage plans—Part C. Retrieved from http://www.medicare-consumerguide.com/medicare-part-c.html
9. AARP. (2016). *Medicare supplemental insurance plans*. Retrieved from https://www.aarpmedicaresupplement.com/
10. Centers for Medicare & Medicaid Services. (2011, May 6). Pub 100-02 Medicare benefit policy: Home health therapy services. Retrieved from http://www.cms.gov/transmittals/downloads/R144BP.pdf
11. Centers for Medicare & Medicaid Services. (2012, April 5). Manuals. Retrieved from http://www.cms.gov/Manuals/IOM/list.asp#TopOfPage
12. Who is covered by Medicaid? (n.d.). Retrieved from http://www.medicaidwebsites.com/whoiscoveredbmedicaid.php
13. Program of all-inclusive care for the elderly (PACE). (n.d.). Retrieved from https://www.cms.gov/Medicare/Health-Plans/pace/Overview.html
14. California Department of Industrial Relations. (n.d.). Division of workers' compensation—Answers to frequently asked questions about workers' compensation for employees. Retrieved from http://www.dir.ca.gov/dwc/WCFaqIW.html
15. United States Department of Labor. (2016). Workers' compensation. Retrieved from https://www.dol.gov/general/topic/workcomp
16. Drummond-Dye, R., Elliott, C., & Lee, G. R. (2010, February). *Emerging issues in Medicare, Medicaid, and private insurance.* Presented at the Health Policy & Administration Combined Sections Meeting, San Diego, CA.
17. La Monica, P. R. (2016). Unitedhealthcare to exit most Obamacare exchanges. *CNNMoney*. Retrieved from http://money.cnn.com/2016/04/19/investing/unitedhealthcare-obamacare-exchanges-aca/
18. New Mexico Medical Insurance Pool. (n.d.). Retrieved from http://www.nmmip.org
19. Jackson, J., & Nolen, J. (2010, March 21). Health care reform bill summary: A look at what's in the bill. CBSNews.com. Retrieved from http://www.cbsnews.com/8301-503544_162-20000846-503544.html
20. American Physical Therapy Association. (n.d.) Use of physical therapist assistants (PTAs) under Medicare. Retrieved from http://www.apta.org/Payment/Medicare/Supervision/UseofPTAs/
21. American Physical Therapy Association. (2011). Implementing MDS 3.0: Use of therapy students. Retrieved from http://www.apta.org/search.aspx?q=implementing%20MDS%203.0

CHAPTER FIVE

1. American Physical Therapy Association. (2003). *Guide to physical therapist practice* (2nd ed.). Alexandria, VA: Author.
2. Sahrmann, S. A. (1988). Diagnosis by physical therapist—a prerequisite for treatment. A special communication. *Physical Therapy, 68*, 1703–1786.
3. Scott, R. W. (1994). *Legal aspects of documenting patient care.* Gaithersburg, MD: Aspen.
4. Swanson, G. (1995, December). *Essentials for the future of physical therapy, every therapist's concern. A continuing education course.* Duluth: American Physical Therapy Association, Minnesota Chapter.
5. El-Din, D., & Smith, G. J. (1995, February). *Performance-based documentation: A tool for functional documentation.* Reno, NV: American Physical Therapy Association.
6. HealthIt.gov. (2016). What is an electronic health record? Retrieved from https://www.healthit.gov/providers-professionals/faqs/what-electronic-health-record-ehr
7. WebPT. (n.d.). Retrieved from http://www.webpt.com
8. ReDoc. (n.d.). Retrieved from http://www.rehabdocumentation.com
9. Therapy charts. (n.d.). Retrieved from http://www.therapycharts.com
10. Clinicient. (n.d.). Retrieved from http://www.clinicient.com
11. HealthWyse. (n.d.). Retrieved from http://www.healthwyse.com
12. American Physical Therapy Association. (2016, May 8). Electronic health records: Guide to understanding and adopting electronic health records. Retrieved from http://www.apta.org/EHR/Guide/Decision/
13. Martin, K. D. (1990). Individualized educational program and individualized family service plan. In American Physical Therapy Association, *Physical therapy practice in educational environments: Policies and guidelines* (p. 61). Alexandria, VA: Author.
14. Centers for Medicare & Medicaid Services. (n.d.). Hospital center. Retrieved from http://www.cms.hhs.gov/center/hospital.asp

CHAPTER SIX

1. American Physical Therapy Association. (2014). *Guide to physical therapist practice* (3rd ed., Chapter 1). Alexandria, VA: Author. Retrieved from http://guidetoptpractice.apta.org
2. American Physical Therapy Association. (2014). Underlying concepts. In *Guide to physical therapist practice* (3rd ed., Chapter 1). Alexandria, VA: Author. Retrieved from http://guidetoptpractice.apta.org/content/current
3. American Physical Therapy Association. (2014). Defensible documentation for patient/client management. In *Guide to physical therapist practice* (3rd ed., Chapter 1). Alexandria, VA: Author. Retrieved from http://www.apta.org/Documentation/DefensibleDocumentation

CHAPTER SEVEN

1. Health Insurance Portability and Accountability Act (HIPAA). (n.d.). Retrieved from http://www.hhs.gov/hipaa/index.html
2. Family Educational Rights and Privacy Act (FERPA). (2011). Retrieved from http://www2.ed.gov/policy/gen/guid/fpco/ferpa/index.html
3. The Privacy Rule. (n.d.). Retrieved from http://www.hhs.gov/hipaa/for-professionals/privacy/index.html
4. Cherry, K. (2016). What is informed consent? Retrieved from https://www.verywell.com/what-is-informed-consent-2795276
5. Hilton, D. (Ed.). (1988). *Documentation: A clinical pocket manual* (p. 135). Springhouse, PA: Springhouse.

CHAPTER EIGHT

1. Kasprak, J. (n.d.). *Patient access to medical records.* Retrieved from http://www.cga.ct.gov/2006/rpt/2006-r-0599.htm
2. *Student record storage.* (2005). Retrieved from http://www.psea.org/uploadedFiles/Publications/Professional_Publications/Advisories/StudentRecords07.pdf
3. Health Information Privacy. (2003, February 20). *Summary of the HIPAA Security Rule.* Retrieved from http://www.hhs.gov/hipaa/for-professionals/security/laws-regulations/index.html
4. Healthcare Providers Service Organization. (2012). *Professional liability insurance—Individual coverage through HPSO.* Retrieved from http://www.hpso.com/professional-liability-insurance/coverage-description.jsp
5. Healthcare Providers Service Organization. (2016). *PT professional liability exposures: 2016 claim report webinar.*
6. Deposition. (2016). In *Nolo's plain-English law dictionary.* Retrieved from http://www.nolo.com/dictionary/deposition-term.html
7. American Physical Therapy Association. (2003). *Guide to physical therapist practice* (2nd ed.). Alexandria, VA: Author.
8. American Physical Therapy Association. *Standards of ethical conduct for the physical therapist assistant.* Retrieved from http://www.apta.org/uploadedFiles/APTAorg/About_Us/Policies/HOD/Ethics/Standards.pdf
9. American Physical Therapy Association. (2011). *Professionalism.* Retrieved from http://www.apta.org/Professionalism
10. American Physical Therapy Association. (2010). *APTA guide for the conduct of the physical therapist assistant.* Retrieved from http://www.apta.org/uploadedFiles/APTAorg/Practice_and_Patient_Care/Ethics/GuideforConductofthePTA.pdf

CHAPTER NINE

1. Rubric. (2011). In *Merriam-Webster's online dictionary.* Retrieved from http://www.merriam-webster.com/dictionary/rubric

CHAPTER TEN

1. Subjective. (2011). In *Merriam-Webster's online dictionary.* Retrieved from http://www.merriam-webster.com/dictionary/subjective

CHAPTER ELEVEN

1. Objective. (2011). In *Merriam-Webster's online dictionary.* Retrieved from http://www.merriam-webster.com/dictionary/objective
2. Tinetti Assessment Tool. (n.d.). Retrieved from http://www.bhps.org.uk/falls/documents/TinettiBalanceAssessment.pdf
3. The Peabody Developmental Motor Scales—2nd Edition (PDMS-2). (n.d.). Retrieved from http://www.proedinc.com/customer/productView.aspx?ID=1783
4. The Barthel Index. (n.d.). Retrieved from http://www.strokecenter.org/wp-content/uploads/2011/08/barthel.pdf
5. Functional Independence Measure (FIM). (n.d.). Retrieved from http://www.rehabmeasures.org/Lists/RehabMeasures/DispForm.aspx?ID=889
6. Baeten, A. M., Moran, M. L., & Phillippi, L. M. (1999). *Documenting physical therapy: The reviewer perspective.* Boston, MA: Butterworth-Heinemann.
7. American Physical Therapy Association. (2010). Defensible documentation for patient/client management. Retrieved from http://www.apta.org/Documentation/DefensibleDocumentation

CHAPTER TWELVE

1. Assessment. (2016). In *Merriam-Webster's online dictionary.* Retrieved from http://www.learnersdictionary.com/search/assessment
2. American Physical Therapy Association. (2003). Guidelines for physical therapy documentation. In *Guide to physical therapist practice* (2nd ed.). Alexandria, VA: Author.
3. American Physical Therapy Association. (2003). Documentation for physical therapist patient/client management. In *Guide to physical therapist practice* (2nd ed.). Alexandria, VA: Author.

CHAPTER THIRTEEN

1. Plan. (2011). In *Merriam-Webster's online dictionary.* Retrieved from http://www.merriam-webster.com/dictionary/plan
2. American Physical Therapy Association. (2003). Guidelines for physical therapy documentation. In *Guide to physical therapist practice* (2nd ed.). Alexandria, VA: Author.

CHAPTER FOURTEEN   1. American Physical Therapy Association. (2014). Guidelines for physical therapy documentation. In *Guide to physical therapist practice* (3rd ed.). Alexandria, VA: Author.

CHAPTER FIFTEEN   1. American Physical Therapy Association. (2014). Guidelines for physical therapy documentation. In *Guide to physical therapist practice* (3rd ed., Chapter 1). Alexandria, VA: Author.
2. State of Alaska. (2016, January). *Statutes and regulations for physical therapy and occupational therapy. Standards for practice of telerehabilitation by physical therapy.* 12 AAC 54.530. Retrieved from https://www. commerce.alaska.gov/web/portals/5/pub/pt-otstatutes.pdf
3. State of Kentucky. (2016). *Statutes and regulations for physical therapy practice utilizing telehealth.* KRS 327 200. Retrieved from http://www.lrc.ky.gov/Statutes/statute.aspx?id=31724

Glossary

A **Accountable:** Responsible, capable of explaining oneself.

Accredit: To supply with credentials or authority.

Accreditation: Granting of approval to an institution by an official review board after the institution has met specific requirements.

Adhesive capsulitis: A condition characterized by adhesions and shortening or tightening of the connective tissue sleeve that encases a joint.

Affordable Care Act (ACA): The Patient Protection and Affordable Care Act (PPACA), also known as the Affordable Care Act and generally known as Obamacare, is the health-care reform that was passed into legislation by the 111th Congress and signed into law by President Barack Obama in March 2010.

Ambulate: To walk about.

American Physical Therapy Association: Professional organization representing the physical therapy profession, which in turn consists of professionals and technicians trained to provide the medical rehabilitative service of physical therapy.

Antalgic: Painful or indicating the presence of pain.

Anterior joint capsule: Front portion of the joint connective tissue sleeve.

Assessment: Measurement, quantification, or placement of a value or label on something. *Assessment* is often confused with *evaluation*; an assessment results from the act of assessing.*

Association for the Advancement of Retired Persons (AARP): Nonprofit, nonpartisan membership organization for people age 50 and over that provides a wide range of benefits, products, and services for members, including supplemental insurance.

Ataxia: Condition characterized by an impaired ability to coordinate movement. An ataxic gait is a staggering, uncoordinated walk.

Athetoid: Condition characterized by impaired movement, often marked by slow, writhing movements of the hands.*

Audit: Examination of records to check accuracy and compliance with professional standards.

Authenticate: To verify, to prove, to establish as worthy of belief.

Autonomy: Independent functioning, ability to self-govern.

B **Balance:** Ability to maintain the body in equilibrium with gravity in either a static or dynamic process.*

Biomechanics: Study of mechanical forces and their interaction with living organisms, especially the human body.

C **Capacity qualifier:** Indication of the patient's ability to perform a task or activity within the ICF framework.

Center for International Rehabilitation Research Information and Exchange (CIRRIE): Entity responsible for the development of the ICF Crosswalk database, which provides evidence-based research articles supporting the coding system of the ICF in clinical practice.

Centers for Medicare and Medicaid Services (CMS): Previously known as the Health Care Financing Administration (HCFA), the CMS is a federal agency within the United States Department of Health and Human Services (DHHS) that administers Medicare and Medicaid (in partnership with state governments), the State Children's Health Insurance Program (SCHIP), and Health Insurance Portability and Accountability Act (HIPAA) standards.

Circumduct: To move the joint in a circular manner.

Clinical decision: Determination that relates to direct patient care, indirect patient care, acceptance of patients for treatment, and whether patients should be referred to other practitioners.‡ A diagnosis that leads a therapist to take an action is a form of a clinical decision. Clinical decisions result in actions. When direct supporting evidence for clinical decisions is lacking, such decisions are based on clinical opinions.

Cognition: Act or process of knowing, including both awareness and judgment.*

Collaborate: To work together, to cooperate.

Compensation: The ability of an individual with a disability to perform a task, either by using the impaired limb with an adapted approach or by using the unaffected limb to perform the task; an approach to rehabilitation in which the patient is taught to adapt to and offset a residual disability.*

Concentric contraction: Muscle contraction that moves the muscle from a resting, lengthened position to a shortened position; a muscle contraction in which the insertion and origin move closer together.

Continuum: A coherent whole characterized as a collection, sequence, or progression of values or elements varying by minute degrees.

Contracture: A condition of fixed, high resistance to passive stretching that results from fibrosis and shortening of tissues that support muscles or joints.*

Coordination: Muscle action of the appropriate intensity, timing, and sequencing to produce a smooth, controlled, purposeful movement.

Criteria: Requirements, standards, rules.

Current Procedural Terminology (CPT): A system developed by the American Medical Association for standardizing the terminology and coding used to describe medical serviced and procedures in the health-care setting.

Cyanosis: A bluish or purplish discoloration of the skin due to a severe oxygen deficiency.*

D   **Data:** Raw information, uninterpreted information organized for analysis or used as the basis for a decision.

Débridement: Excision of contused or necrotic tissue from the surface of a wound.*

Deposition: Examination before a trial that provides sworn testimony from a witness outside of a court setting.

Derived classifications: More specialized classifications of diseases or disorders that are derived from broader reference classifications (e.g., the International Classification of Diseases for Oncology, the ICF version for Children and Youth [ICF-CY], The Application of the ICF to Neurology).

Diagnosis: A label encompassing a cluster of signs and symptoms, syndromes, or categories. It is determined as a result of the diagnostic process, which includes (1) evaluating the data obtained during the examination, (2) organizing it into cluster syndromes or categories, and (3) interpreting it.*

Direct access: Legislation that enables the consumer to enter the medical care system by going directly to a physical therapist. The patient needing physical therapy treatment does not need to be referred to a physical therapist by a physician.

Disability: Incapacitated by illness or injury; physically or mentally impaired in a way that substantially limits activity, especially in relation to employment or education.

Discharge evaluation: A document written by the PT containing recommendations and decisions for after treatment is terminated by the PT.

Discharge summary: A document that may be written by the PTA stating the treatments provided and the status of the patient at the time of discharge. If this document contains recommendations or decisions about future treatment, it is considered an evaluation and must be written by the PT.

Documentation: Written information supplying proof; a written record; supporting references.

Duration: Period of time in which something persists or exists.

Dysarthria: A motor disorder that results in impairment of motor speech mechanisms.*

Dysphagia: Difficulty in swallowing.*

Dyspnea: Shortness of breath; subjective difficulty or distress in breathing frequently manifested by rapid, shallow breaths; usually associated with serious diseases of the heart or lungs.*

E **Eccentric contraction:** A muscle contraction that moves the muscle from a shortened position to its lengthened or resting position; muscle contraction in which the insertion and origin move away from each other.

Edema: Swelling; accumulation of fluid in the tissues.

Efficacy: Effectiveness, ability to achieve results.

Electronic Health Record (EHR): A digital version of a patient's paper chart that provides medical information in real time and is usually available in an online format through a web-based medical program and is provided in a secure manner to authorized users.

Episode of care: All physical therapy services that are (1) provided by a physical therapist or under the direction and supervision of a physical therapist, (2) provided in an unbroken sequence, and (3) related to the physical therapy interventions for a given condition or problem or related to a request from the patient/client, family, or other health-care provider.§

Erythema: Describing an abnormal redness of the skin.*

Evaluation: Judgment based on a measurement; often confused with assessment and examination. Evaluations are judgments of the value or worth of something. A dynamic process in which the physical therapist makes clinical judgments based on data gathered during the examination.§

Examination: Test or a group of tests used for the purpose of obtaining measurements or data.* The process of obtaining a history, performing relevant systems reviews, and selecting and administering specific tests and measurements.§

Extension: Movement of a joint in which the angle between the two adjoining bones increases.

Exudation: Process of expressing material through a wound, usually characterized as oozing.

F **Facilitate:** To enhance or help an action or function.

Family Educational Rights and Privacy Act (FERPA): The procedure, similar to HIPAA, of protecting the confidentiality of medical information related to students enrolled in an education institution.

Femur: Thigh bone.

Flexion: Movement of a joint in which the angle decreases between the two adjoining bones.

Fractured: Broken. Typically refers to broken bones.

Fremitus: Sensation felt when placing a hand on a body part that vibrates during speech or deep breathing.*

Frequency: Number of times something occurs, number of repetitions, number of treatment sessions.

Function: Those activities identified by an individual as essential to support physical, social, and psychological well-being and to create a personal sense of meaningful living.*

Functional limitation: Restriction of the ability to perform a physical action, activity, or task in an efficient, typically expected, or competent manner.§

Functional Outcomes: A measureable goal that helps a patient perform specific activities related to daily living and their ability to function in the most appropriate manner.

Functional Outcome Reports (FOR): A structured reporting system to identify the functional assessment and outcomes related to patient care in a health-care setting.

G **Gait:** Walking pattern; the manner in which a person walks.

Gait patterns:*

Two-point gait: Assistive device and contralateral lower extremity advance and meet the floor simultaneously.

Three-point gait: Assistive devices and one weight-bearing lower extremity maintain contact with the floor.

Four-point gait: In sequential order of contact: the left crutch is advanced, followed by the right lower extremity, then the right crutch is advanced prior to the left lower extremity.

Swing-to gait: Pattern in which both crutches (or other assistive device) are advanced, and then bilateral lower extremities advance parallel to the plane of the assistive device.

Swing-through gait: Pattern in which both crutches (or other assistive device) are advanced, and then bilateral lower extremities advance anterior to the placement of the device.

Tandem walk: Heel-to-toe pattern in which the heel is placed in front of the toe of the opposite extremity; pattern is repeated with each lower extremity.

Braiding/grapevine gait: Pattern in which the left lower extremity is adducted anterior to the right lower extremity, the right lower extremity is abducted, the left lower extremity is adducted posterior to the right lower extremity, and the right lower extremity is abducted to complete the sequence. Sequence may be repeated with the right lower extremity initiating.

Girth: Distance around something, circumference.

Goal: Statement(s) that defines the patient's expected level of performance at the end of the rehabilitation process; the functional outcomes of therapy, indicating the amount of independence, supervision, or assistance required and the equipment or environmental adaptation necessary to ensure adequate performance. Desired outcomes may be stated as long-term or short-term as determined by the needs of the patient and the setting.*

Goniometry: Procedure for measuring the range-of-motion angles of a joint.

H **Health Insurance Portability and Accountability (HIPPA):** A United States law that provides privacy standards to protect patients' medical records and other health information provided to health plans, doctors, hospitals and other health-care providers.

Hamstrings: Common name for the group of three muscles located on the posterior thigh.

Handicap: As defined by the World Health Organization, the disadvantage resulting from an impairment or disability that limits or prevents fulfillment of a role that is normal, depending on age, sex, and social and cultural factors. *Handicap* describes the social and economic roles of impaired or disabled persons that place them at a disadvantage when compared with others (e.g., inability to use public transportation, inability to work, social isolation).*

Health maintenance organization (HMO): A type of managed care organization that provides health-care options to individuals who meet specific requirements and requires those individuals to follow the organization's guidelines to receive health care.

Health status: Level of an individual's physical, mental, affective, and social functions. Health status is an element of well-being.*

Hemianopsia: Loss of vision in one-half of the visual field of one or both eyes.*

Hip extensors: Common name for the group of muscles that produce extension motion of the hip joint.

Homonymous hemianopsia: Defective vision or blindness affecting the right or left half of the visual fields of both eyes.*

House of Delegates (HOD): Governing body of the American Physical Therapy Association; responsible for setting guidelines for the professional practice of physical therapists and physical therapist assistants.

Hypertonus: Excessive muscle tone or prolonged muscle contraction.

I **ICD-10 Codes:** The international classification system used by all health-care providers to classify and code all diagnoses, procedures and symptoms related to patient care.

Impairment: A loss or abnormality of physiological, psychological, or anatomical structure or function.§

Incident: Distinct occurrence; an event inconsistent with usual routine or treatment procedure; an accident.

Incident report: Documentation required when an unusual event occurs in a clinical or medical facility.

Individual educational program (IEP): Written statement outlining the goals and objectives of the services provided to meet a disabled child's educational needs.

Informed consent: Permission or agreement for medical treatment provided with full knowledge of the treatment.

Initial and mid swing: Portions of the walking pattern when the heel and then the toes leave the ground and the leg swings to the point where the hip is at 0° flexion or extension.

Instrumental activities of daily living (IADL): Activities that are important components of maintaining independent living (e.g., shopping, cooking).*

Internship: Period of time during which a medical professional in training provides clinical care under supervision.

Intervention: The purposeful and skilled interaction of the physical therapist with the patient/client and, when appropriate, with other individuals involved in care, using various methods and techniques to produce changes in the patient's/client's condition.§

J   Joint Commission on Accreditation of Healthcare Organizations: Agency responsible for ensuring that hospitals and medical centers follow federal and state regulations and meet the standards necessary for the provision of safe and appropriate health care.

Joint integrity: Conformance of the joints to expected anatomical, biomechanical, and kinematic norms.*

Joint mobility: Ability to move a joint; takes into account the structure and shape of the joint surface as well as characteristics of tissue surrounding the joint.*

K   Kinesthesia: The awareness of the body's or a body part's movement.*

L   Laceration: Torn, jagged wound.

Lag: To fall behind, not keep up, develop slowly, weaken, or slacken.

Lower extremity: Area that includes the thigh, lower leg, and foot.

M   Managed care organization (MCO): Network-based organization responsible for monitoring and providing reduced-cost health-care benefits to members of the general population who meet specific guidelines.

Medicaid: Health-care program for certain people and families with low incomes and resources, jointly funded by state and federal governments and managed by individual states.

Medical diagnosis: Identification of a systemic disease or disorder on the basis of the findings from a physician's examination and diagnostic tests.

Medicare: A national health insurance program, founded in 1965, that is administered by the United States federal government and that guarantees access to health insurance for Americans ages 65 and older, younger people with disabilities, and people with end-stage renal disease.

Mobilization techniques: Manual techniques or procedures used by physical therapy professionals to increase a joint's range of motion.

Modality: Method of therapy or treatment procedure.

Motor function: The ability to learn or demonstrate the skillful and efficient assumption, maintenance, modification, and control of voluntary postures and movement patterns.*

Fine motor function: Refers to relatively delicate movements, such as using a fork or tying a shoelace.

Gross motor function: Refers to larger-scale movements, such as assuming an upright position or carrying a bag.

Muscle spasms: Persistent, involuntary contractions of a muscle or certain groups of fibers within the muscle.

Muscle tone: The velocity-dependent resistance to stretch that muscle exhibits.*

Flaccidity: Total loss of muscle tension or responsiveness to stimulation.

Hypotonia: Reduced muscle tension with a slowed response to stimulation.

Hypertonia: Increased muscle tension resulting in resistance to movement, with increased speed and effort of movement.

Mild: A slight resistance to movement, with full ROM when the movement is performed slowly (not apparent at rest).

Moderate: A resistance to movement with limitation to the variety and smoothness or response to stimulation that is affected by positioning and the speed of movement.

Severe: Observed posturing at rest, with limitation in ROM and resistance to movement regardless of the position or speed of stimulation.

N **Nagi model:** Model that provides a definitive summary of an active pathology and its relationship to the resulting impairment, functional limitation, and disability.

Negligence: State of being extremely careless or lacking in concern.

Neuromusculoskeletal: Pertaining to the nervous system, the muscular system, and the skeletal system.

O **Objective:** Measurable statement of an expected response or outcome; something worked toward or striven for; a statement of direction or desired achievement that guides actions and activities.*

Occupational therapist: Trained health-care professional who provides occupational therapy.

Occupational therapy assistant: Trained health-care technician who provides occupational therapy under the supervision of an occupational therapist.

Orthopedics: Branch of medicine devoted to the study and treatment of the skeletal system and its joints, muscles, and associated structures.

Orthostatic hypotension: Lowering of systolic blood pressure >10 mm Hg with a change of body position from supine to erect, which may or may not be accompanied by clinical signs.*

Outcomes: Outcomes are the result of patient/client management. They are related to remediation of functional limitations and disabilities, primary or secondary prevention, and optimization of patient/client satisfaction.*

Outcomes analysis: A systematic examination of patient/client outcomes in relation to selected patient/client variables; outcomes analysis may be used in a quality assessment, economic analysis or practice, and other processes.*

Oxygen saturation: The degree to which oxygen is present in a particular cell, tissue, organ, or system.*

P **Palpable:** Able to be felt or touched, as in touching with the hands.

Parameters: Limits or boundaries; a value or constant used to describe or measure a set of data representing a physiological function or system.

Paraparesis: Partial paralysis or extreme weakness.

Pathokinesiologic: Pertaining to the study of movements related to a given disorder.

Pathological: Pertaining to a condition that is caused by or involves a disease.

Pathology: Study of the characteristics, causes, and effects of disease.

Percussion (diagnostic): Procedure in which the clinician taps a body part manually or with an instrument to estimate its density.*

Performance qualifier: Indication of what a patient can do in his or her current environment within the ICF framework.

Perseveration: Involuntary and pathological persistence of the same verbal response or motor activity regardless of the type of stimulus or its duration.*

Physical function: Fundamental component of health status describing the state of those sensory and motor skills necessary for mobility, work, and recreation.*

Physical therapist assistant: A technically educated health-care provider who assists the physical therapist in the provision of physical therapy. The physical therapist assistant, under the direction and supervision of the physical therapist, is the only paraprofessional who provides physical therapy interventions. The physical therapist assistant is a graduate of a physical therapist assistant degree program accredited by the Commission on Accreditation in Physical Therapy Education (CAPTE).§

Physical therapy: The treatment of impairments and functional limitations by physical means, such as exercise, education and training, heat, light, electricity, water, cold, ultrasound, massage, and manual therapy to improve or restore the patient's ability to function in his or her environment. Physical therapy is provided by trained persons who have graduated from accredited physical therapy and physical therapist assistant programs.

Physical therapy practice act: State legislation that defines and regulates the practice or provision of physical therapy services.

Physical therapy problem: Identification of the neuromusculoskeletal dysfunction and resulting functional limitation that is treatable with physical therapy.

Physician assistants: Trained technicians providing medical care under the supervision of a physician.

Plan of care: Statements that specify the anticipated long-term and short-term goals and the desired outcomes, predicted level of optimal improvement, specific interventions to be used, duration and frequency of the intervention required to reach the goals and outcomes, and criteria for discharge.*

Points of service (POS) organization: A type of managed care organization that provides health-care options to individuals who meet specific guidelines and requires individuals to follow the organization's requirements to receive health care. The points of service plan has levels of progressively higher patient financial participation as the patient moves away from the more managed features of the plan.

Preferred provider organization (PPO): A type of managed care organization that provides options for health care to individuals who meet specific guidelines and requires those individuals to follow the organization's rules to receive health care.

Prevention:*

Primary: Preventing disease in a susceptible or potentially susceptible population through specific measures, such as general health-promotion efforts.
Secondary: Decreasing duration of illness, severity of disease, and sequelae through early diagnosis and prompt intervention.
Tertiary: Limiting the degree of disability and promoting rehabilitation and restoration of function in patients with chronic and irreversible diseases.

Primary care physician (PCP): The physician responsible for managing the patient's care within a health maintenance organization or preferred provider system to keep patient-care costs at a minimum.

Problem-oriented: Based on or directed toward the problem, as when the medical record is organized around the identification of the medical problems.

Professional Liability Insurance: Insurance that provides protection against litigation for malpractice in the medical setting.

Prognosis: Determination of the level of optimal improvement that might be attained by the patient/client and the amount of time needed to reach that level.*

Program of All-Inclusive Care for the Elderly (PACE): A service under both Medicare and Medicaid, offered in certain states, that provides comprehensive medical and social services in noninstitutional settings for individuals.

Progress/Daily Note: A record of the treatment provided for each problem, the patient's reaction to the treatment procedures, progress towards goals and outcomes, and any changes in the patient's condition.

Prone: Horizontal with the face downward. Opposite of supine.

Proprioception: The reception of stimuli from within the body; includes position sense and kinesthesia.*

Psoriasis: Common, chronic, inheritable skin disorder characterized by circumscribed red patches covered by thick, dry, silvery, adherent scales.

Q   **Quadriparesis (tetraplegia):** Partial paralysis or extreme weakness of the arms, legs, and trunk resulting from injury to spinal nerves in the cervical spine.

Quality assurance: Name of the department in health-care facilities that reviews medical charts to identify when regulations and standards are not being met or when unsafe or inappropriate medical care is being provided.

Quality assurance committee: Group that performs chart reviews.

R   **Range of motion:*** The space, distance, or angle through which movement occurs at a joint or a series of joints.

Passive (PROM): 100% therapist- or assistant-performed movement through the available excursion of the joint or body segment.

Active (AROM): 100% self-performed movement through the available excursion of the joint or body segment.

Active assistive (AAROM): Partial self-performed movement with external assistance provided to complete the desired available excursion of the joint or body segment.

Reference classifications: Classifications of health-care issues affecting an individual's ability to function, including the International Classification of Diseases (ICD) and the International Classification of Functioning, Disability, and Health (ICF).

Rehabilitation facilities: Clinics or institutions that provide rehabilitation services, such as physical therapy, occupational therapy, speech pathology, psychological services, social services, orthotics and prosthetics, and patient and family education.

Rehabilitation types:*

Acute: Term used by some sources to denote intense rehabilitation in an inpatient rehabilitation facility or designated unit.

Comprehensive: Rehabilitation involving a full array of services and disciplines.

Intense: Generally interpreted to mean rehabilitation involving three or more hours of acute physical, occupational, psychological, or speech and language therapy per day, five or more days per week.

Rehabilitation hospital: Free-standing hospital that is organized and staffed to provide intense and comprehensive inpatient rehabilitation.

Rehabilitation unit: Distinct part of an acute-care hospital or skilled nursing facility that is organized and staffed to provide intense and comprehensive inpatient rehabilitation.

Subacute care: Goal-oriented, comprehensive inpatient care that is designed for an individual who has had an acute illness, injury, or exacerbation of a disease process and that is rendered immediately after, or instead of, acute hospitalization.

Reimbursement: Payment for services.

Related classifications: Classifications that describe aspects of health not commonly addressed otherwise or related to specific diseases or disabilities (e.g., the International Classification of Primary Care [ICFPC]).

Release-of-information form: Document that the patient signs to give permission for the person(s) named in the document to receive information about the patient's medical condition and treatment.

Reliable: Dependable, reproducible.

Retrospective: Looking back on, contemplating, or directed to the past.

Rule of confidentiality: The principle that information about patients should not be revealed to anyone not authorized to receive the information.

S   **Signs:** Characteristics or indications of disease or dysfunction determined by objective tests, measurements, or observations.

Social Security Disability Insurance (SSDI): A payroll tax–funded federal insurance program administered by the United States government. It is managed by the Social Security Administration and is designed to provide income supplements to people who are restricted in employment because of a specific disability.

Source-oriented: Organized around the source of the information, as when the medical record is organized according to the various disciplines providing and documenting the care.

Speech pathologist: Trained professional who diagnoses and treats abnormalities in speech.

Standardized Functional Assessments: Tools with set protocols and procedures, clear instructions, and methods to score a patient's level of function.

Status quo: No change in a specified state or condition.

Strengthening:[*]

> *Active:* Form of strength-building exercise in which the therapist applies resistance through the range of motion of active movement.
>
> *Assistive:* Form of strength-building exercise in which the therapist assists the patient/client through the available range of motion.
>
> *Resistive:* Any form of active exercise in which a dynamic or static muscular contraction is resisted by an outside force. The external force can be applied manually or mechanically.
>
> *Isometric exercise:* Active contraction of a muscle or group of muscles against a stable force without joint movement.
>
> *Isokinetic exercise:* Active movement performed at an established fixed speed against an accommodating resistance.

Symptoms: Subjective characteristics or indications of disease or dysfunction as perceived by the patient.

Systemic: Pertaining to the whole body.

Systems review: A brief or limited examination that provides additional information about the patient's general health to help the physical therapist formulate a diagnosis and select an intervention program.[*]

T Tactile: Pertaining to the sense of touch.

Telerehabilitation/Telehealth: An interactive audio, video or other electronic media to deliver health care to a patient in a different physical location form the treating health-care provider.

Third-party payer: A medical reimbursement agency, such as Medicare, Medicaid, managed care organizations, indemnity insurers, and businesses that contract for services. Each type of payer has its own reimbursement policies.

Transfers/position:[*]

> *Dependent transfer:* Patient/client relies totally on external support for transfer and exerts no physical assistance in transfer.
>
> *Sliding board/transfer board:* Patient/client transfers with assistance of board placed under ischial tuberosities; the board bridges two opposing surfaces.
>
> *Depression transfer:* Patient/client transfers by depressing scapulae with upper extremity pressure against surface and lifting pelvis laterally or anteroposteriorly.
>
> *Stand pivot:* Patient/client transfers by pushing to stand and pivoting with one or both lower extremities.
>
> *Supported sitting:* Sitting position maintained with external support and/or use of the patient's/client's upper extremities.
>
> *Unsupported sitting:* Sitting position maintained without external support or use of the patient's/client's upper extremities.
>
> *Quadruped:* Position where weight-bearing occurs on extended upper extremities and on flexed hips or knees; upper extremities placed at 90° should flexion with 0° to 10° abduction and full elbow extension, and lower extremities are placed on 90° hip-knee flexion with lower legs resting parallel to floor.
>
> *Long sitting:* Sitting with hips at 90° angle and bilateral lower extremities extended fully on a supported surface.

U Ulcers:[*]

> *Stage I:* Nonblanchable erythema of intact skin reversible with intervention.
>
> *Stage II:* Tissue loss involving the epidermis and dermis that may present as an abrasion, blister, or a shallow crater, with a wound base that is moist, pink, painful, and free of necrotic tissue.

Stage III: Damage or actual necrosis of subcutaneous tissue that may extend down to but not through the fascial layer; may include necrotic tissue; wound base not usually painful.

Stage IV: Tissue loss extending to the level of bone, muscle, tendon, or other supporting structure; involves necrotic tissue; wound base usually not painful.

V   Vital signs: Measurements of pulse rate, respiration rate, body temperature, and blood pressure.

W   Weight-bearing status:*

Non–weight-bearing (NWB): No weight on involved extremity.

Toe-touch/touchdown/foot-flat weight-bearing (TTWB, TDWB, FFWB): Extremity may rest on floor (is unloaded); negligible weight is placed on extremity. Status used primarily for balance or stability during gait and transfers.

Partial weight-bearing (PWB): Prescribed, measured percentage of weight is allowed.

Weight-bearing as tolerated (WBAT): As much weight as is tolerated within pain limits is allowed.

Full weight-bearing (FWB): 100% of body weight, with or without assistive devices, is allowed.

Workers' compensation Insurance: State- and business-funded health insurance that manages and funds medical care for persons injured on the job.

World Health Organization (WHO): The authority on global health matters and on health-care issues within the United Nations system. WHO developed a family of international classifications that may be used to compare health information internationally as well as nationally.

WHO Family of International Classifications (WHO-FIC): A classification system used in health-care settings worldwide.

---

*Task Force on Standards for Measurement in Physical Therapy. (1991). Standards for tests and measurement in physical therapy practice. *Physical therapy, 71,* 589. Retrieved from http://ptjournal.apta.org/content/71/8/589.full.pdf

‡-This definition is modified from the one presented by Charles Magistro at a conference on clinical decision-making held under APTA auspices in October 1988 in Lake of the Ozarks, MO.

§Retrieved from www.Merriam-Webster.com

Appendix A

Abbreviations

A

ā	before
A:	assessment data
Ⓐ	assist
A/	active
AA/	active assist
AAROM	active assistive range of motion
abd	abduction
ABI	acquired brain injury
Abn	abnormal
a.c.	before meals
ACA	anterior cerebral artery, Affordable Care Act
AC joint	acromioclavicular joint
ACCE	Academic Coordinator of Clinical Education
ACL	anterior cruciate ligament
AD	Assistive Device
ADA	American with Disabilities Act; American Diabetes Association
add.	adduction
ADL	activities of daily living
ad lib	at discretion
AE	above elbow
AFO	ankle foot orthoses
AIIS	anterior inferior iliac spine
A/K	above knee
AKA	above knee amputation
AKS	arthroscopic knee surgery
AKFO	ankle knee foot orthosis
AMA	against medical advice
amb	ambulation
amt	amount
ant	anterior
ante	before
AOTA	American Occupational Therapy Association
A-P	anterior-posterior
appt, appts	appointment(s)
APTA	American Physical Therapy Association
AROM	active range of motion
ASAP	as soon as possible
ASHA	American Speech Language Hearing Association
ASIS	anterior superior iliac spine
assist.	assistance
ATNR	asymmetrical tonic neck reflex
ax. cr	axillary crutches

B

Ⓑ	bilateral, both
BBFA	both bone forearm (fractures)
b/c	because
BE	below elbow
bid	twice a day
bil.	Bilateral
biw	twice a week
B/K	below knee
BKA	below knee amputation
BLE	both lower extremities
BMI	body mass index
BOS	base of support
BP	blood pressure
bpm	beats per minute
BUE	both upper extremities
BR	bedrest
B/S, B.S.	beside; bedside

C

c̄	with
CAPTE	Commission on Accreditation in Physical Therapy Education
CARF	Commission on Accreditation of Rehabilitation Facilities

C/C, CCs	chief complaint; chief complaint		DOA	dead on arrival
cc	cubic centimeter		DOB	date of birth
CCCE	Center Coordinator of Clinical Education		DOD	date of discharge
			DPT	Doctor of Physical Therapy
C & DB	cough and deep breathing		drsg	dressing
CGA	contact guard assist		DRGs	Diagnosis-Related Groups
CHD	congenital heart disease; congenital hip dislocation		DTR	deep tendon reflex
			DSD	dry sterile dressing
CHI	closed head injury		DVT	deep venous thrombosis
CI	Clinical Instructor		Dx	diagnosis
CiTx	cervical intermittent traction			
cm	centimeter(s)		**E**	
c/o	complains of, complaint(s) of		ECF	extended care facility
COG	center of gravity		Elec.	electrical
coord	coordination		EMG	electromyogram
CP	compression pump; cerebral palsy		EOB	edge of bed
			equip.	equipment
CPM	continuous passive motion machine		ER	emergency room ED
			E.S. E-stim	electrical stimulation
CMS	Centers for Medicare & Medicaid Services		ex.	exercise
			ext.	extension
CN	cranial nerve		Ev, ev	eversion
cont	continue		Eval	evaluation
CORF	Comprehensive Outpatient Rehabilitation Facility			
			F	
COTA	certified occupational therapist assistant		F	female, fair muscle strength grade
CPM	continuous passive motion		Ⓕ	father
CPR	cardiopulmonary resuscitation		FAQ	full arc quads
			FAROM	functional active range of motion
CPT	Current Procedural Terminology; chest PT		FERPA	Family Educational Rights and Privacy Act
CRA	Certified Rehabilitation Agency		FES	functional electrical stimulation
CRF	chronic renal failure		FIM	Functional Independence Measure
CSF	cerebral spinal fluid			
CT scan	computerized axial tomography		Flex, ✓	flexion
			FLR	Functional Limitation Reporting
CVA	cerebral vascular accident			
CW	continuous wave		FOR	functional outcome report
CX	cancel		FRC	functional residual capacity
c/w	consistent with		FS	Functional Scale; use with *lower extremity (LEFS)*
D			ft	foot, feet
D_1, D_2	diagonal 1, diagonal 2 (PNF patterns)		FTP	failure to progress
			FTSG	full thickness skin graft
d/c	discharged, discontinued		F/U	follow up
DEP	data, evaluation, performance goals		FWB	full weight-bearing
			FWW, fw/w	front-wheeled walker
Dept	department		Fx, fx	fracture(d)
DIP	distal interphalangeal joint			
DF	dorsiflexion		**G**	
DJD	degenerative joint disease		G	good (muscle strength, balance)
DME	Durable Medical Equipment			
DNR	do not resuscitate		GA	gestational age

gastrocs	gastrocnemius muscles	ICIDH	International Classification of Impairments, Disabilities, and Handicaps
GBS	Guillain-Barré syndrome		
GCS	Glasgow Coma Scale		
GI	gastrointestinal	ICIDH-2	International Classification of Functioning and Disability
gluts.	gluteals		
gm	gram		
GMT	gross muscle test	ICP	intracranial pressure; intermittent compression pump
gt.	gait		
GXT	graded exercise test		
		ICU	intensive care unit
H		IE	Initial Evaluation
Ⓗ	husband	I/E ratio	inspiratory/expiratory ratio
HBP	high blood pressure		
HCFA	Health Care Financing Administration	IEP	individualized education plan
h, hr.	hour	IFC	Interferential Current; use with *H/S (high sweep)* or *L/S (low sweep)*
H & P	history and physical		
HA, H/A	headache		
Hemi	hemiplegia	IFSP	individual family service plan
HEP	home exercise program	IM	intramuscular
HHA	hand held assist; home health aide; home health agency	in.	inches
		inf.	inferior
		IP	inpatient, interphalangeal
HI	head injury	IPA	Individual Practice Association
HMO	Health Maintenance Organization		
		int.	internal
HNP	herniated nucleus pulposus	IS	incentive spirometer
h/o	history of	IV	intravenous
HO	heterotopic ossification		
HOB	head of bed	**J**	
horiz.	horizontal; use with *abd, add*	JCAHO	The Joint Commission on Accreditation of Healthcare Organizations
HP	hot pack		
HPSO	Health-care Provider Service Organization	*JAMA*	*Journal of the American Medical Association*
HR	heart rate	JRA	juvenile rheumatoid arthritis
hr	hour	jt.	joint
h.s.	at bedtime		
HS	hamstring(s)	**K**	
ht.	height	K	potassium
HWR	hardware removal	Kcal	kilocalories
HX, Hx, hx	history	kg	kilogram
I		**L**	
Ⓘ	Independent	Ⓛ lt.	left
ICBG	iliac crest bone graft	L., l.	liter
ICD-9	International Classification of Diseases, Ninth Revision	L5	5th lumbar vertebra
		lat.	lateral
ICD-10	International Classification of Diseases, Tenth Revision	LAQ	long arc quads
		lb	pound
ICD-11	International Classification of Diseases, Eleventh Revision	LBBB	left bundle branch block
		LBP	low back pain
		LE	lower extremity
ICH	intracranial hemorrhage	lg	large
ICHI	International Classification of Health Interventions	lic	license
		LL	long leg braces

LLC	long leg cast	nn	nerve
LLE	left lower extremity	noc	night, at night
LLL	left lower lobe	NPO	nothing by mouth
LMN	lower motor neuron	NWB	non–weight-bearing
LOA	leave of absence		
LOB	loss of balance	**O**	
LOC	loss of or level of consciousness	O:	objective data
		OA	osteoarthritis
LP	lumbar puncture	OASIS	Outcome and Assessment Information Sets
LPN	licensed practical nurse		
LTC	long-term care	OBS	organic brain syndrome
LTG	long-term goals	occ	occasional
LUE	left upper extremity	OD	overdose
		OM	otitis media
M		OOB	out of bed
M	male	OOT	out of town
Ⓜ	mother	O.P.	outpatient
man.	manual	O.R.	operating room
m., mm	muscle	ORIF	open reduction, internal fixation
max.	maximum		
MCA	motorcycle accident	ortho	orthopedics
MCO	Managed Care Organization	OT	occupational therapy
MD	muscular dystrophy	OTR	registered occupational therapist
MDS	Minimum Data Set		
mech	mechanical	oz	ounce
MED	minimal erythemal dose		
Meds.	medications	**P**	
mg	milligram	p̄	post, after
MH	moist heat	P	poor (muscle strength, balance)
MHz	megahertz		
min	minutes	P/	passive
min.	minimum, minimal	P:	plan (treatment plan)
mm.	muscles	P.H., PH, PMH	past history, past medical history
mm Hg	millimeters of mercury		
MMT	manual muscle test	PA	Physician Assistant
mo	month	para	paraplegia
mod.	moderate	p.c.	after meals
MP, MCP	metacarpophalangeal	PC	pressure control
MS	multiple sclerosis	PCA	patient-controlled analgesia
mtr.	motor		
MVA	motor vehicle accident	PCL	posterior cruciate ligament
		PCP	Primary Care Physician
N		PD	postural drainage
N	normal (muscle strength)	PE	pulmonary embolus
N/A	not applicable	peds	pediatrics
NAD	no acute distress	PEEP	positive end expiratory pressure
NBQC	narrow-based quad cane		
NCV	nerve conduction velocity	PF	plantarflexion
NICU	Newborn Intensive Care Unit	PFT	pulmonary function test
		PHO	Physician/Hospital Organizations
NIDRR	National Institute on Disability and Rehabilitation Research		
		PIP	proximal interphalangeal
		PiTx	pelvic intermittent traction
NKA	no known allergies		
nl	normal	PLOF	prior level of function

PNF	proprioceptive neuromuscular facilitation		qw	once weekly
PO	by mouth		quad	quadriplegic
POC	plan of care		quads	quadriceps
POD	post-op day			
POE	prone on elbows		**R**	
polio	poliomyelitis		Ⓡ	right
POMR	problem-oriented medical record		RA	rheumatoid arthritis
			RAD	reactive airway disease
			RBBB	right bundle branch block
POS	Point of Service Plan		RBC	red blood cells
post.	Posterior		R.D.	registered dietician
post	after		RDS	respiratory distress syndrome
post-op	after surgery; operation		re:	regarding
PPACA	Patient Protection and Affordable Care Act		re-ed	re-education
			REM	rapid eye movement
PPO	Preferred Provider Organization		reps	repetitions
			resist.	resistance
pps	pulses per second		ret.	return
PPS	Prospective Payment System		RLE	right lower extremity
PQRS	Physician Quality Reporting System		RLL	right lower lobe
			rm	room
Pr	problem		RN	registered nurse
PRE	progressive resistive exercise		R/O, R.O	rule out
pre-op	before surgery; operation		ROM	range of motion
prn, PRN	whenever necessary, as needed		rot.	rotation
			rr	respiratory rate
PROM	passive range of motion		RROM	resistive range of motion
pro time	prothrombin time		RT	respiratory therapist
prox.	proximal		RUE	right upper extremity
Prx	prognosis		RUGs	Resource Utilization Groups
PSIS	posterior superior iliac spine			
PSP	problem, status, plan		RUL	right upper lobe
PSPG	problem, status, plan, goals		Rx	therapy, treatment
PT	physical therapy, physical therapist			
			S	
Pt., pt.	patient		S:	subjective data
pt	protime		s̄	without
PTA	physical therapist assistant; prior to admission		S	supervision
			SAH	subarachnoid hemorrhage
PUW	pick up walker (standard walker)		SAQ	short arc quads
			SB	spontaneously breathing
PVD	peripheral vascular disease		SBA	standby assist
pw	power; use with *w/c*		SCI	spinal cord injury
PWB	partial weight-bearing		SDH	subdural hematoma
			SEC	single-end cane
Q			sec	second(s)
q̄	every		SGA	small for gestational age
qcane	quad cane		shld	shoulder
qd	every day		SICU	surgical intensive care unit
qh	every hour		SLB	short leg brace
qhs	at bedtime		SLC	short leg cast
qid	four times a day		SLP	speech language pathologist
qm	every minute		SLR	straight leg raise
qod	every other day		SNF	Skilled Nursing Facility
qt	quart		SO	significant other

SOAP	subjective, objective, assessment, plan	UED1	upper extremity diagonal 1
SOB	shortness of breath	UEFI	Upper Extremity Functional Index
SOMR	source-oriented medical record	UMN	upper motor neuron
S/P	status post	U/S, US	ultrasound
SPC	single point cane	UTI	urinary tract infection
SPTA	student physical therapist assistant; physical therapist assistant student	UV	ultraviolet
		V	
stat.	immediately, at once	v.c.	verbal cues
STG	short-term goal	VC	vital capacity
str.	strength	vent	ventilator
STSG	split thickness skin graft	VMO	vastus medialis oblique
sup.	Superior	VO	verbal order
SV	supervisory visit	VO₂	oxygen consumption
SWD	shortwave diathermy	VRS	verbal rating scale
Sx	symptoms	v.s.	vital signs
		VSU	venous stasis ulcer
T		**W**	
T	trace muscle strength	Ⓦ	wife
TBI	traumatic brain injury	w/	with
TCO	total contact orthosis	WB	weight-bearing
TDD	tentative discharge date	WBAT	weight-bearing as tolerated
TDP	tentative discharge plan	WBQC	wide-based quad cane
TDWB	touch down weight-bearing	WC, w/c	wheelchair
TEDS	antiembolitic stockings	w/cm²	watts per square centimeter
temp	temperature	WFL	within functional limits
TENS	transcutaneous electrical nerve stimulation	WHO	World Health Organization
TFs	transfers	WHO-FIC	WHO Family of International Classifications
Ther. Ex.	therapeutic exercise	WNL	within normal limits
THR (THA)	total hip replacement (total hip arthroplasty)	wlp	whirlpool
TIA	transient ischemic attack	w/o	without
tid.	three times daily	wt.	weight
TKE	terminal knee extension	**X**	
TKR (TKA)	total knee replacement (total knee arthroplasty)	x	number of times performed
TLC	total lung capacity	XR	x-ray
TLSO	thoracic lumbar sacral orthotic	xfer (transf)	transfer
TO	telephone order	**Y**	
tol.	Tolerate	YO, y/o	years old
train., trng.	training	yr.	year
TT	tilt table	**Z**	
TTP	tender to palpation; to the point; thrombotic thrombocytopenic purpura	Z	zero

Other Common Symbols

↔	to/from
↑	up, upward, increase
↓	down, downward, decrease
→	to, progressing forward, approaching
⊥	perpendicular

U	
UE	upper extremity
TTWB	toe touch weight-bearing
TWB	touch weight-bearing
tx	treatment
Tx	traction

//	parallel or parallel bars (// bars)	~	approximately
@, /	per	+, pos.	plus, positive
&	and	−, neg.	minus, negative
'	feet	=	equals
"	inches	≥	greater than
#	number, pounds	≤	less than
Ω	resistance	Δ	change
1°	primary	♀	female
2°	secondary, secondary to	♂	male
		∴	therefore

Appendix B

Defensible Documentation Elements and Documentation Review Sample Checklist

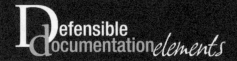 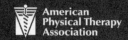

TOP 10 TIPS

1. **Limit use of abbreviations.**
2. **Date and sign all entries.**
3. **Document legibly.**
4. **Report functional progress towards goals regularly.**
5. **Document at the time of the visit when possible.**
6. **Clearly identify note types, eg, progress reports, daily notes.**
7. **Include all related communications.**
8. **Include missed/cancelled visits.**
9. **Demonstrate skilled care and medical necessity.**
10. **Demonstrate discharge planning throughout the episode of care.**

Documenting Skilled Care

- Document clinical decision making/ problem-solving process.
- Indicate why you chose the interventions/ why they are necessary.
- Document interventions connected to the impairment and functional limitation.
- Document interventions connected to goals stated in plan of care.
- Identify who is providing care (PT, PTA, or both).
- Document complications of comorbidities, safety issues, etc.

Documenting Medical Necessity

- Services are consistent with nature and severity of illness, injury, medical needs.
- Services are specific, safe, and effective according to accepted medical practice.
- There should be a reasonable expectation that observable and measurable improvement in functional ability will occur.
- Services do not just promote the general welfare of the patient/client.

Tips for Documenting Evidence-Based Care

- Keep up-to-date with current research through journal articles and reviews, Open Door, Hooked on Evidence at www.apta.org.
- Include valid and reliable tests and measures as appropriate.
- Include standardized tests and measures in clinical documentation.

Documentation Format

INITIAL EXAMINATION

History – May include:

○ Pertinent medical/surgical history	○ Cultural preferences
○ Social history	○ General health status
○ Growth and development	○ Previous and current functional status/activity level
○ Living environment	○ Medication and other clinical tests
○ Work status	○ Current condition(s)/chief complaint(s)

Systems Review – Brief, limited exam to rule out problems in the musculoskeletal, neuromuscular, cardiovascular/pulmonary, and integumentary systems that may/ may not be related to the chief complaint and may require consultation with others. Also may include:

○ Communication skills	○ Factors that might influence care
○ Cognitive abilities	○ Learning preferences

Tests and Measures – Used to prove/ disprove the hypothesized diagnosis or diagnoses. Includes:

○ Specific tests and measures: increased emphasis placed on standardized tests/measures, eg, OPTIMAL
○ Associated findings/outcomes

Evaluation – A thought process leading to documentation of impairments, functional limitations, disabilities, and needs for prevention. May include:

○ Synthesis of all data/findings gathered from the examination highlighting pertinent factors
○ Should guide the diagnosis and prognosis
○ Can use various formats: problem list, statement of assessment with key factors influencing status

Diagnosis – Should be made at the impairment and functional limitation levels. May include:

○ Impact of condition on function
○ Common terminology, eg ICD-9 CM coding or Preferred Physical Therapist Practice Patterns

Prognosis – Conveys the physical therapist's professional judgment. May include:

○ Predicted functional outcome
○ Estimated duration of services to obtain functional outcome

Plan of Care – May include:

○ Overall goals stated in measurable terms for the entire episode of care
○ Expectations of patient/client and others
○ Interventions/treatments to be provided during the episode of care
○ Proposed duration and frequency of service to reach goals
○ Predicted level of improvement in function
○ Anticipated discharge plans

Tips for Documenting Progress

- Update patient/client goals regularly.
- Highlight progress toward goals.
- Clearly indicate if this is a progress report by demonstrating patient/client improvement.
- Show comparisons from previous date to current date.
- Show a focus on function.
- Re-evaluate when clinically indicated.

Avoid

- "Patient/client tolerated treatment well"
- "Continue per plan"
- "As above"
- Unknown/confusing abbreviations – use abbreviations sparingly

Other Tips

Confidentiality

- Keep patient/client documentation in a secure area.
- Keep charts face down so the name is not displayed.
- Patient/client charts should never be left unattended.
- Do not discuss patient/client cases in open/public areas.
- Follow HIPAA requirements: http://www.cms.hhs.gov/HIPAAGenInfo/

Coding Tips

- Have a current CPT, ICD-9, and HCPCS book.
- Review code narrative language.
- Select codes that accurately describe the impairment or functional limitations that you are treating.
- Use the most specific code that accurately describes the service.
- Know when a modifier is necessary and accepted by a payer.

Additional Resources:

- State Licensing Boards: http://www.fsbpt.org/licensing/index.asp
- Joint Commission: http://www.jointcommission.org/
- CARF: http://www.carf.org/
- CMS: http://www.cms.hhs.gov/
- Physical Fitness: http://www.apta.org/pfsp

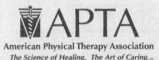

American Physical Therapy Association
The Science of Healing. The Art of Caring.

For additional information on Defensible Documentation, please visit **www.apta.org/documentation**

RE-EXAMINATION

Is provided to evaluate progress and to modify or redirect intervention. Should occur whenever there is:

- An unanticipated change in the patient's/client's status
- A failure to respond to physical therapy intervention as expected
- The need for a new plan of care and/or time factors based on state practice act, or other requirements

○ Includes findings from repeated or new examination elements

VISIT/ENCOUNTER NOTES

Document implementation of the plan of care established by the physical therapist.

Includes:

○ Changes in patient/client status	○ Variations and progressions of specific interventions used
○ Patient/client/caregiver report	
○ Interventions/equipment provided	○ Frequency, intensity, and duration as appropriate
○ Patient/client response to interventions	

○ Communication/collaboration with other providers/patient/client/family/ significant other

○ Factors that modify frequency/intensity of intervention and progression of goals

○ Plan for next visit(s): including interventions with objectives, progression parameters, precautions, if indicated

DISCHARGE SUMMARY

Required following conclusion of physical therapy services, whether due to discharge or discontinuation.

May include:

○ Highlights of a patient/client's progress/lack of progress towards goals/discharge plans

○ Conveyance of the outcome(s) of physical therapy services

○ Justification of the medical necessity for the episode of care

Top 10 Payer Complaints about Documentation (Reasons for Denials)

1. Poor legibility.
2. Incomplete documentation.
3. No documentation for date of service.
4. Abbreviations – too many, cannot understand.
5. Documentation does not support the billing (coding).
6. Does not demonstrate skilled care.
7. Does not support medical necessity.
8. Does not demonstrate progress.
9. Repetitious daily notes showing no change in patient status.
10. Interventions with no clarification of time, frequency, duration.

Supplement to PT Magazine

Documentation Review Sample Checklist

APTA
American Physical Therapy Association
The Science of Healing. The Art of Caring...

REVIEW FOR MEDICAL RECORDS DOCUMENTATION
Physical Therapy

Note: This is meant to be a sample documentation review checklist only. Please check payer, state law, and specific accreditation organization (i.e., Joint Commission, CARF, etc) requirements for compliance.

Therapist reviewed: Privileged and Confidential

PT Initial Visit Elements for Documentation Date:	N/A	Yes	No
Examination:			
1. Date/time			
2. Legibility			
3. Referral mechanism by which physical therapy services are initiated			
4. History – medical history, social history, current condition(s)/chief complaint(s), onset, previous functional status and activity level, medications, allergies			
5. Patient/client's rating of health status, current complaints			
6. Systems Review – Cardiovascular/pulmonary, Integumentary, Musculoskeletal, Neuromuscular, communication ability, affect, cognition, language, and learning style			
7. Tests and Measures – Identifies the specific tests and measures and documents associated findings or outcomes, includes standardized tests and measures, e.g., OPTIMAL, Oswestry, etc.			
Evaluation:			
1. Synthesis of the data and findings gathered from the examination: A problem list, a statement of assessment of key factors (e.g., cognitive factors, co- morbidities, social support, additional services) influencing the patient/client status.			
Diagnosis:			
1. Documentation of a diagnosis - include impairment and functional limitations which may be practice patterns according to the Guide to Physical Therapists Practice, ICD9-CM, or other descriptions.			
Prognosis:			
1. Documentation of the predicted functional outcome and duration to achieve the desired functional outcome			
Plan of Care:			
1. Goals stated in measurable terms that indicate the predicted level of improvement in function			
2. Statement of interventions to be used; whether a PTA will provide some interventions			
3. Proposed duration and frequency of service required to reach the goals (number of visits per week, number of weeks, etc)			
4. Anticipated discharge plans			
Authentication:			
1. Signature, title, and license number (if required by state law)			

PT Daily Visit Note Elements for Documentation Date:	N/A	Yes	No
1. Date			
2. Cancellations and no-shows			
3. Patient/client self-report (as appropriate) and subjective response to previous treatment			
4. Identification of specific interventions provided, including frequency, intensity, and duration as appropriate			
5. Changes in patient/client impairment, functional limitation, and disability status as they relate to the plan of care.			
6. Response to interventions, including adverse reactions, if any.			
7. Factors that modify frequency or intensity of intervention and progression toward anticipated goals, including patient/client adherence to patient/client-related instructions.			
8. Communication/consultation with providers/patient/client/family/ significant other.			
9. Documentation to plan for ongoing provision of services for the next visit(s), which is suggested to include, but not be limited to: The interventions with objectives Progression parameters Precautions, if indicated			
10. Continuation of or modifications in plan of care			
11. Signature, title, and license number (if required by state law)			

PT Progress Report Elements for Documentation * Date:	N/A	Yes	No
1. Labeled as a Progress Report/Note or Summary of Progress			
2. Date			
3. Cancellations and no-shows			
4. Treatment information regarding the current status of the patient/client			
5. Update of the baseline information provided at the initial evaluation and any needed reevaluation(s)			
6. Documentation of the extent of progress (or lack thereof) between the patient/client's current functional abilities/limitations and that of the previous progress report or at the initial evaluation			
7. Factors that modify frequency or intensity of intervention and progression toward anticipated goals, including patient/client adherence to patient/client-related instructions.			
8. Communication/consultation with providers/patient/client/family/ significant other			
9. Documentation of any modifications in the plan of care (i.e., goals, interventions, prognosis)			
10. Signature, title, and license number (if required by state law)			

** The physical therapist may be required by state law or by a payer, such as Medicare, to write a progress report. The daily note is not sufficient for this purpose unless it includes the elements listed above.

PT Re-examination Elements for Documentation Date:	N/A	Yes	No
1. Date			
2. Documentation of selected components of examination to update patients/client's impairment, function, and/or disability status.			
3. Interpretation of findings and, when indicated, revision of goals.			
4. Changes from previous objective findings			
5. Interpretation of results			
6. When indicated, modification of plan of care, as directly correlated with goals as documented.			
7. Signature, title, and license number (if required by state law)			

PT Discharge/Discontinuation/Final Visit Elements for Documentation Date: Note: discharge summary must be written by the PT and may be combined with the final visit note if seen by the PT on final visit	N/A	Yes	No
1. Date			
2. Criteria for termination of services			
3. Current physical/functional status.			
4. Degree of goals and outcomes achieved and reasons for goals and outcomes not being achieved.			
5. Discharge/discontinuation plan that includes written and verbal communication related to the patient/client's continuing care.			
6. Signature, title, and license number (if required by state law)			

PTA Visit Note Elements for Documentation Date:	N/A	Yes	No
1. Date			
2. Cancellations and no-shows			
3. Patient/client self-report (as appropriate) and subjective response to previous treatment			
4. Identification of specific interventions provided, including frequency, intensity, and duration as appropriate			
5. Changes in patient/client impairment, functional limitation, and disability status as they relate to the interventions provided.			
6. Subjective response to interventions, including adverse reactions, if any			
7. Continuation of intervention(s) as established by the PT or change of intervention(s) as authorized by PT			
8. Signature, title, and license number (if required by state law)			

Appendix C

SOAP Note Rubric

Section	25	20	15	10	5	0
Subjective	For **25** points, this section must include information and parameters reported to the treating therapist by the patient, family, or a coworker. For example: "My daughter's pain level following exercises this morning increased from a 5/10 prior to exercise to a 7/10."	For **20** points, the student may not state the parameters of the subjective statement. For example: "My father reported that his pain was better following the treatment session yesterday"; "My ROM was increased from the session last week."	For **15** points, the student may not state parameters or that the patient reported anything to the treating therapist that was appropriate for treatment. For example: "I went bowling last night and hurt my neck."	For **10** points, the student may not state parameters or report the patient stated anything about the last treatment session that is appropriate for the current treatment. For example: "My mother slept well last night."	For **5** points, the student may simply make a statement not relayed by the patient at all. For example: "The plan of care was changed last session."	The student did not complete this section satisfactorily.
Objective	For **25** points, this section must include information about the activity the patient engages in to increase his or her level of function, range, strength, and so on. Activities should be reproducible by anyone treating the patient and should include level of assistance, number of repetitions, number of sets, equipment involved, distance or time parameters, positioning, type of range of motion, and strength measures. For example: "The patient completed (1) ambulation 100 feet, 2X on an even surface during the session."	For **20** points, the student may not state all of the parameters of the activities and may forget to list **one** specific item, such as the level of assistance, number of reps and sets, amount of weight, and so on.	For **15** points, the student may not state all of the parameters of the activities and may forget to list **two** specific items, such as the level of assistance, number of reps and sets, amount of weight, and so on.	For **10** points, the student may not state all of the parameters of the activities and may forget to list **three** specific items, such as the level of assistance, number of reps and sets, amount of weight, and so on.	For **5** points, the student may not state all of the parameters of the activities and may forget to list **four** specific items, such as the level of assistance, number of reps and sets, amount of weight, and so on. The student may state only the activity and give none of the appropriate parameters for duplication of the activity.	The student did not complete this section satisfactorily.

Continued

Section	25	20	15	10	5	0
Assessment	For **25** points, this section must include a summary of the subjective and objective sections. It should include any information that demonstrates the patient's progress and state if there is no progress or if the patient is stable with the exercise program. For example: "The patient was able to ambulate 200 feet on an even surface using a SPC with SBA, 1X as compared with ambulating 100 feet on an even surface using a FWW with CGA at the last session on January 10, 2017."	For **20** points, this section may not include a summary of the subjective and objective sections or demonstrate progress through a comparison with another treatment session. For example: "The patient was able to ambulate 200 feet on an even surface using a SPC with SBA, 1x today." No comparison is given to a prior treatment session.	For **15** points, this section must include a summary of information in the subjective and objective sections that relates to the treatment session. For example: "The patient performed 10 reps of shld flex, in a seated position." The statement does not provide a comparison with an earlier treatment session and does not report the exact activity the patient completed.	For **10** points, this section must include a summary of information in the subjective and objective sections that relates to the treatment session. For example: "The patient is independent in walking." This statement does not provide all of the parameters of the actual activity nor a comparison with an earlier treatment session.	For **5** points, this section must include a summary of information in the subjective and objective sections that relates to the treatment session. For example: "The patient walked today." This statement gives no parameters for the activity or a comparison with an earlier treatment session.	The student did not complete this section satisfactorily.
Plan	For **25** points, this section must include information that tells the reader what is going to happen, what the plan is for the patient, and if any other medical services or equipment are required. It also states when the PT's supervisory visit will be (by date, day of week, or following which visit). For example: "The patient will continue to be seen 3x/week until the next PT supervisory visit on January 30, 2017."	For **20** points, this section may not include information about one of the following: what is going to happen, what the plan is for the patient, and if any other medical services or equipment are required. It also must state when the PT's supervisory visit will be (by date, day of week, or following which visit).	For **15** points, this section may not include information about two of the following: what is going to happen, what the plan is for the patient, and if any other medical services or equipment are required. It also must state when the PT's supervisory visit will be (by date, day of week, or following which visit).	For **10** points, this section may not include information about three of the following: what is going to happen, what the plan is for the patient, and if any other medical services or equipment are required. It also must state when the PT's supervisory visit will be (by date, day of week, or following which visit).	For **5** points, this section may not include information about four of the following: what is going to happen, what the plan is for the patient, referrals to another discipline, and if any other medical equipment might be required. It also states when the PT's supervisory visit will be (by date, day of week, or following which visit).	The student did not complete this section satisfactorily.

Appendix D

Documenting Interventions

SUGGESTED
INTERVENTION
DOCUMENTATION
STYLE

Documenting interventions thoroughly enough that they can be reproduced by another PTA or PT while still keeping the progress note as brief as possible is not easy. What follows is a method for providing the appropriate information in a concise format. In this "formula" style for documenting interventions, the information is placed in a continuous line and separated by slashes. A list of information that should be included for the intervention to be reproducible is provided in Chapter 11.

The information is documented as illustrated here but does not have to be placed in this order: Type of intervention/dosage or intensity/treatment area/time/patient position/frequency/purpose

EXAMPLES:

- Direct contact US/3 MHz/mild heat at (0.5 w/cm^2)/right TMJ/5 min/sitting/to decrease inflammation
- Direct contact US/1 MHz/(1w/cm^2)/ left middle trapezius & rhomboid/7 min/prone/to relax spasm
- Direct contact US/1 MHz/(1.5 w/cm^2)/(L) shoulder, anterior capsule/5 min/sitting/to prepare for stretching
- Induction SWD/large pad/dose III/vigorous heat/L1 to S2/20 min/prone/to prepare for stretching
- Intermittent cervical traction/15 lb/Saunders halter/30 sec on, 10 sec off/supine/20 min/to stretch C1-C4 cervical extensors
- Immersion US/1 MHz/(2 w/cm^2)/10 min/right deltoid ligament/sitting/to prepare for stretching
- Static pelvic traction/100 lb/L4-L5/10 min. max or until pain centralizes/prone/to reduce disc bulge
- Ice massage/standard procedure/R wrist extensors tendons at origin/to numbing response/sitting, shoulder abd 90°, elbow flexed 90° on pillow/after exercise/to minimize inflammatory response
- Hot packs/12 towel layers/R biceps femoris muscle belly/20 min/prone/to increase circulation for healing
- Foot whirlpool/110/decubitus on L lateral malleolus/20 min/sitting in wheelchair/for mechanical débridement
- ICP/50 lb/RUE/30 sec on, 10 sec off/supine, elevated 45/3 hr/to decrease edema
- FES/monopolar; one channel, three leads; two 2-inch square electrodes; origin & insertion; nontreatment electrode under ® thigh/(L) anterior tibialis/15 min/pt. semi-sitting/30 pps motor response/for muscle re-education and AAROM

INDEX

Note: Page numbers followed by "b," "f," and "t" indicate boxes, figures, and tables, respectively.

283